MODERN TECHNOLOGIES IN HEALTHCARE

This book comprehensively explores the latest technological advancements in healthcare, with a particular focus on the application of cutting-edge technologies, such as artificial intelligence (AI), computer vision, and robotics. The focus extends across crucial domains, such as disease diagnosis and monitoring, medical imaging, and the facilitation of remote healthcare services.

The book provides a comprehensive overview of AI techniques for intelligent diagnoses, discussing how machine learning and deep learning models enhance accuracy and speed in medical imaging, diagnostics, and patient care. It also delves into the integration of AI with other disciplines, such as data science, computer vision, edge computing, robotics, and web development, to tackle complex medical challenges. Moreover, it highlights current trends and future prospects in surgery, rehabilitation, neuroscience, and automated healthcare systems, offering valuable insights into the future of technology-driven healthcare solutions. The chapters are authored by researchers and professionals from every region of the globe, including Africa, Asia, the Americas, Europe, and Oceania. This global contribution highlights the versatility and broad perspectives of the shared insights and conclusions presented in the book.

This book is an essential guide for healthcare professionals, researchers, and enthusiasts eager to understand and actively contribute to shaping the future of healthcare through the integration of AI and other disciplines.

Temitope Emmanuel Komolafe is an Assistant Professor at the Collaborative Research Centre, Shanghai University of Medicine and Health Sciences. His research focuses on intelligent medicine, medical imaging processing, and precision rehabilitation robotics. He has published many research articles in peer-reviewed international journals.

Patrice Monkam is an Assistant Professor at Northeastern University, China. His research interests include image processing and analysis, medical imaging, and deep learning and its applications. He has authored over 20 research articles in leading peer-reviewed journals and at top-tier conferences.

Blessing Funmi Komolafe is a Lecturer at the College of International Education, Shanghai University of Medicine and Health Sciences. Her research focuses on pre-service physics teacher training, curriculum, pedagogy, medical education, and AI-based teaching. She has published extensively in international journals.

Nizhuan Wang is a Research Assistant Professor at the Hong Kong Polytechnic University, China. His research interests include brain-machine interface, neural computation, neuroimaging, neuroscience, and neurolinguistics. He has authored over 90 research articles in peer-reviewed top-tier journals and at conferences.

Analytics and AI for Healthcare

Artificial Intelligence (AI) and analytics are increasingly being applied to various healthcare settings. AI and analytics are salient to facilitate better understanding and identifying key insights from healthcare data in many areas of practice and enquiry including at the genomic, individual, hospital, community and/or population levels. The Chapman & Hall/CRC Press Analytics and AI in Healthcare Series aims to help professionals upskill and leverage the techniques, tools, technologies and tactics of analytics and AI to achieve better healthcare delivery, access, and outcomes. The series covers all areas of analytics and AI as applied to healthcare. It will look at critical areas including prevention, prediction, diagnosis, treatment, monitoring, rehabilitation and survivorship.

About the Series Editor

Professor Nilmini Wickramasinghe is Professor of Digital Health and the Deputy Director of the Iverson Health Innovation Research Institute at Swinburne University of Technology, Australia and is inaugural Professor – Director Health Informatics Management at Epworth HealthCare, Victoria, Australia. She also holds honorary research professor positions at the Peter MacCallum Cancer Centre, Murdoch Children's Research Institute and Northern Health. For over 20 years, Professor Wickramasinghe has been researching and teaching within the health informatics/digital health domain. She was awarded the prestigious Alexander von Humboldt award in recognition of her outstanding contribution to digital health.

For more information about this series, please visit: https://www.routledge.com/analytics-and-ai-for-healthcare/book-series/Aforhealth

MODERN TECHNOLOGIES IN HEALTHCARE

AI, Computer Vision, Robotics

*Edited by Temitope Emmanuel Komolafe,
Patrice Monkam, Blessing Funmi Komolafe
and Nizhuan Wang*

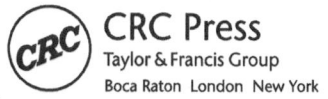

CRC Press
Taylor & Francis Group
Boca Raton London New York

CRC Press is an imprint of the
Taylor & Francis Group, an **informa** business

First edition published 2025
by CRC Press
2385 NW Executive Center Drive, Suite 320, Boca Raton FL 33431

and by CRC Press
4 Park Square, Milton Park, Abingdon, Oxon, OX14 4RN

CRC Press is an imprint of Taylor & Francis Group, LLC

Library of Congress Cataloging-in-Publication Data
Names: Komolafe, Temitope Emmanuel, editor. | Monkam, Patrice, editor. | Komolafe, Blessing Funmi, editor. | Wang, Nizhuan, editor.
Title: Modern technologies in healthcare : AI, computer vision, robotics / edited by Temitope Emmanuel Komolafe, Patrice Monkam, Blessing Funmi Komolafe, and Nizhuan Wang.
Other titles: Analytics and AI for healthcare
Description: First edition. | Boca Raton, FL : CRC Press, 2025. |
Series: Analytics and AI for healthcare | Includes bibliographical references and index.
Identifiers: LCCN 2024053814 (print) | LCCN 2024053815 (ebook) |
ISBN 9781032772332 (hardback) | ISBN 9781032772325 (paperback) |
ISBN 9781003481959 (ebook)
Subjects: MESH: Artificial Intelligence | Delivery of Health Care |
Biomedical Technology
Classification: LCC RA971.6 (print) | LCC RA971.6 (ebook) |
NLM W 26.55.A7 | DDC 362.10285--dc23/eng/20250210
LC record available at https://lccn.loc.gov/2024053814
LC ebook record available at https://lccn.loc.gov/2024053815

ISBN: 978-1-032-77233-2 (hbk)
ISBN: 978-1-032-77232-5 (pbk)
ISBN: 978-1-003-48195-9 (ebk)

DOI: 10.1201/9781003481959

Typeset in Sabon
by KnowledgeWorks Global Ltd.

CONTENTS

SERIES EDITOR FOREWORD

This book, *Modern Technologies in Healthcare: AI, Computer Vision, Robotics*, edited by Temitope Emmanuel Komolafe, Patrice Monkam, Blessing Funmi Komolafe, and Nizhuan Wang serves to explore the latest technological advancements in healthcare, with a particular focus on the application of cutting-edge technologies such as artificial intelligence (AI), robotics, and computer vision. The focus extends across crucial domains such as disease diagnosis and monitoring, medical imaging, and the facilitation of remote healthcare services.

Today, given the immense challenges facing healthcare delivery globally, especially in OECD countries, including escalating costs, an aging population that is living longer, workforce shortages and pressures, the rapid rise of chronic conditions, and the impact COVID 19 has had on healthcare delivery workforce, it is clear technology holds the key to addressing this Gordian knot. However, knowing technology holds the key and having precise and specific understanding of how to design, develop, and deploy technological solutions to ameliorate the current challenges are not one and the same thing. Thus, this book fills a key void, by enabling the reader to develop a full and deep appreciation and understanding around how to employ advances in technology such as AI and robotics to enable superior, patient centered, high value care that leads to better clinical outcomes to ensure. I am confident that all healthcare stakeholders who read this book will be wiser and more empowered to effect and support superior healthcare delivery enhanced with the latest technological advances.

CONTRIBUTORS

Mohammad Foad Abdi holds bachelor's and master's degrees in computer science, specializing in machine learning with a focus on sequential data processing and bioinformatics. His research explores machine learning algorithms for applications in signal processing, natural language processing, and speech processing. He has hands-on industry experience in various machine learning projects, contributing to the development and implementation of innovative solutions. He is actively involved in academic research and has published several papers in his field.

Mary Adedoyin is a Senior Lecturer in the Department of Electronic and Computer Engineering, Lagos State University, Nigeria. Her research interests include wireless and mobile networks, electronics, medical wearables, and robotic devices. She earned a PhD in electrical engineering at the University of Cape Town (UCT), South Africa, in 2018. Dr. Adedoyin worked as a Research Assistant at the Center of Excellence (CoE) for Broadband Networks and Applications, UCT, South Africa, from 2016 to 2018. She has authored numerous research articles in peer-reviewed journals and conference proceedings. She is a recipient of several grants and best paper awards.

Hamed Ahmadyani is a sixth-year medical student at Kermanshah University of Medical Sciences, Iran. In addition to his practical medicine and medical internship, his research interests include cognitive/systems neuroscience and medical imaging, particularly CT and MR imaging. Hamed is working on a tissue engineering project, aiming to advance medical treatments through innovative research. His dedication to both clinical practice and research highlights his commitment to improving healthcare outcomes.

Olanrewaju James Awoniya is a dynamic scholar who earned a BSc in physics and electronics at the prestigious Adekunle Ajasin University, Akungba Akoko. He is pursuing a master's degree in the Department of Information Technology at the National Open University of Nigeria, Abuja. His research interests include the application of artificial intelligence in medical imaging. He has also co-authored publications in peer-reviewed journals.

Ayub Bokani is a Lecturer and Research Scientist at Central Queensland University (CQU), Sydney, Australia. His research spans video coding, content streaming, interactive multimedia communications, and AI applications. He earned a PhD in computer science and engineering at the University of New South Wales (UNSW), Sydney. Dr. Bokani has published numerous peer-reviewed papers and received several best paper awards. He served as Discipline Leader of Mobile and Computing Apps at CQU and received the CQU Student Voice Award (2021).

Debasish Borah is pursuing a BTech at Manipal University Jaipur in the Department of IoT and Intelligent Systems. His research interests include medical image processing, machine learning, and deep learning in image processing.

Adanze Nge Cynthia is a public health professional specializing in health education and policy in the Global South. She has worked across East, West, and Central Africa, focusing on health advocacy. She holds an MPH from the University of Buea (2018) and a PhD from Dokuz Eylul University (2024). Dr. Nge has collaborated with various organizations on research and advocacy and has published in multiple peer-reviewed journals. Her research interests include the ethical application of AI in public health, particularly in areas such as resource allocation and health communication. She runs the "Sankofa Career Accelerator Program," where she mentors young public graduates and early-career health professionals.

Sweta Soundarya Das is pursuing a BTech in Computer Science and Engineering (specialization in data science) at the School of Computer Science and Engineering, Vellore Institute of Technology, India. Her research areas include data analytics, mobile app development, and deep learning research.

Arvind Dhaka earned a PhD in Computer Science and Engineering at NIT Hamirpur, India in 2018. Since then he has been an Associate Professor in the Department of Computer and Communication Engineering at Manipal University Jaipur. His research interests include wireless communication, wireless sensor networks, ad-hoc networks, medical image processing, machine learning, and deep learning in image processing. He has published one book with IET publishers related to medical image processing. He has more than 40 research papers, of which 30 are in top-rated SCI indexed journals. He completed one research project funded by DST New Delhi in 2023.

Ebenezer Juliet Selwyn is an Associate Professor in the School of Computer Science and Engineering at Vellore Institute of Technology, India. Her research interests include medical image processing, health analytics, and computer vision. She earned a PhD in computer science and engineering at Manonmaniam Sundaranar University, India, in 2013. Dr. Ebenezer has authored numerous research articles in peer-reviewed journals and conferences. She is a lifetime member of professional bodies such as ISTE, IE, and IETE.

Diako Ebrahimi is a leading researcher in quantitative biology, heading a cross-disciplinary program that integrates genetics, virology, cancer research, evolution, bioinformatics, mathematics, and statistics. His lab focuses on identifying and quantifying molecular processes in viral and cancer immunity and evolution. Dr. Ebrahimi's research aims to uncover population-specific virus-host interaction mechanisms, delineate the genetic and mechanistic basis of antiviral and cancer immunity, and develop quantitative biology methods to deconvolute complex biological processes. With over a decade of experience in quantitative biology and genomics, Dr. Ebrahimi employs multi-omics analysis and systems biology to address critical questions in his field.

Rezwan Firuzi is a PhD student in health science at the University of Köln, supervised by Prof. Kurt Pfankuche. His research focuses on bioinformatics and regenerative medicine. Rezwan earned a DVM at Urmia University and specializes in gene editing, single-cell RNA sequencing, spatial transcriptomics, and proteomics.

Jahan Hassan is a Senior Lecturer at Central Queensland University, Australia, with a PhD from the University of New South Wales and a bachelor's from Monash University in computer science. She serves as Area Editor for Elsevier's Ad Hoc Networks and has guest-edited many Q1 journals. Her research includes civilian drone applications, IoT and AI. As an IEEE Senior Member, she has served on the TPC for many conferences and promotes women in technology, co-chairing N2Women at IEEE WoWMoM 2024 and chairing the Women in Technology workshop at IEEE ITNAC 2020. She is also co-chair of the 2024 DroneSense-AI workshop.

Oluwagbenga P. Idowu is an AI/ML and Data Engineer at NVIT IT Solutions and Consulting, USA. Before this role, he served as Postdoctoral Research Associate at the University of Calgary and Alberta Children's Hospital in Canada from 2022 to 2024. He earned a PhD in pattern recognition and intelligent systems at the University of Chinese Academy of Sciences, China, in 2021. He has published numerous research articles in peer-reviewed journals and holds the position of Reviewer Editor. As an active member of the BCI Society and an IEEE EMBS Ambassador, he is dedicated to advancing his field.

Oluwaremilekun O. Idowu is an experienced data analyst and software quality assurance professional with a strong interest in healthcare and real estate. She holds a degree in mechanical engineering from Lagos State University and a mini-MBA from Tekedia Institute, USA. An accomplished author, she has notably contributed to the research titled "Neuro-Evolutionary Approach for Optimal Selection of EEG Channels in Motor Imagery-Based BCI Application," published in the *Journal of Biomedical Signal Processing and Control*. She is a software quality assurance specialist at HomeTrumpeter, USA. Her interests lie in leveraging emerging technologies and data-driven strategies to drive innovation in healthcare.

Blessing Funmi Komolafe is a Lecturer at the College of International Education, Shanghai University of Medicine and Health Sciences. She previously worked at the Department of Science Education, Adekunle Ajasin University, Nigeria. Her research focuses on pre-service physics teacher training, curriculum development, pedagogy, medical education, and AI-based teaching methods. She earned a PhD in curriculum and pedagogy at Zhejiang Normal University, China, in 2021. Dr. Komolafe has published extensively in international journals and serves as a reviewer for peer-reviewed journals as well as an article editor for Sage Open.

Temitope Emmanuel Komolafe is an Assistant Professor at the Collaborative Research Centre, Shanghai University of Medicine and Health Sciences. His research interests include intelligent medicine, medical imaging processing, and precision medical rehabilitation robotic devices. He earned a PhD in biomedical engineering at the University of Science and Technology of China, Hefei, in 2021. He worked as a postdoctoral researcher at the School of Biomedical Engineering, Shanghai Tech University, from 2021 to 2023. He has authored numerous research articles in peer-reviewed journals and serves as a reviewer editor for *Data Mining and Management* (Frontiers in Big Data) and as book reviewer and Editor for Taylor & Francis Group.

Li Liu is an Associate Professor at Great Bay University and the Dongguan Great Bay Institute for Advanced Study, Dongguan, China. His research focuses on intelligent medicine. Liu earned a PhD in biomedical engineering at the University of Bern, Switzerland, in 2016. From 2020 to 2024, he worked as Research Assistant Professor in the Department of Electronic Engineering at the Chinese University of Hong Kong. Dr. Liu has chaired publications for IEEE ICIA and served as Program Chair for ICIA 2019, as well as reviewing for multiple journals and programs.

Marwa Mohammed is an Assistant Professor in the Department of Physiotherapy at the Faculty of Allied Medical Sciences, Applied Science Private University, Amman, Jordan. She earned her PhD in Rehabilitation Medicine and Physical Therapy from Nanjing Medical University, China, in 2022. Dr. Mohammed has authored numerous peer-reviewed research and review articles in leading international journals. Her research interests encompass cardiopulmonary rehabilitation, geriatric robotics, AI in rehabilitation, cancer research, exercise physiology, neurorehabilitation, sarcopenia, frailty, and cachexia. She also serves as a peer reviewer for journals such as IGI Global, Frontiers in Neurology, and the Journal of Cachexia, Sarcopenia, and Muscle.

Vivens Mubonanyikuzo is a graduate student at the University of Shanghai for Science and Technology in Shanghai, China. He is a researcher at the Collaborative Research Center at Shanghai University of Medicine and Health Sciences. His research focuses on deep learning and medical imaging processing. He has authored numerous research articles in peer-reviewed journals.

Dana Naderi is a PhD student in statistics at CEREMADE, Université Paris Dauphine-PSL, and INSA de Lyon, under the supervision of Prof. Christian Robert and Dr. Kaniav Kamary. His research focuses on statistical methodologies, particularly Bayesian analysis. Dana's work aims to develop and apply advanced statistical techniques to solve complex problems in various fields. He is actively involved in academic research and has contributed to several projects and publications in the area of Bayesian statistics.

Amita Nandal earned a PhD in Electronics and Communication Engineering at SRM University, Chennai, in 2014. Since 2018, she has been an Associate Professor in the Department of IoT and Intelligent Systems, Manipal University Jaipur. Her research interests include digital signal processing, machine learning and deep learning for medical image processing, wireless communication, and circuit systems. She has published a book with IET publishers, *Machine Learning in Medical Imaging and Computer Vision*, related to medical image processing. She has written more than 50 research papers, of which 30 are in top-rated SCI-indexed journals. She completed one research project funded by DST New Delhi in 2023.

Charles Oretomiloye is a clinical student at Lethbridge Polytechnic in Alberta, Canada. He has worked with Gem Health Care, Shannex Healthcare,

Maquerries Pharmaceuticals, and VON Canada. He currently works on a casual basis with Alberta Health Services at Chinook Regional Hospital in a clinical capacity. Charles completed his clinical placement at MacDonald Geriatrics Hospital in Antigonish, Nova Scotia, where he provided palliative and long-term care for patients. He has received extensive training in pathophysiology, including experience with MRI and CT scans for cancer diagnosis. Additionally, Charles is licensed in the care of dementia and Alzheimer's disease. He also has a background in human nutrition and dietetics in the Faculty of Medical Sciences, Obafemi Awolowo University, Ile-Ife, Southwest, Nigeria. He is experienced in providing care for clients with different disease conditions. He is continuing his medical education and training.

Gadewar Gayatri Pandurang is pursuing a BTech in computer science and engineering (specialization in data science) at the School of Computer Science and Engineering, Vellore Institute of Technology, India. Her research areas include artificial intelligence, big data analytics, and mobile app development.

Yizhao Qian earned a BS in electronic engineering at Beijing University of Technology, Beijing, China, in 2020 and an MS in control engineering at Beijing Institute of Technology, Beijing, China, in 2023. He is currently pursuing a PhD in the Department of Electronic Engineering at the Chinese University of Hong Kong. His research interests include control systems in medical robotics.

Olapeju A. Sam-Oyerinde earned a Bachelor of Medicine and a Bachelor of Surgery (MBBS) at the College of Medicine, University of Lagos, Nigeria. She earned an MS in ophthalmology, with distinction, at University College London and is currently studying applied clinical research at McMaster University, Canada. Olapeju has served as an Outreach Research Coordinator at the Canadian National Institute for the Blind (CNIB). Her research focuses on the role of artificial intelligence in diagnostics and treatments in clinical medicine, particularly in retina and glaucoma. She has authored numerous peer-reviewed articles and presented her findings at both national and international conferences.

Arpit Kumar Sharma is an Assistant Professor in the Department of Computer and Communication Engineering at Manipal University Jaipur, Jaipur, India. He earned a PhD in brain tumor detection using machine learning and image processing at Manipal University Jaipur, India. Dr. Sharma completed his master's degree in computer science engineering at MDSU, Ajmer. With more than 5 years of academic teaching experience, he has published more than 25 papers in reputable, peer-reviewed national and international journals and conferences. His research interests medical image processing, data science, and machine learning experts to integrate machine learning and deep learning into other areas. He has a professional membership in ACM. Additionally, Dr. Sharma has served as a reviewer and editorial member for various academic journals.

Yuhu Shi is an Associate Professor at the Information Engineering College, Shanghai Maritime University, China. His research interests include artificial intelligence and machine learning, image processing, and pattern recognition as well as neural computing and biological information mining. He earned a PhD in management at the Shanghai Maritime University, China, in 2018. He has authored numerous research articles in peer-reviewed journals.

Yuchi Tian is a Senior Scientist at the Institute of Artificial Intelligence and Clinical Innovation, Neusoft Medical Systems Co., Ltd. His research focuses on AI-assisted diagnosis, medical image processing, deep learning, and machine learning. He earned a PhD in biomedical engineering at Fudan University in Shanghai in 2023. Following the completion of his doctorate, he joined Neusoft Medical Systems as a Senior Scientist, where he has been contributing since 2023. Dr. Tian has published numerous research articles in peer-reviewed journals, showcasing his expertise in the field.

Anmol Tiwari is pursuing a BTech in Computer Science and Engineering at the School of Computer Science and Engineering, Vellore Institute of Technology, India. His interests include health record analytics, mobile app development, and deep learning research.

Raj Vardhan is pursuing a BTech in Computer Science and Engineering (specialization in blockchain technology) at the School of Computer Science and Engineering, Vellore Institute of Technology, India. His research interests include machine learning, information security, and mobile app development.

Nizhuan Wang is a Research Assistant Professor with the Department of Chinese and Bilingual Studies, Hong Kong Polytechnic University, China. His research interests include brain-machine interface, neural computation, neuroimaging, neuroscience, and neurolinguistics. He earned a PhD in communications, information engineering and control at the Shanghai Maritime University, China in 2016. He has authored over 80 research articles in leading journals such as *Journal of Medical Internet Research*, *Human Brain Mapping*, *IEEE Transactions on Biomedical Engineering*, *IEEE Journal of Biomedical and Health Informatics*, as well as top-tier conferences like AAAI and MICCAI. Dr Wang is a senior member of the Chinese Biomedical Engineering Society and serves on the Board of the Shanghai Association for Noetic Science.

Wenxiu Zhang is a senior research collaboration expert at Neusoft Medical Systems Co., Ltd. Her research interest covers intelligent medical image processing and analysis as well as AI-assisted diagnosis of brain diseases and chronic respiratory diseases. She earned a master's degree in biomedical engineering at Beijing University of Technology in 2022. Since 2022, Zhang has been engaged in research work at Neusoft Medical Systems Co., Ltd., where she has established cooperation relationships with multiple top domestic hospitals and published numerous research papers in peer-reviewed journals. Additionally, she has successfully applied for several national, provincial, and municipal scientific research projects.

Weiming Zeng is a Professor at the Information Engineering College, Shanghai Maritime University, China. His research interests include medical image analysis and processing, brain science, artificial intelligence, and computational neuroscience. He earned a PhD in biomedical engineering at the Southeast University, China, in 2005. He has authored numerous research articles in peer-reviewed journals.

1

A DEEP LEARNING METHOD FOR IDENTIFICATION OF PNEUMONIA FROM CHEST X-RAYS

Debasish Borah, Amita Nandal, and Arvind Dhaka

1.1 Introduction

When it comes to quick treatment and improved patient outcomes, a correct diagnosis is very necessary. Chest X-rays are often used in the process of diagnosing pneumonia. On the other hand, chest X-ray interpretation may be challenging, particularly in circumstances when resources are limited or when radiologists lack the necessary experience [1, 2]. A diagnosis that is either delayed or wrong may be the consequence of a failure to recognize minor abnormalities or uncommon presentations. Especially in economically disadvantaged areas, there is a shortage of qualified radiologists, which makes the problem even worse. Deep learning algorithms, particularly convolutional neural networks (CNNs), have shown remarkable success in medical imaging applications in recent years, particularly in the areas of sickness diagnosis and categorization. As a result of their ability to automatically learn key properties from raw picture data, CNNs lend themselves very well to the interpretation of medical images. X-rays of chests are analyzed in this study to see whether or not deep learning can detect pneumonia.

Radiology specialists may be able to identify pneumonia from chest X-rays with the use of deep learning, particularly in youngsters. Due to the fact that children are more likely to experience severe repercussions and quick course of their sickness, timely and precise detection of pneumonia is essential. Through the use of deep learning and vast datasets, this work has the potential to improve pneumonia screening in areas with limited resources. It is possible that radiologists may utilize the model as a decision support tool in order to lessen the number of missed diagnoses and identify pneumonia [3–6].

DOI: 10.1201/9781003481959-1

When it comes to medical photo identification, the complexity of the work that has to be done necessitates the use of a system that is not only efficient but also successful. Deep learning is one of the methods that may be used for the purpose of training medical image datasets via the use of various methodologies. As a matter of fact, there are additional methods that may also be applied. Within the scope of the research endeavor, a deep learning model that was composed of RestNet-101 and RestNet-50 was used with the intention of determining whether or not the individual was suffering from pneumonia [7–10]. Despite the fact that these strategies have been taken into consideration, it has led to a variety of outcomes, which vary according to the characteristics of each person who is being considered. In order to compensate for this disparity, an efficient deep learning technique was developed. This strategy incorporates the numerous approaches that have been discussed here in order to get the desired results. This action was taken in order to make up for the inequality that existed. A dataset consisting of 14,863 X-ray pictures was used in order to achieve the objectives of this experiment. As a consequence, the accuracy achieved was 96%. There is a great degree of accuracy that can be obtained from the model; however, it does have certain limits that need to be taken into consideration. These constraints are the consequence of the difficulty of combining the RestNet models, which may have an impact on the accuracy of the findings when a bigger dataset is taken into consideration in a real-time situation [11–13]. The underlying reason for these limits is the difficulty of merging the RestNet models. In order to demonstrate how deep learning models may be used for the purpose of diagnosing certain illnesses, this experiment was carried out [14, 15].

Within the framework of this specific instance, the deep neural network was used to provide help in the identification of 14 different condition types.

The following provides a full explanation of the approach, data preparation, model design, and training. The results of the investigation and an evaluation of the effectiveness of the proposed model are then presented in detail, along with an analysis of examples that were correctly and incorrectly classified. In conclusion, the implications and applications of this study are examined, which paves the way for further developments in artificial intelligence (AI)-assisted medical picture analysis.

1.2 Literature review

The development of neural networks and the challenges they face in the diagnosis of pneumonia are the subjects of this literature review. Pneumonia diagnosis is an important area of healthcare that brings together technology and diagnostic medicine in order to improve accuracy and patient care. Over the course of the last ten years, a large number of researchers have been using deep learning in order to acquire the capability of autonomously diagnosing lung infections and other ailments based on chest X-rays. By demonstrating that deep learning models had the capacity to diagnose pneumonia from chest X-rays, a substantial contribution was made to the field under investigation [16, 17]. Their proposed method's ability to outperform previously established techniques in medical imaging represents a significant achievement in the field. In the period that has passed since then, there have been further major advancements in the field. Because of its resemblance to other lung disorders, pneumonia is a disease that is often misdiagnosed, particularly in young patients. This is especially true in respiratory diseases. The study presented in ref. [18] examined the challenges faced by medical professionals in identifying pneumonia. This study not only achieves remarkable sensitivity and area under the curve (AUC) metrics but also demonstrates the effectiveness of CNN ensembles in distinguishing between normal, viral, and bacterial pneumonia in chest X-ray images. This is accomplished by utilizing the power of seven CNN models that have already been trained. With the help of this study, the diagnosis accuracy for pneumonia in children has been significantly improved, which is a big step forward. In ref. [19], the authors underlined the critical necessity for a timely and accurate diagnosis of pneumonia, particularly for vulnerable pediatric populations. They emphasized the importance of this diagnosis. In addition to providing a simpler deep learning strategy that took use of MobileNet, they were able to make significant gains in terms of accuracy, recall, and F-score for their solution. A big step forward in the process of enhancing early pneumonia diagnosis and intervention is represented by the efficacy of the model, which is shown by the fact that it requires a shorter amount of time to train and has a lower demand for processing. The study that was published in [20] made an effort to find a solution to the issue of the limited availability of annotated computed tomography (CT) images for the diagnosis of pneumonia. This was accomplished by proposing a novel three-level optimization technique. In order to compensate for the absence of labeled scans in the target domain, this method brings about an improvement in the performance of deep learning models. This is accomplished by leveraging CT data from the source domain. As a consequence of this, it successfully reduces the weight of low-quality source data in order to reduce the amount of validation loss, and it also greatly enhances the accuracy of pneumonia diagnosis. Pneumonia-Plus is a one-of-a-kind deep learning system that was developed with the goal of accurately diagnosing the many types of pneumonia by making use of a variety of CT scans. The system is discribed in ref. [21]. A great diagnostic performance is shown by the model, as seen by the AUC values of 0.816, 0.715, and 0.934 for viral, fungal, and bacterial pneumonia, respectively.

In this study, the authors investigate neural network techniques for pneumonia identification, with a particular emphasis on the ChestX-ray14 dataset for consistency. According to the findings of the study, computer-aided diagnostic techniques have the potential to bridge the diagnostic gap, especially in economically disadvantaged areas [22]. An innovative approach to the diagnosis of pneumonia is presented in the paper titled "A Deep Convolutional Neural Network for Pneumonia Detection in X-ray Images with Attention Ensemble." The combination of EfficientNetB0 and DenseNet121 results in a deep CNN that offers improvements in terms of attention processes. This model has the potential to be used in clinical settings since it has an accuracy of 95.19%.

Deep learning in chest radiography is helpful in evaluating chest X-ray findings and measuring their stability over time; nevertheless, it lacks accuracy in categorizing discoveries, which limits its capabilities in comparison to those of radiologists [23].

An Enhanced Convolutional Neural Network was used for pneumonia detection, leveraging deep learning methods like VGG-19 and ResNet-50. The model achieved a 92.4% accuracy rate, surpassing both ensemble methods and state-of-the-art approaches [24].

The CheXNet-based pneumonia identification on chest X-rays using the deep learning algorithm is superior to the majority of radiologists in its ability to identify pneumonia from chest X-rays. With the ChestX-ray14 dataset serving as its training ground, it is able to provide state-of-the-art findings on all 14 diseases, therefore showing its diagnostic potential [25].

There is a significant improvement in accuracy when using deep convolutional networks for large-scale image recognition [26]. To properly identify patients who were suffering from pneumonia in the past, medical practitioners depended on a range of approaches, such as clinical exams, medical histories, and chest X-rays [27–30]. These methods included a variety of diagnostic procedures. Because of substantial technological breakthroughs, particularly in the field of biomedical equipment, the price of chest X-rays has been steadily decreasing in recent years. This is a direct result of the advancements that have occurred in the field, particularly in the area of radiation therapy. An X-ray of the chest is often used for the purpose of identifying lung disorders such as pneumonia, which is a common application [31–33]. The issue of an insufficient number of specialists may be addressed in a number of ways, one of which is by using a number of different computer-aided diagnostic procedures. AI technology has made great strides in recent years, and these advancements have shown its potential applications in the field of disease diagnostics. As an example, for the purpose of classifying chest X-rays and distinguishing between the presence of pneumonia and other illnesses, methods such as CNN are used. A number of significant studies have been carried out in a variety of sectors, including the identification of anomalous patterns, the recognition of biometrics, the evaluation of the degree of injuries, the prevention of airport accidents, the prediction of information efficiency via the use of artificial neural networks, and the diagnosis of bone disease. On the other hand, the fact that there is a greater degree of variation in the characteristics of the picture has an impact on the accuracy of the reconstruction [34–41].

1.3   Materials and methods

1.3.1   Dataset

The dataset used in this study is taken from the Kaggle online repository [28]. The images were organized into three main folders: "train," "test," and "val" (validation). Within each folder, the images were further sorted into two subfolders labeled "Pneumonia" and "Normal." Figure 1.1 presents the interpretation of pneumonia. Figure 1.2 shows example of chest X-ray images. All of the chest radiographs were originally checked for quality control, and any scans that were of poor quality or were illegible were removed from the dataset after the thorough curation process. The diagnoses for the photographs were then assessed by two specialists in the field of medicine, and the assessment set was examined once again by a third specialist in order to determine whether or not there were any flaws in the grading process.

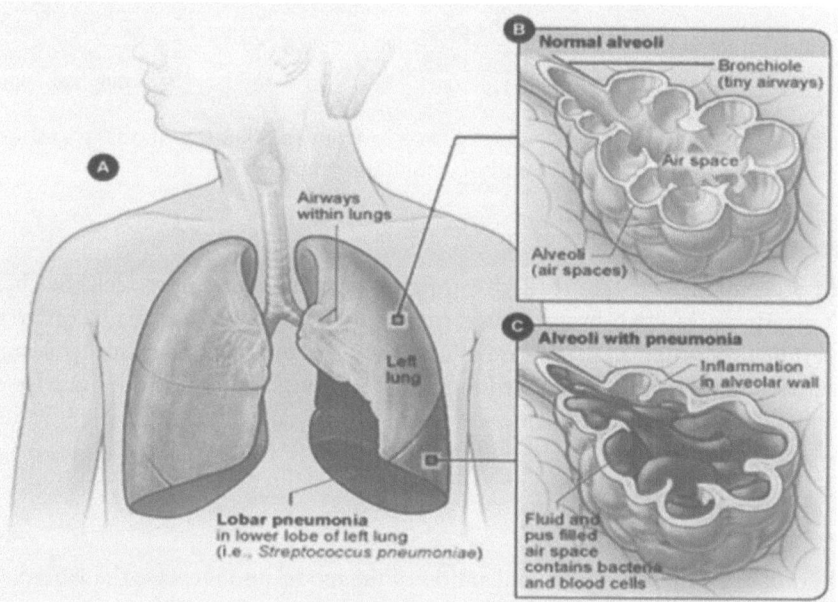

FIGURE 1.1   Interpretation of pneumonia.

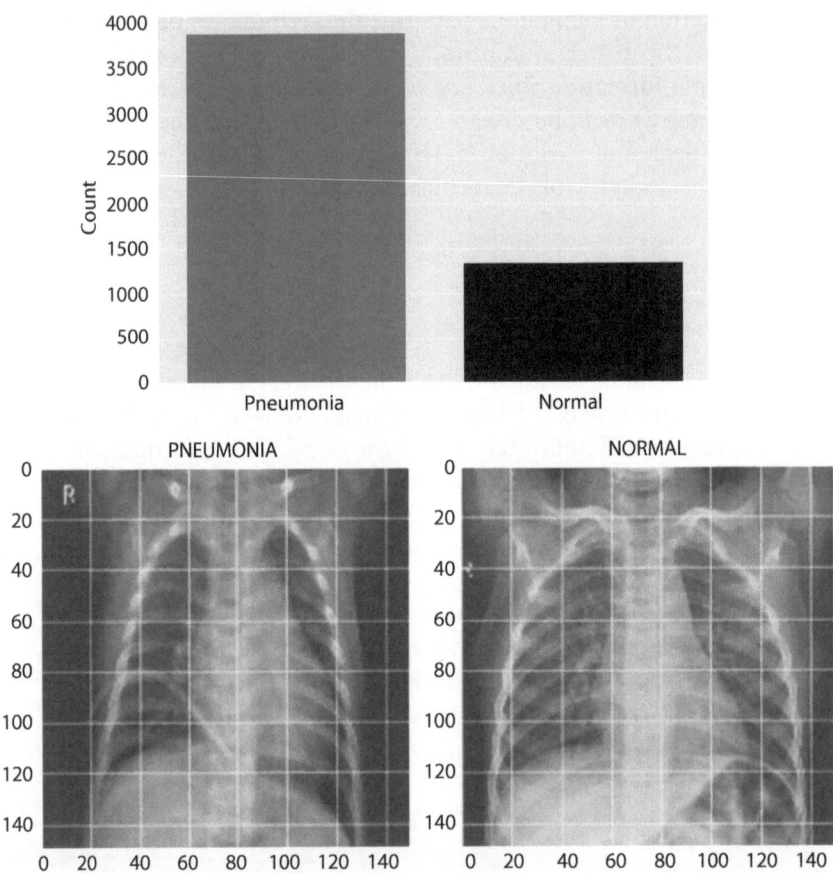

FIGURE 1.2 Example of chest X-ray images from the dataset, showing cases of pneumonia (left) and normal lungs (right).

1.3.2 The preprocessing of data

In order to get the data ready for training the deep learning model, the chest X-ray pictures were preprocessed into their respective formats. In order to permit processing that is more effective, the photos were shrunk to a constant dimension of 150 pixels long and 150 pixels wide. For the purpose of enhancing convergence during the process of model training, the pixel values were also normalized to fall within the range of 0 to 1.

1.3.3 Data augmentation

In order to enhance the generalization of the model and increase the variety of the training data, data augmentation approaches were used. Through the application of a variety of changes to the already existing photos while maintaining their labels, these strategies were able to artificially increase the dataset significantly. Alterations such as random rotations up to 30 degrees, magnification up to 20%, horizontal and vertical shifts up to 10% of the picture dimensions, and horizontal flipping were included in the collection of transformations.

1.3.4   Architecture of the model

The deep learning model that was used in this investigation was a CNN architecture. Its purpose was to automatically learn pertinent characteristics from chest X-ray pictures in order to identify pneumonia. A number of convolutional, pooling, and dropout layers, in addition to batch normalization layers, were included in the model in order to enhance the stability and convergence performance of the training process.

Additionally, the pooling layers were responsible for reducing the spatial dimensions and providing translational invariance. The convolutional layers were responsible for extracting low-level and high-level characteristics from the input pictures. Through the process of training, the dropout layers used a random deactivation of a portion of the neurons, which served to minimize overfitting.

1.3.5   Training for models

For the purpose of training the CNN model, the dataset was preprocessed and then supplemented. Additionally, the binary cross-entropy loss function and the RMSprop optimizer were used. Monitoring the training process was accomplished via the use of a learning rate reduction strategy known as ReduceLROnPlateau. This technique was utilized to dynamically alter the learning rate depending on the validation accuracy, thus preventing the model from being trapped in local minima. The model was trained for a total of 12 epochs, during which time the ModelDataGenerator was used to augment both the training data and the validation data on the fly. The performance of the model was tested using a test set that was held back, and metrics such as accuracy, loss, precision, recall, and F1-score were computed along with other metrics.

The findings that were produced from the trained model are described in the following sections. These results include its performance metrics, visualizations, and an analysis of instances that were successfully categorized and examples that were mistakenly classified.

1.4   Experimental results

1.4.1   Model performance

When it came to differentiating pneumonia cases from normal chest X-rays, the CNN model that had been trained obtained a high level of accuracy. When applied to the test set that was held out, the model achieved an accuracy of

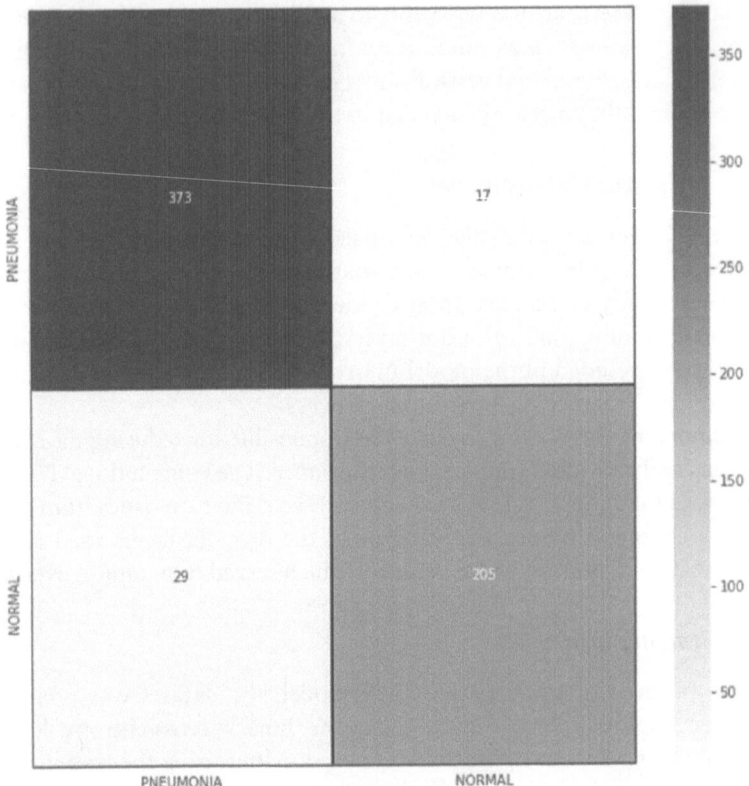

FIGURE 1.3 Confusion matrix for the pneumonia detection model.

[X] while suffering a loss of [Y]. A further evaluation of the performance of the model was carried out by using accuracy, recall, and F1-score measures, as shown in the result.

The confusion matrix, which depicts the number of true positives, true negatives, false positives, and false negatives, provided insights into the model's predictions. Figure 1.3 presents a confusion matrix for the pneumonia detection model.

1.4.2 Training and validation curves

The progression of the model's training and validation accuracy and loss over the epochs was monitored to assess its performance and identify potential overfitting or underfitting issues. The training and validation curves exhibited a steady increase in accuracy and a decrease in loss, indicating that the model was able to learn relevant features from the data and generalize well to unseen examples. Figure 1.4 presents training and validation accuracy and loss curves over epochs.

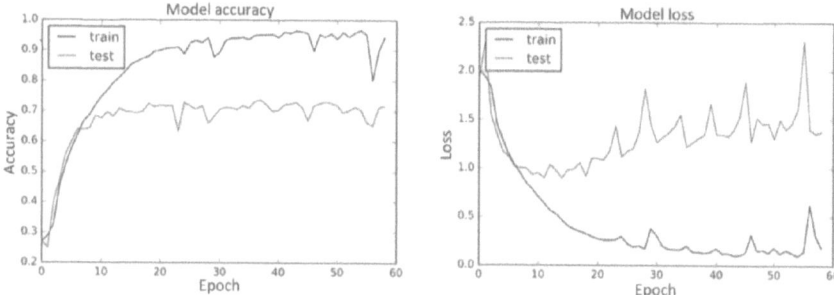

FIGURE 1.4 Training and validation accuracy (left) and loss (right) curves over epochs.

1.4.3 Correctly and incorrectly classified examples

To gain insights into the model's strengths and limitations, correctly and incorrectly classified examples from the test set were analyzed and visualized. Figures 1.5 and 1.6 show examples of correctly and incorrectly predicted pneumonia, respectively.

The instances that were successfully categorized provide evidence that the model is able to effectively detect typical patterns that are linked with pneumonia as well as normal lung diseases. The instances that were mistakenly categorized, on the other hand, bring to light difficult situations in which the model had difficulty. This might be due to a number of causes, including

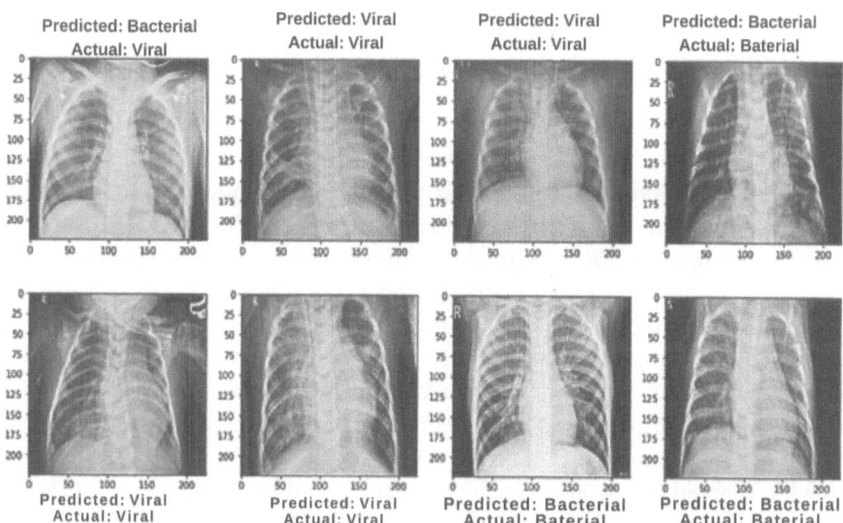

FIGURE 1.5 Examples of correctly predicted pneumonia (top row) and normal (bottom row) cases.

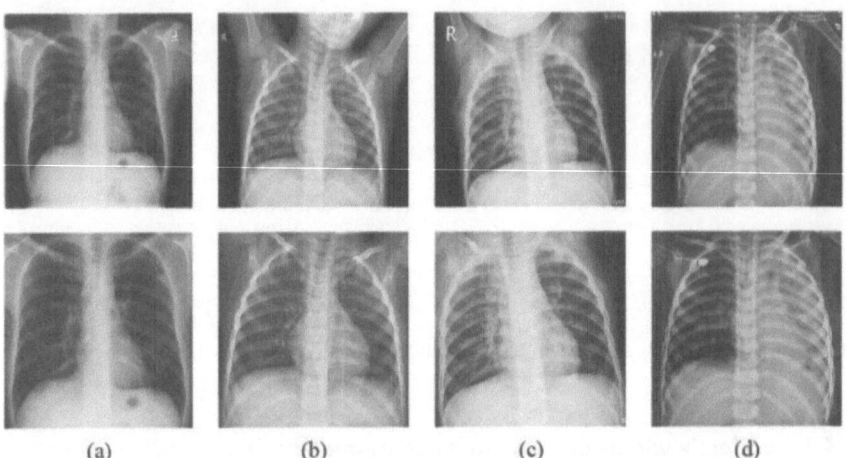

(a)   (b)   (c)   (d)

FIGURE 1.6   Examples of incorrectly predicted pneumonia (top row) and normal (bottom row) cases.

unusual presentations, minor anomalies, or traits that overlapped between the two groups.

These findings provide important insights into the effectiveness of the deep learning model for the identification of pneumonia in pediatric chest X-rays due to the fact that they give vital insights. In order to increase the accuracy of the model, especially in difficult instances, as well as to boost its resilience and generalizability over a wide range of patient groups and imaging settings, further analysis and optimization may be necessary.

1.5   Conclusion

The purpose of this study was to address the important need for prompt and accurate diagnosis, particularly for those who are more susceptible to severe sequelae. To this end, we suggested a deep learning technique for the accurate identification of pneumonia from pediatric chest X-ray images. To further analyze the performance of the model, multiple metrics such as accuracy, precision, recall, and F1-score were used. The results of these evaluations indicated that the model is successful in the automated identification of pneumonia. A number of data augmentation approaches were used in order to improve the generalization capabilities of the model, and meticulous preprocessing was utilized in order to guarantee that the input photos were of a constant quality.

The results of our research are consistent with those of other studies that have highlighted the promise of deep learning, and more specifically CNNs, in the field of illness identification and medical picture analysis. The model that was built has the potential to act as a helpful decision support tool for radiologists. It may assist in the early detection of pneumonia cases and reduce the risk of missed diagnoses, particularly in settings that are restricted in resources or in regions that have a dearth of qualified healthcare personnel.

Nevertheless, in spite of the very encouraging outcomes, there remain obstacles that need to be overcome. Considering how well the model performs in difficult situations, it is clear that more optimization and refinement are required. In order to give useful assistance to healthcare practitioners, further research efforts should concentrate on refining the robustness of the model, improving its generalizability over a wide range of patient demographics, and integrating it into clinical workflows.

In conclusion, this research highlights the enormous potential of deep learning methods in increasing the diagnosis of pediatric pneumonia and the delivery of healthcare. This study also paves the way for future advancements in AI-assisted medical imaging and diagnostic systems. As the technological landscape continues to undergo transformations, it will be necessary for academics, physicians, and industry stakeholders to work together in order to fully capitalize on the potential of AI to enhance patient care and outcomes.

References

1 Hassan MM, Billah MAM, Rahman MM, Zaman S, Shakil MMH, Angon JH. Early Predictive Analytics in Healthcare for Diabetes Prediction Using Machine Learning Approach. In: 2021 12th international conference on computing communication and networking technologies (ICCCNT). IEEE, pp. 1–5, 2021.

2 Selitskaya N, Seliski S, Jakaite L, Schetinin V, Evance F, Conrad M, Sant P. Deep learning for biometric face recognition: experimental study on benchmark data sets. In: Jiang R, Li C, Crookes D, Meng W, Rosenberger C (eds) Deep biometrics. Cham: Springer, pp. 71–970, 2020. https://doi.org/10.1007/978-3-030-32583-1

3 Schetinin V, Jakaite L, Krzanowski W. Bayesian averaging over decision tree models: an application for estimating uncertainty in trauma severity scoring. Int J Med Inform. 2018;112:6–14. https://doi.org/10.1016/j.ijmedinf.2018.01.009

4 Kabiraj S, Akter L, Raihan M, Diba NJ, Podder E, Hassan MM. Prediction of recurrence and non-recurrence events of breast cancer using bagging algorithm. In: 2020 11th international conference on computing, communication and networking technologies (ICCCNT). IEEE, pp. 1–5, 2020.

5 Hassan MM, Peya ZJ, Mollick S, Billah MAM, Shakil MMH, Dulla AU (2021) Diabetes prediction in healthcare at early stage using machine learning approach. In: 2021 12th international conference on computing communication and networking technologies (ICCCNT). IEEE, pp. 1–5, 2021.

6 Rejwan Bin S, Schetinin V. Deep neural-network prediction for study of informational efficiency. In: Arai K (ed) Intelligent systems and applications. IntelliSys 2021. Lecture notes in networks and systems, vol. 295. Springer, Cham, 2022. https://doi.org/10.1007/978-3-030-82196-8_34

7 Jakaite L, Schetinin V, Hladuvka J, Minaev S, Ambia A, Krzanowski W. Deep learning for early detection of pathological changes in X-ray bone microstructures: case of osteoarthritis. Sci Rep. 2021. https://doi.org/10.1038/s41598-021-81786-4

8 Abbas A, Abdelsamea MM, Gaber MM. DeTrac: transfer learning of class decomposed medical images in convolutional neural networks. IEEE Access. 2020;8:74901–13. https://doi.org/10.1109/ACCESS.2020.2989273

9 Pandey P, Pallavi S, Pandey SC. Pragmatic medical image analysis and deep learning: an emerging trend. In: Advancement of machine intelligence in interactive medical image analysis. Singapore: Springer Singapore, pp. 1–18, 2019.

10 Khatri A, Jain R, Vashista H, et al. Pneumonia identification in chest X-ray images using EMD. In: Trends in communication, cloud, and big data: Proceedings of 3rd national conference on CCB, 2018, Singapore: Springer; pp. 87–98, 2020.

11 Yang Z-Y, Zhao Q. A multiple deep learner approach for X-ray image-based pneumonia detection. In: 2020 international conference on machine learning and cybernetics (ICMLC), pp. 70–75, 2020. https://doi.org/10.1109/ICMLC51923.2020.9469043

12 Sarada N, Rao K. A neural network architecture using separable neural networks for the identification of "pneumonia" in digital chest radiographs. IjeC. 2021;17:89–100. https://doi.org/10.4018/IJeC.2021010106

13 Artemi M, Liu H. Image optimization using improved gray-scale quantization for content based image retrieval. In: 2020 IEEE 6th international conference on optimization and applications (ICOA), IEEE, pp. 1–6, 2020.

14 Deepal DAA, Fernando TGI. Convolutional neural network approach for the detection of lung cancers in chest X-ray images. In Deep learning for cancer diagnosis. Singapore: Springer Singapore, pp. 203–226, 2020.

15 Guan Q, Huang Y, Zhong Z, et al. Thorax disease classification with attention guided convolutional neural network. Pattern Recognit Lett. 2020;131:38–45. https://doi.org/10.1016/j.patrec.2019.11.040

16 Bhandary A, Prabhu GA, Rajinikanth V, et al. Deep-learning framework to detect lung abnormality—a study with chest X-ray and lung CT scan images. Pattern Recognit Lett. 2020;129:271–8. https://doi.org/10.1016/j.patrec.2019.11.013

17 Lee S, Seo J, Yun J, et al. Deep learning applications in chest radiography and computed tomography: current state of the art. J Thoracic Imaging. 2019;34:75–85. https://doi.org/10.1097/RTI.0000000000000387

18 Huang S, Lee F, Miao R, et al. A deep convolutional neural network architecture for interstitial lung disease pattern classification. Med Biol Eng Comput. 2020;58:725–37. https://doi.org/10.1007/s11517-019-02111-w

19 Ye W, Yao J, Xue H, Li Y. Weakly supervised lesion localisation with probabilistic-cam pooling. 2020. http://arxiv.org/abs/2005.14480

20 Huang X, Fang Y, Lu M, et al. Dual-ray net: automatic diagnosis of thoracic diseases using frontal and lateral chest X-rays. J Med Imaging Health Inform. 2020;10:348–55. https://doi.org/10.1166/jmihi.2020.2901

21 Tilve A, Nayak S, Vernekar S, et al. Pneumonia detection using deep learning approaches. In: 2020 international conference on emerging trends in information technology and engineering (ic-ETITE). IEEE, pp. 1–8, 2020.

22 Alapat DJ, Menon MV, Ashok S. A review on detection of pneumonia in chest X-ray images using neural networks. J Biomed Phys Eng. 2022;12(6):551–8. https://doi.org/10.31661/jbpe.v0i0.2202-1461

23 An Q, Chen W, Shao W. A deep convolutional neural network for pneumonia detection in X-ray images with attention ensemble. Diagnostics 2024;14(4):390. https://doi.org/10.3390/diagnostics14040390

24 Singh R, Kalra MK, Nitiwarangkul C, Patti JA, Homayounieh F, et al. Deep learning in chest radiography: detection of findings and presence of change. PLOS ONE 2018;13(10):e0204155. https://doi.org/10.1371/journal.pone.0204155

25 Aljawarneh SA, Al-Quraan R. Pneumonia detection using enhanced convolutional neural network model on chest X-ray images. 2022. doi: 10.1089/big.2022.0261

26 Rajpurkar, P. "CheXNet: Radiologist-Level Pneumonia Detection on Chest X-Rays with Deep Learning." ArXiv abs/1711 5225 (2017).

27 Simonyan K, Zisserman A. Very deep convolutional networks for large-scale image recognition. 2014. https://doi.org/10.48550/arXiv.1409.1556

28 https://www.kaggle.com/datasets/paultimothymooney/chest-xray-pneumonia

29 Hegedűs I, Danner G, Jelasity M. Decentralized learning works: an empirical comparison of gossip learning and federated learning. J Parallel Distrib Comput. 2021;148:109–24. https://doi.org/10.1016/j.jpdc.2020.10.006

30 Vyas J, Han M, Li L, et al. Integrating blockchain technology into healthcare. In Proceedings of the 2020 ACM southeast conference, ACM, pp. 197–203, 2020.

31 Maleh Y, Shojafar M, Alazab M, Romdhani I Blockchain for cybersecurity and privacy. Milton: CRC Press; 2020.

32 Yadav P, Menon N, Ravi V, Vishvanathan S. Lung-GANs: unsupervised representation learning for lung disease classification using chest CT and X-ray images. IEEE Trans Eng Manag. 2021. https://doi.org/10.1109/TEM.2021.3103334

33 Xie Y, Wu Z, Han X, et al. Computer-aided system for the detection of multicategory pulmonary tuberculosis in radiographs. J Healthc Eng. 2020;2020:1–12. https://doi.org/10.1155/2020/9205082

34 Yi P, Kim T, Lin C. Generalizability of deep learning tuberculosis classifier to COVID-19 chest radiographs: new tricks for an old algorithm? J Thoraic Imaging. 2020;35:W102–4. https://doi.org/10.1097/RTI.0000000000000532

35 Hegedűs I, Danner G, Jelasity M. Decentralised learning works: an empirical comparison of gossip learning and federated learning. J Parallel Distrib Comput. 2021;148:109124.

36 Pal K, Patel BV. Data classification with k-fold cross validation and holdout accuracy estimation methods with 5 different machine learning techniques. In: 2020 fourth international conference on computing methodologies and communication (ICCMC), pp. 83–87, 2020. https://doi.org/10.1109/ICCMC48092.2020. ICCMC-00016

37 Oi H, Kawakami R, Nacmura T. Analysis of evaluation metrics with the distance between positive pairs and negative pairs in deep metric learning. In: 2021 17th international conference on machine vision and applications (MVA), pp. 1–5, 2021. https://doi.org/10.23919/MVA51890.2021.9511393

38 Hossain MY, Sayeed A. A comparative study of motor imagery (MI) detection in electroencephalogram (EEG) signals using different classification algorithms. In: 2021 international conference on automation, control and mechatronics for Industry 4.0 (ACMI), pp. 1–6, 2021. https://doi.org/10.1109/ACMI53878. 2021.9528276

39 Singla J, Nikita K. Comparing ROC curve based thresholding methods in online transactions fraud detection system using deep learning. In: 2021 international conference on computing, communication, and intelligent systems (ICCCIS), pp. 9–12, 2021. https://doi.org/10.1109/ICCCIS51004.2021.9397167

40 Chen K-C, Yu H-R, Chen W-S, et al. Diagnosis of common pulmonary diseases in children by X-ray images and deep learning. Sci Rep. 2020;10:17374. https://doi. org/10.1038/s41598-020-73831-5

41 Sharma AK, Nandal A, Dhaka A, et al. Brain tumor classification using the modified ResNet50 model based on transfer learning. Biomed. Signal Process. Control. 2023;86:105299. https://doi.org/10.1016/j.bspc.2023.105299

2

RECENT DEVELOPMENT AND APPLICATIONS OF DEEP LEARNING IN MEDICAL IMAGING

Olanrewaju James Awoniya, Vivens Mubonanyikuzo, and Temitope Emmanuel Komolafe

2.1 Introduction

In recent years, the rapid advancement of information technology and digital innovation has increased the application of medical imaging within the healthcare field. Medical imaging is gaining greater recognition and demand as a crucial diagnostic tool. To meet diverse diagnostic needs, various types of imaging technologies have emerged.

In the field of medical imaging, various modalities are used, which include nuclear medicine, positron emission tomography (PET), magnetic resonance imaging (MRI), X-ray computed tomography (CT), optical coherence tomography (OCT), single-photon emission computed tomography (SPECT), medical ultrasound, infrared thermography, radiography, fluoroscopy, interventional radiology, photofluorography, and echocardiography (Figure 2.1). Each modality enhances the diagnostic capabilities of medical practitioners, enabling them to differentiate between healthy and diseased organs with greater precision. Today, medical imaging has become an integral part of the diagnostic and treatment planning process. Non-invasive techniques like CT and MRI are widely used, facilitating the detection of abnormalities within bodily cavities and providing crucial insights for organ diagnosis.

As computer technology advances alongside modern medical imaging, there has been a significant increase in both the size and complexity of medical image data. Effectively harnessing computer technology for processing such large data presents a formidable challenge. Medical institutions regularly generate vast amounts of high-resolution imaging data, demanding substantial time and expertise from healthcare professionals for analysis. However, subjective interpretation often prevails, potentially impacting

DOI: 10.1201/9781003481959-2

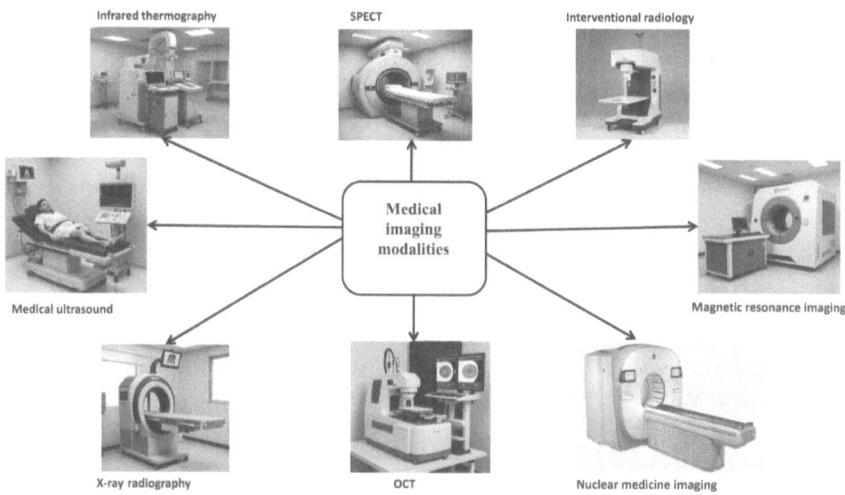

FIGURE 2.1 Overview of medical imaging modalities (SPECT: single-photon emission computed tomography; OCT: optical coherence tomography). These medical imaging modalities includes traditional methods like X-ray and ultrasound, advanced techniques such as MRI and CT scans, and specialized modalities like SPECT and OCT for precise disease diagnostics.

diagnostic accuracy. In both medical research and clinical practice, the ability to swiftly and accurately identify disease types and detect lesions is paramount in medical image analysis and processing. Here, the role of detection algorithms cannot be overemphasized. A robust algorithmic framework enhances diagnostic efficiency, minimizes misdiagnosis rates, and facilitates the development of targeted treatment plans for patients. Ultimately, this fosters improvements in public health outcomes while propelling advancements in medical science. Using big data and deep learning (DL) technology, medical staff can formulate more precise treatment plans and provide personalized medical services, thereby improving treatment effects and patient survival rates. Ultimately, the integration of big data analytics and DL technology into clinical practice not only enhances treatment outcomes but also drives advancements in medical science. By continuously refining predictive models and treatment algorithms based on real-world data, healthcare systems can adapt and evolve to meet the evolving needs of patients and society at large. This iterative process fosters innovation, improves public health outcomes, and paves the way for transformative breakthroughs in medical research and patient care.

This chapter explores the cutting-edge developments in DL techniques applied to diverse areas such as medical image registration, disease detection, classification, segmentation, and reconstruction. By leveraging DL algorithms, researchers and practitioners have achieved remarkable progress in automating and enhancing these critical tasks in medical imaging. From accurately registering medical images to detecting and classifying diseases with precision, the DL algorithm has revolutionized diagnostic and analytical processes. Additionally, segmentation algorithms powered by DL enable the precise delineation of anatomical structures and pathological regions, facilitating targeted treatment planning. Furthermore, DL-based reconstruction techniques have shown promise in enhancing image quality and reducing noise, thereby improving the overall interpretability of medical images.

2.2 Recent advances in deep learning for medical image registration

2.2.1 Introduction of medical image registration

Image registration is the process of aligning diverse images through geometric transformations into a unified coordinate system, despite variations in sources, sensors, or acquisition details [1]. The goal of image registration is to determine the optimal geometric transformation that maps the coordinates from one image space to another, allowing for the alignment of corresponding points or features across the images or datasets. This alignment enables the integration, analysis, and fusion of information from multiple sources into a coherent representation. Image registration finds applications in various domains, including remote sensing, computer vision (CV), medical imaging, and computer graphics. It is a crucial step in tasks such as image stitching, change detection, multimodal data fusion, atlas construction, and image-guided surgery, among others [2]. Accurate image registration is essential for combining complementary information, compensating for differences in acquisition conditions, and enabling meaningful comparison or analysis across multiple datasets.

Medical image registration is used for a variety of clinical applications, including image guidance, motion tracking, segmentation, dose accumulation, and image reconstruction [3, 4]. DL methods play a pivotal role in enhancing the accuracy and efficiency of image registration tasks in medical imaging (see Figure 2.2). By harnessing DL algorithms, researchers can achieve more precise alignment and fusion of medical images from different modalities or time points. This capability enables healthcare professionals to better analyze and interpret complex medical data, ultimately improving diagnostic accuracy and treatment planning [5]. The integration of DL-based image registration techniques holds promise for advancing medical imaging technologies and enhancing patient care. The image registration process typically consists of four major components: (1) feature detection and extraction, (2) feature matching, (3) transformation model estimation, and (4) image resampling

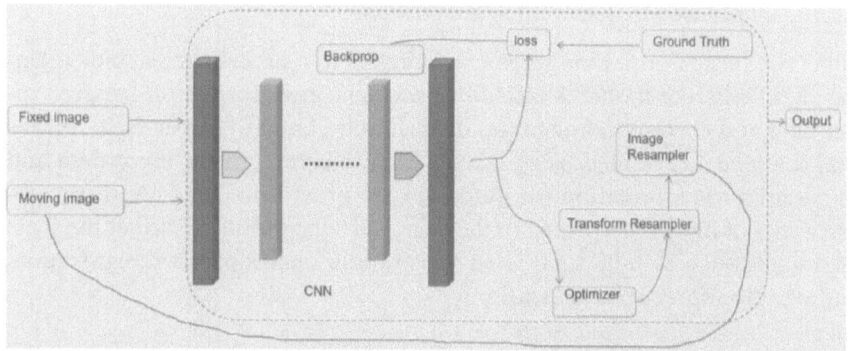

FIGURE 2.2   Represent the visualization of the registration pipeline for works that use deep learning.

and transformation [6]. The specific algorithms and approaches used may vary based on the image properties, accuracy, and computing capabilities.

However, a common formulation of DL-based registration involves using convolutional neural networks (CNNs) to learn the transformation parameters that align reference images (I_1) and images to be transformed (I_2).

$$\Theta = argmin_\Theta\, L\left(I_1, T_\Theta\left(I_2\right)\right) \tag{2.1}$$

where Θ denotes the parameters of DL made up of weights and biases of CNN, $T_\Theta(I_2)$ represents the transformed images I_2 with transformation parameterized by Θ, and L denotes the defined loss function which computes the dissimilarity between the transformed image and the reference image I_2. It is noteworthy that the most common loss functions are mean squared error (MSE), cross-entropy loss, or structural similarity index measure (SSIM) loss [7]. In practice, the optimization of Θ is typically performed using gradient-based optimization methods such as stochastic gradient descent (SGD) [8] or Adam optimizer [9], where the gradients of the loss function with respect to the model parameters are computed through backpropagation.

DL-based registration methods can be classified according to the characteristics of the DL models, such as network training architectures, training process, inference types (iterative, one-shot prediction), output types, and so on [10]. In the following subsections, we have classified DL-based medical image registration methods based on their methods, functions, and popularity into five categories [11]: (a) supervised transformation prediction, (b) unsupervised transformation prediction, (c) GAN in medical image registration, (d) deep similarity-based methods, and (e) reinforcement learning-based registration.

2.2.1.1 Supervised transformation predication

Supervised transformation "prediction" refers to a process in machine learning (ML) where a model is trained to predict a transformation between input data and corresponding target data. In this context, "supervised" means that the model is trained using labeled data, where both the input data and the desired transformation (or outcome) are provided. There are three subcategories of models according to the degree of supervision utilized at the stage of training such as fully supervised registration, dual-supervised registration, and weakly supervised registration.

2.2.1.2 Unsupervised registration

It is desired to develop unsupervised image registration methods to overcome the lack of training datasets with known transformations. However, it is difficult to define the proper loss function of the network without ground truth transformations [12]. In 2015, Jaderberg et al. [13] proposed a spatial transformer network (STN) that explicitly allows spatial manipulation of data within the network. Importantly, the STN was a differentiable module that could be inserted into existing CNN architectures. The work of STN has inspired many unsupervised image registration methods since STN enables image similarity loss calculation during the training process. A typical unsupervised transformation prediction network for deformable image registration (DIR) takes an image pair as input and directly output dense deformable vector field (DVF), which was used by STN to warp the moving image to generate warped images. The warped images were then compared to fixed images to calculate image similarity loss. DVF smoothness constraint was normally used to regularize the predicted DVF.

2.2.1.3 Generative adversarial networks (GANs) in medical image registration

The GANs, consisting of a generator (G) and discriminator (D), operate adversarially to enhance medical image registration. The generator crafts deformation fields, striving to replicate real images, while the discriminator discerns between generated and actual data, thereby assessing registration quality. This approach offers benefits such as unsupervised learning for high-quality deformation fields, crucial when ground truth data is lacking, and capturing intricate image features for enhanced accuracy [14]. GANs address label noise and significant motions, common hurdles in medical image registration. Elmahdy et al. [15] utilized a shallow discriminator for prostate CT DIR and segmentation, showcasing efficacy of GANs in challenging registration tasks. Liu et al. [16] introduced a dual-image discriminator to mitigate matching difficulties. Challenges remain, including refining loss functions and discriminator architecture for realistic deformation fields. Future endeavors should explore synergies with other DL techniques like attention mechanisms and cycle-consistency loss to bolster GAN-based registration models.

2.2.1.4 Deep similarity-based registration

Deep similarity-based registration refers to a method of registering or aligning images using DL techniques, specifically by leveraging the concept of image similarity. In traditional image registration, the goal is to find the spatial transformation that aligns two images such that they are in the same coordinate space [17]. This transformation is typically found by optimizing a similarity metric, such as mutual information or normalized cross-correlation, to measure the overlap or correspondence between the images. In deep similarity-based registration, DL models, such as CNNs, are trained to directly predict the transformation parameters between two images based on their visual similarity [18]. Instead of relying on handcrafted similarity metrics, the model learns to extract relevant features from the images and estimate the transformation that maximizes their similarity. Deep similarity-based registration can be applied to both unimodal and multimodal registration tasks. In both cases, it aims to learn the relationship between image pairs and their corresponding transformations based on visual similarity.

2.2.1.5 Reinforcement learning-based registration

One drawback of previous registration methods is the need for an iterative and time-consuming process. It is desirable to develop a method that can predict transformations in a single step. However, predicting transformations in one shot is challenging due to the high dimensionality of the output parameter space. Recently, reinforcement learning has gained significant attention for its ability to achieve human-level performances in various domains. Inspired by its success, researchers have proposed combining reinforcement learning with CNN to decompose the registration task into a series of classification problems. This approach involves finding a sequence of actions, such as rotations and translations along specific axes by specific values, to iteratively improve image alignment.

In summary, recent advances in DL techniques have significantly improved the field of medical image registration, enabling the development of accurate and efficient algorithms for aligning and integrating multimodal imaging data. DL-based methods have shown significant improvements in registration accuracy and robustness compared to traditional feature-based and intensity-based registration techniques. The incorporation of DL models into clinical practice has the potential to improve diagnostic accuracy, enhance patient care, and facilitate personalized medicine. Furthermore, the development of DL-based registration algorithms has opened up new avenues for research in medical imaging, including the creation of robust and adaptive registration methods and the integration of multimodal imaging data. Overall, the integration of DL techniques into medical image registration is poised to transform the field and improve patient outcomes.

2.3 Recent advances in deep learning for disease detection and classification

2.3.1 Introduction to disease detection and classification

The DL for disease detection and classification refers to the application of DL techniques, which are a subset of ML methods based on artificial neural networks, to identify and categorize various diseases or medical conditions [19]. The primary objective of CV in medical imaging is the classification of medical images. This involves differentiating between malignant and benign lesions or identifying specific diseases from input images. Over the past decade, the integration of DL into medicine has paved the way for more accurate, efficient, and cost-effective disease detection and classification [20]. As datasets and computational power continue to grow, we expect further breakthroughs in this field, leading to improved patient outcomes and a more personalized approach to healthcare. However, the performance of deep neural networks is heavily reliant on the availability of a substantial amount number of annotated images, which can be a challenge for many medical image datasets [5]. To address the scarcity of large annotated datasets, various DL techniques have been employed [21], with transfer learning emerging as the most prominent paradigm. Apart from transfer learning, other learning paradigms such as unsupervised image synthesis [22], self-supervised learning [23], and semi-supervised learning [24] have exhibited great potential in enhancing performance when annotated data is limited. Herein we discuss the three categories of image classification based on learning methods.

2.3.1.1 Supervised learning

Supervised image classification is a technique used in ML and CV where a model is trained to classify images into predefined categories or classes. The process is called "supervised" because the model learns from a labeled dataset, meaning each image in the dataset is associated with a specific label or category.

The landscape of image classification has undergone a remarkable evolution since the introduction of AlexNet by Krizhevsky et al. in 2012 [25], marking a pivotal moment in the field. This breakthrough was succeeded by a series of increasingly sophisticated models that delved deeper and expanded their representational capabilities. Prominent models include the VGG model proposed by Simonyan and Zisserman [26] in 2014, GoogleLeNet proposed by Szegedy et al. [27] in 2015, the ResNet architecture proposed by He et al. [28] in 2016, and the DenseNet framework proposed by Huang et al. [29] in 2017. Collectively, these innovations have not only raised the benchmark for CV systems but also significantly influenced the broader field of medical image processing. In the specialized domain of medical image classification, there has been a notable introduction of cutting-edge models specifically tailored for medical imaging tasks. Furthermore, EfficientNet has demonstrated its utility in this domain [30]. This collection of CNN architectures, known for setting new efficiency and performance standards in image classification, has been effectively applied to medical image classification tasks, achieving competitive results with more optimized computational resource usage. And lastly is the ResNeXt, which is an extension of the ResNet model. ResNeXt introduces a cardinality parameter that segments the transformations within each residual block into multiple groups, offering greater flexibility in model design [31]. This approach has been shown to enhance performance across a spectrum of image classification tasks, including those in medical image classification.

2.3.1.2 Unsupervised learning

Unsupervised DL in medical image classification refers to the application of DL techniques without the need for labeled data to classify and analyze medical images [32]. Traditional DL methods rely on supervised learning, where models are trained on labeled datasets. However, in medical imaging, labeled data can be scarce and expensive to obtain due to the need for expert annotation. Unsupervised DL methods offer an alternative approach by allowing models to learn representations directly from unlabeled medical image data [33]. Here are some DL approaches and techniques used in unsupervised medical disease classification and detection from medical images: Autoencoders, Variational Autoencoders (VAEs), and Generative Adversarial Networks (GANs).

2.3.1.3 Semi-supervised learning

Semi-supervised DL in medical image classification and detection combines elements of both supervised and unsupervised learning approaches to leverage the benefits of labeled and unlabeled data [34]. In medical imaging, acquiring labeled data can be expensive and time-consuming due to the need for expert annotations. Semi-supervised learning offers a solution by utilizing a small amount of labeled data along with a larger pool of unlabeled data to train DL models.

In medical image classification, semi-supervised DL addresses the challenge of limited labeled data by effectively utilizing both labeled and unlabeled images [35]. Recently techniques like pseudo-labeling, where models like Mean Teacher and self-training incorporate the model's high-confidence predictions on unlabeled data as additional labels for training [36], improve model performance. Consistency-based regularization methods like Anti-Curriculum Learning and Temporal Ensembles further enhance this process by enforcing consistent predictions even with slight variations in the unlabeled data, prompting the model to learn the underlying data patterns [37]. Even generative models like GANs can be employed. In GANs, a generative network learns to produce realistic images, and a discriminative network distinguishes real images from the generated ones [38]. Unlabeled data can be used to train the generative network, which in turn creates synthetic data to augment the labeled data for classification.

In summary, by leveraging the powerful feature learning capabilities of deep neural networks, these models can automatically extract relevant features and patterns from the input data, potentially improving the accuracy and efficiency of disease detection and classification processes compared to traditional methods that rely on manually engineered features or rule-based systems.

The application of DL in disease detection and classification has shown promising results in various medical domains, including radiology, dermatology, ophthalmology, genomics, and drug discovery, among others. However, it is important to note that these models should be carefully validated and integrated with human expertise to ensure safe and effective deployment in clinical settings.

2.4 Recent advances in deep learning for medical image segmentation

2.4.1 Introduction to deep learning-based medical image segmentation

Medical image segmentation is a core task in the analysis of medical images, as it involves identifying and delineating relevant structures (e.g., organs, tumors, tissues) within the images. However, due to the variability in image modalities (e.g., MRI, CT, ultrasound), image acquisition settings, anatomical objects, and the presence of noise, the application DL to new medical imaging tasks often requires the creation of domain-specific training datasets [39]. These datasets must be annotated with ground truth labels to train accurate DL models. This annotation process is highly resource-intensive and costly, as it typically requires domain expertise from trained biomedical professionals to ensure the accuracy and reliability of the labels [40]. The accuracy of medical

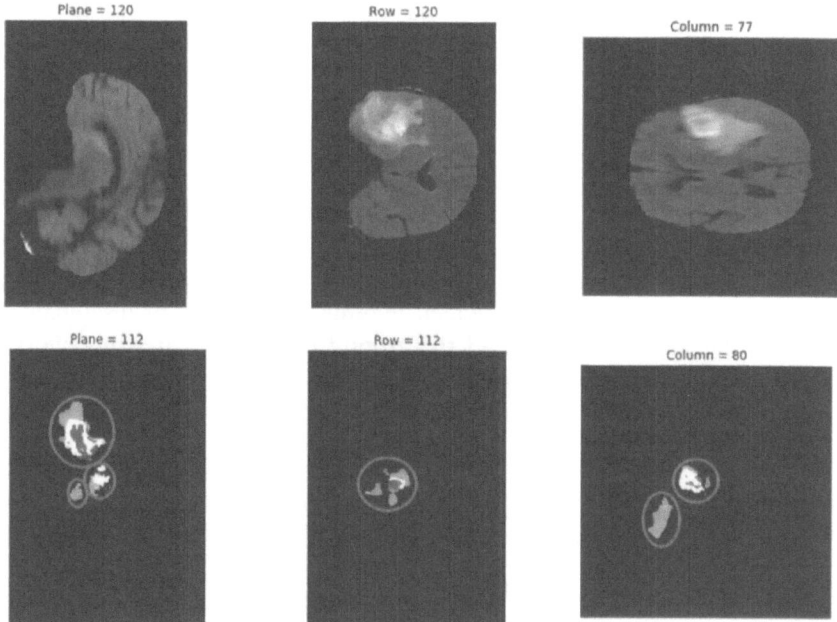

FIGURE 2.3   The brain tumor segmentation in MRI images. Row 1 shows the sample output of the images included in the dataset. Row 2 shows the results predicted by the model that correspond to the actual images.

image segmentation is crucial for clinical diagnosis and treatment. Inaccurate segmentation may decrease the model's credibility from a clinical perspective and lead to significant changes in subsequent computer-generated diagnoses. Therefore, there is a need to design more effective image segmentation architectures to capture detailed information about target objects in medical images.

The role of DL is paramount in medical image segmentation, given its high accuracy and broad applicability (see Figure 2.3). The DL has shown promising results in many biomedical image segmentation benchmarks [41]. However, due to the substantial variations in biomedical images, using DL in new applications requires new training datasets. The advantages of DL in medical image segmentation lie in its accuracy and widespread applicability [33, 42], but it also faces challenges in acquiring sufficient training data and the difficulty and high cost of annotation work.

This section delves into the latest breakthroughs in leveraging DL models used for medical image segmentation. The content within this section serves as a valuable resource for researchers and medical workers helping them identify potential areas for future exploration and stay abreast of emerging trends in this domain. By doing so, it encourages ongoing development and innovation in the integration of DL techniques within image segmentation applications.

Generally, the optimization formula for image segmentation using DL involves minimizing a loss function which can be obtained by using a CNN, and it can be represented as follows:

$$\min_{\Theta} \sum_{i=1}^{N} L_{\text{Seg}}\left(f_{\Theta}(x_1), y_1\right) \tag{2.2}$$

where Θ denotes parameters of CNN, $f_{\Theta}(x_1)$ is the output of the CNN model, x_1 and y_1 are input and ground truth segmentation masks, respectively, L_{Seg} is the loss function which minimizes the value of discrepancies between the predicted mask and the ground truth mask. It is noteworthy that L_{Seg} can be minimized using cross-entropy loss (L_{CE}), dice loss (L_{Dice}), and intersection over union loss as shown below:

$$L_{\text{CE}}(p,q) = -\sum_{m=1}^{M} p_m \log(q_m) \tag{2.3}$$

$$L_{\text{Dice}}(p,q) = \frac{1 - 2\sum_{m=1}^{M} p_m q_m}{\sum_{m=1}^{M} p_m + \sum_{m=1}^{M} q_m} \tag{2.4}$$

$$L_{\text{IoU}}(p,q) = \frac{1 - \sum_{m=1}^{M} p_m q_m}{\sum_{m=1}^{M} p_m + \sum_{m=1}^{M} q_m - \sum_{m=1}^{M} p_m q_m} \tag{2.5}$$

where p and q are probabilities representing ground truth and predicted over classes m.

2.4.2 Recent deep learning models for medical image segmentation

2.4.2.1 Fully convolutional network (FCN)

Early DL image segmentation initially used the sliding window method, which is inefficient due to redundant regions and computational intensity, impacting accuracy and efficiency. However, in 2015, Long et al. [43] proposed a FCN. This innovation in image segmentation replaces the sliding window with FCNs. FCNs replace traditional CNN fully connected layers with convolutional layers, preserving spatial information lost in standard CNNs.

FCN preserves spatial information by using only convolutional layers, allowing it to accept input images of arbitrary size while maintaining the resolution of the original image at the output. The network is typically composed of two main parts: the encoder and the decoder. The encoder extracts high-level features from the input image, while the decoder is responsible for reconstructing the spatial details from these features [44]. After processing by convolutional and pooling layers, the spatial dimensions of the image are gradually reduced but at the same time important information is retained. While the decoder part up-samples these output feature maps and restores them to the same dimensions as the input image. In this process, the decoder is responsible for mapping the extracted high-level features to each pixel of the final feature map, enabling pixel-level segmentation of the image. This architecture allows the network to capture details and thus be more precise and accurate when performing image segmentation [45]. The advantage of FCN over classical CNN networks is that there is no restriction on the size of the image input to the network [46]. However, FCNs also have some disadvantages that cannot be ignored. First, FCN employs pixel-by-pixel classification, disregarding the interrelations between individual pixels and overlooking global contextual cues. Second, during the up-sampling phase, only a single zoom operation is performed to directly expand the feature map by 8, 16, or 32 times. This approach risks discarding intricate details within the image, potentially resulting in blurrier segmentation outcomes.

2.4.2.2   The U-Net

Another classical network in the field of medical image segmentation is U-Net proposed by Ronneberger et al. [47] and has been widely used in medical image segmentation tasks. U-Net improves upon FCN with a similar structure but uses convolutional and pooling layers instead of fully connected layers. It incorporates jump connections between encoder and decoder layers to preserve information across different resolutions and recover fine details. In addition, U-Net employs more feature maps to provide more contextual information, which helps to better understand the global structure of the image. The structure of the U-Net network allows it to perform well in medical image segmentation [48]. It excels in detailed segmentation and context preservation, widely preferred for medical and cellular image processing tasks. The variants of U-Net are improvements and extensions of the original architecture, designed to enhance performance in image segmentation tasks, improve generalization capabilities, or adapt to various application scenarios [49]. Table 2.1 shows some common variants of U-Net and their main features.

TABLE 2.1 Some common variants of U-Net and their main features

Common variants of U-Net	Main features
U-Net++ (U-Net Plus Plus) [50]	A multi-scale feature fusion mechanism is introduced to improve feature representation by stacking multiple U-Net structures. Each U-Net structure operates at a different resolution, making the network more robust by fusing these features
Attention U-Net [51]	An attention mechanism is introduced to enable the network to pay more attention to regions that are important to the task. The learned weights are used to dynamically adjust the features at different locations to improve perception, which is especially suitable for dealing with complex scenes
Residual U-Net [52]	The idea of Residual Networks (ResNet) is combined to alleviate the gradient vanishing problem and speed up the training process by introducing residual connections. This contributes to a deeper network structure
V-Net [53]	It is a three-dimensional (3D) extension of U-Net, which is mainly applied to the task of 3D segmentation of medical images, such as segmentation of MRI or CT body data
Recurrent U-Net [54]	Introducing the structure of recurrent neural networks (RNNs) or long short-term memory networks (LSTMs) to handle image segmentation tasks with temporal information

2.4.2.3 The segmentation network (SegNet)

The SegNet is a deep CNN for semantic segmentation proposed by Badrinarayanan et al. [55] in 2015 at the University of Cambridge. SegNet aims for accurate pixel-level classification, handling varied image sizes. Its innovative decoder uses maximum pooling indices for nonlinear up-sampling, simplifying the process, enhancing boundary definition, and reducing parameters. In addition, compared to some other network structures, SegNet is relatively lightweight and suitable for use when computational resources are limited [55].

2.4.2.4 The DeepLab

The DeepLab algorithm uses a variety of methods such as dilated convolution, spatially pooled pyramids, and fully connected conditional random fields (CRFs) to improve the efficiency and accuracy of image segmentation [56]. In addition, probabilistic graphical models such as Markov random fields (MRFs) or CRFs have also been used to improve image segmentation, especially in edge refinement [57].

2.4.2.5 *The segment anything model (SAM)*

The SAM is a DL architecture designed for semantic segmentation tasks. Unlike traditional segmentation models that are trained to segment specific object classes or categories, SAM aims to segment anything present in an image without prior knowledge of specific object classes [58]. While SAM is generally effective in segmentation tasks, its performance tends to degrade in medical image segmentation. The Medical SAM Adapter (MSA) integrates medical domain knowledge for enhanced segmentation performance across diverse medical image types. It pre-trains with mixed medical datasets using self-supervised learning and adapts the SAM architecture for medical cues, surpassing existing methods in various tasks and modalities. However, general-purpose segmentation models still face certain challenges in medical applications, such as data imbalance, noise interference, and interpretability of algorithms [59]. To address these issues, researchers should continue to explore and improve DL models to better meet the practical needs of the medical field.

2.4.3 *Applications in medical image segmentation*

DL has demonstrated significant success in various medical imaging modalities. It is widely used in image segmentation for MRI, CT, and ultrasound modalities adopted in various organs of interest such as brain, lung, liver, bone, spine, breast, etc. for diagnosis of diseases, surgical planning, etc. U-Net and its variants are commonly used for the segmentation of these images. Techniques such as jump connections and attention mechanisms are introduced to capture multi-scale information and improve the perceptual ability of the network.

In summary, DL has made a number of important achievements in the field of medical image segmentation, bringing significant advances in medical imaging, disease diagnosis, and treatment planning [64]. DL enables highly accurate organ segmentation, tumor and lesion detection, multimodal image fusion, and fast and automated segmentation.

DL also has some drawbacks; deep models typically require large amounts of labeled medical image data for training. When this data is insufficient, the model's ability to generalize is limited. For medical and clinical decision-making, the explanatory nature of the model is crucial, especially in healthcare environments where models need to be held accountable for their predictions, but DL models have difficulty explaining the reasons for their predictions. Although challenges remain, ongoing research efforts promise to address these issues and drive further innovation in the critical field of medical imaging [65]. For more detailed information on deep learning methods for medical image segmentation, refer to Table 2.2.

TABLE 2.2 Various applications of DL techniques in the segmentation of medical images

Organ of interest	Deep-learning architecture	Applications
Brain Segmentation [60]	U-Net and its variants, such as 3D U-Net, are used for high-resolution brain structure segmentation. The introduction of jump connections helps to preserve detailed information (see Figure 2.3)	DL is widely used for brain segmentation in MRI images, including segmentation of gray matter, white matter, and cerebrospinal fluid
Lung Segmentation [61]	U-Net and its improved versions are widely used in lung segmentation tasks. Deep learning can help automate the identification and segmentation of lung regions	In CT images, lung segmentation can be used to analyze lung structure, evaluate lesions (e.g., lung cancer), and more
Breast Segmentation [62]	U-Net and its variants, such as Attention U-Net, can be used for breast segmentation. Deep learning can help physicians identify and localize abnormal areas more accurately	In mammography and breast MRI images, segmentation helps in quantitative analysis of breast tissue and early detection of breast cancer
Cardiac Segmentation [63]	U-Net, DeepLab, and models combining convolutional neural networks and recurrent neural networks (e.g., recurrent U-Net) are applied to heart segmentation tasks	Segmentation of cardiac structures in MRI images helps in assessing the function of the heart and detecting cardiac lesions

2.5 Recent advances in deep learning for medical image reconstructions

2.5.1 Introduction to deep learning for medical image reconstructions

Image reconstruction refers to the process of computationally creating or estimating an image from incomplete or degraded data or measurements, which is a crucial step in various imaging modalities like X-ray projections radiography, CT, PET, SPECT, and so on, useful in astronomy, remote sensing, and non-destructive testing. In medical imaging, it involves reconstructing an image of the internal structure of the body from the measured data acquired by the imaging device, such as CT, MRI, or gamma ray emissions (PET/SPECT).

The reconstruction process solves an inverse problem, using mathematical algorithms and models that account for the physics of the imaging process, noise, and other degrading factors, to estimate the original image or object. The main objectives are accurate representation of the underlying anatomical or functional information, high spatial and temporal resolution, noise reduction, and computational efficiency [66]. Successful image reconstruction is crucial for accurate diagnosis, treatment planning, and research, making it an active area of research focused on advanced algorithms, computational methods, and hardware acceleration techniques [67].

DL-based reconstruction methods leverage neural networks to learn the mapping between acquired data (e.g., raw sensor measurements) and the desired high-quality images. These neural networks are trained on a large number of examples, allowing them to learn the intricate relationships and patterns present in the data. By incorporating prior knowledge and regularization techniques [68], DL models can effectively denoise, super-resolve, and reconstruct images from sparse or incomplete data, potentially leading to improved diagnostic accuracy and reduced radiation exposure for patients. These architectures have demonstrated remarkable performance in tasks like low-dose CT reconstruction, accelerated MRI reconstruction, and PET image denoising, among others [69].

In this sub-section, we delve into the latest advancements in DL architectures that have demonstrated exceptional performance in medical imaging, particularly in image reconstruction. Recent developments in CNNs and GANs-based models have shown remarkable results in reconstructing high-quality images from incomplete or noisy data as shown in Figure 2.4. These

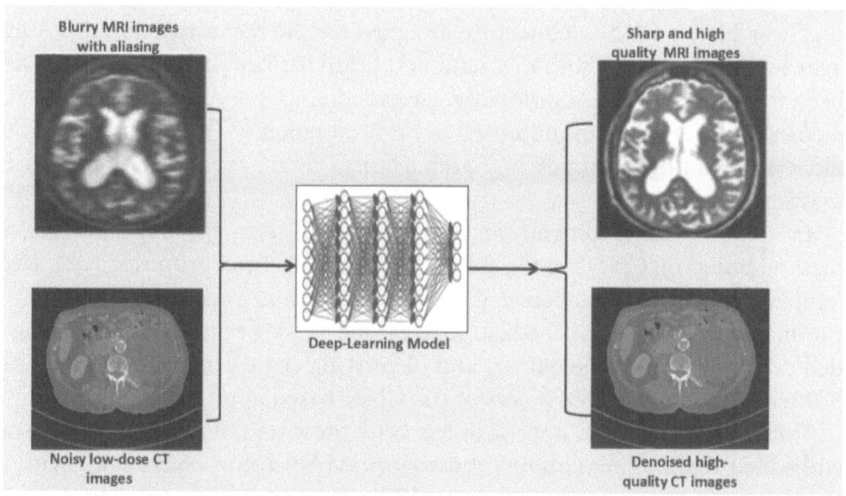

FIGURE 2.4   The blurry image with noise is reconstructed by DL to get the high-quality image.

innovative approaches have the potential to revolutionize medical imaging, enabling faster and more accurate diagnoses. By exploring these recent architectures, we can gain insights into the future of medical imaging and its applications.

2.5.2 Convolutional neural networks

The CNNs have made significant strides in the field of medical image reconstruction. By utilizing convolutional and pooling layers, CNNs have demonstrated their ability to extract meaningful features from medical images and produce high-quality reconstructed images. However, several challenges persist, including the necessity for ample large-scale data to mitigate overfitting and the optimization of network structures to enhance overall performance [70].

Recent studies have employed phantom data for quantitative validation, confirming the robust denoising capabilities of CNNs for static portions of medical images while preserving temporal fidelity [71, 72]. Notably, CNN's performance was comparable to that of regularized iterative reconstruction using the split Bregman method [73]. The implementation of a software solution could produce the reconstruction of high-resolution (HR) images from low-resolution (LR) medical X-ray images [74]. A mechanism based on granular-level features for HR grayscale medical X-ray image reconstruction from LR counterparts has been introduced, representing a valuable contribution to the ongoing efforts to harness DL methods for enhancing medical imaging quality. The CNNs have consistently demonstrated state-of-the-art performance in the field of CV, and their application in medical image processing has garnered increasing attention in recent years [75].

The Y-Net, a CNN architecture designed for the reconstruction of PA images by incorporating both raw data and beam formed images as inputs, has been introduced [76]. Additionally, cascaded CNNs specifically tailored for medical image super-resolution have been designed [77], exploring various filter sizes and optimizing CNN architectures to enhance the complexity of existing techniques.

In another development, an efficient medical image super-resolution method based on CNNs in the shearlet domain has been proposed [78]. Recognizing the disparities between imaging mechanisms optimized for natural images and those for medical images, the work began by constructing a dedicated medical image dataset and identifying critical areas to significantly bolster the training effectiveness of the CNN-based approach.

Furthermore, a novel approach has been presented, in which a CNN was embedded within a maximum a posteriori (MAP) reconstruction algorithm, forming an integral part of the prior [79]. This deviation from the conventional post-processing application of CNNs enabled a more robust representation of images within the reconstruction framework.

2.5.3 Generative adversarial networks

GANs have been widely used for medical image reconstruction. GANs are capable of generating high-quality medical images through adversarial learning of generators and discriminators, but their training process is complex and stability is still a challenge, while the generated images may be affected by noise [80].

Recent studies have proposed novel frameworks for medical image-to-image translation, operating on the image level in an end-to-end manner [81]. Additionally, GANs have been used for the reduction of streaking artifacts and the improvement of PET image quality. GANs and their extensions have carved open many exciting ways to tackle well-known and challenging medical image analysis problems [82].

The application of DL techniques, GANs, has shown significant promise in the field of medical image reconstruction. These techniques have demonstrated the ability to extract meaningful features from medical images and produce high-quality reconstructed images. However, several challenges persist, including the necessity for ample large-scale data to mitigate overfitting and the optimization of network structures to enhance overall performance.

In summary, the recent advancements in DL techniques have significantly impacted the field of medical image reconstruction, enabling the development of accurate and efficient algorithms for reconstructing high-quality images from limited or noisy data. Comparative studies have demonstrated that deep-learning-based methods exhibit significant improvements in image quality and reconstruction accuracy compared to traditional iterative reconstruction techniques. The integration of deep-learning models into clinical practice holds great promise for enhancing diagnostic accuracy, reducing radiation exposure, and improving patient care. Furthermore, the development of DL-based reconstruction algorithms has opened up new avenues for research in medical imaging, including the creation of personalized reconstruction models and the integration of multimodal imaging data. Overall, the integration of DL techniques into medical image reconstruction is poised to revolutionize the field and have a profound impact on patient outcomes.

2.6 Generative model future of deep learning medical imaging

2.6.1 Brief introduction of generative model

A generative model is a type of statistical model that learns the underlying structure of a dataset in order to generate new data that is similar to the original. In other words, it tries to understand how data is generated and then uses that understanding to create new, realistic samples.

The diffusion model is a specific type of generative model that focuses on modeling the evolution of data over time. It assumes that data at each time step is a diffusion (or mixture) of previous data points, capturing dependencies and correlations within the data sequence.

The diffusion model has gained popularity due to its effectiveness in various applications such as segmentation, registration, detection, classification, and reconstruction. In segmentation tasks, the diffusion model can help identify distinct regions or objects within an image or dataset by modeling the spatial relationships between pixels or data points. In registration, the model can be used to align multiple images or datasets by learning the transformations that best align them with each other. For detection and classification, the diffusion model can learn the characteristics of different classes or categories within a dataset, enabling accurate identification and labeling of new data points. Finally, in reconstruction tasks, the diffusion model can fill in missing or corrupted parts of data, effectively "reconstructing" the original signal or image.

Overall, the diffusion model's versatility and ability to capture complex dependencies make it a powerful tool in various fields; in this section we will focus on the application of diffusion models in different medical tasks.

2.6.2 Application of diffusion model for medical image registration

Diffusion models are being explored for medical image registration tasks. For instance, in 2022, the paper by Kim et al. [83] proposed DiffuseMorph, a diffusion-based method for DIR. This method employs two main networks – a diffusion network and a deformation network – both trained end-to-end to score the deformation between moving and fixed images and to estimate the deformation field, respectively. The model is capable of providing both image registration and generation tasks, demonstrating high accuracy in registering both 2D facial expressions and 3D medical images. DiffuseMorph uses a diffusion network and a deformation network, both trained end-to-end. The diffusion network scores the deformation between moving and fixed images, while the deformation network uses this scoring to estimate the deformation field. The model generates deformation fields along a continuous trajectory from the moving to the fixed image. The moving image is then transformed into a deformed image using the generated deformation fields and a spatial transformation layer (STL).

2.6.3 Application of diffusion model for disease detection and classification

Diffusion models have been utilized for disease detection and classification in medical imaging. A paper by Wolleb et al. [84] proposed a weakly supervised learning method based on denoising diffusion implicit models (DDIMs) for medical anomaly detection. The method translates an input image of a healthy or diseased subject into a healthy one and then identifies anomaly regions by subtracting the output image from the input. This approach has shown superiority over both VAE and GAN models on datasets like BraTS2020 (Brain Tumor Segmentation Challenge 2020 dataset) and CheXpert.

This weakly supervised learning method is based on DDIMs. It performs image-to-image translation to convert an input image into a healthy one. Anomaly regions are identified by subtracting the output image from the input. The process involves encoding the input image into a noisy image with reversed DDIM sampling and guiding the denoising process through a binary classifier trained on healthy and diseased images.

2.6.4 Application of diffusion model for medical image segmentation

In the context of medical image segmentation, diffusion models are being used to synthesize labeled data, thereby reducing the need for pixel-annotated data. A study by Fernandez et al. [85] proposes brainSPADE, a generative model for synthesizing labeled brain MRI images. This model consists of a label generator and an image generator sub-model, which work together to produce synthetic segmentation maps and images based on these labels. The synthesized data can be used to train segmentation models, with the study showing comparable results when using synthetic versus real data. brainSPADE is a generative model that synthesizes labeled brain MRI images. It includes a label generator for creating synthetic segmentation maps and an image generator for synthesizing images based on these labels. The label generator encodes and diffuses the input segmentation map to produce a latent space, which is then used to construct artificial segmentation maps. The image generator employs a VAE-GAN model to decode the output image using the synthetic segmentation map.

2.6.5 Application of diffusion model for medical image reconstruction

Diffusion models are being employed to address the challenge of medical image reconstruction from under-sampled data. For example, Jalal et al. [86] proposed the use of score-based generative models for compressed sensing MRI, training these models on MRI images to use as prior information in the reconstruction process. This approach, referred to as Compressed Sensing Generative Model (CSGM), demonstrated better performance over existing methods in terms of SSIM and peak signal-to-noise ratio (PSNR) metrics for reconstructing realistic MRI data from under-sampled MRI data. The model trains on MRI images to use as prior information in the reconstruction process. This approach, referred to as CSGM, employs Langevin dynamics for a posterior sampling scheme to reconstruct realistic MRI data from under-sampled data in the spatial domain (or k-space).

In sum, these applications highlight the versatility and potential impact of diffusion models in various aspects of medical image analysis, from registration and segmentation to disease detection and image reconstruction. The diffusion models' ability to generate high-quality images and their robustness to distribution shifts make them promising tools for advancing medical imaging techniques.

2.7 Conclusion

In recent years, DL has revolutionized the field of medical imaging, providing powerful tools for tackling challenging tasks across four key areas: image classification, segmentation, reconstruction, and registration. The remarkable success of DL in these domains has been driven by the availability of some public datasets, increased computational power, and advanced algorithmic innovations. In the domain of medical image classification, DL models have demonstrated exceptional performance in detecting and diagnosing various diseases, such as cancer, neurological disorders, and cardiovascular conditions. These models can learn intricate patterns from vast amounts of data, enabling accurate and efficient diagnosis, which can ultimately lead to improved patient outcomes and reduced healthcare costs.

DL has also made significant strides in medical image segmentation, a crucial task for delineating anatomical structures, lesions, and other regions of interest. CNN and their variants have proven highly effective in generating precise segmentation masks, facilitating accurate quantification, treatment planning, and follow-up monitoring.

Another area where DL has had a profound impact is medical image reconstruction. Traditional reconstruction methods often suffer from limitations such as noise, artifacts, and incomplete data. DL techniques have shown remarkable potential in overcoming these challenges, enabling high-quality image reconstruction from sparse or corrupted data, reducing radiation exposure, and improving overall image quality.

Furthermore, DL has played a pivotal role in medical image registration, a critical task for aligning and integrating multimodal imaging data. By leveraging powerful neural networks, DL algorithms can accurately register images from different modalities, time points, or viewpoints, facilitating comprehensive analysis and enabling precise tracking of disease progression or treatment response.

Despite the numerous successes, there are still challenges and limitations that need to be addressed. Ensuring the robustness, interpretability, and generalizability of DL models remains a significant concern, particularly in safety-critical medical applications. Additionally, issues related to data privacy, bias, and ethical considerations must be carefully navigated as these technologies become more widely adopted.

Looking ahead, the future of DL in medical imaging is promising. Ongoing research efforts are focused on developing more efficient and interpretable models, leveraging multimodal data fusion, and exploring advanced techniques such as self-supervised learning, federated learning, and domain adaptation. Moreover, the integration of DL with other cutting-edge technologies, such as radiomics, radiogenomics, and digital pathology, holds the potential to unlock new frontiers in personalized medicine and precision diagnostics.

As DL continues to evolve, its impact on medical imaging will become increasingly profound, enabling more accurate diagnosis, personalized treatment planning, and ultimately improved patient care. However, it is crucial to maintain a balanced perspective, addressing ethical concerns and ensuring responsible development and deployment of these powerful technologies.

References

1 Zitova, B., & Flusser, J. (2003). Image registration methods: A survey. Image and vision computing, 21(11), pp. 977–1000.

2 https://viso.ai/computer-vision/image-registration/

3 Abbasi, S., et al. (2022). Medical image registration using unsupervised deep neural network: A scoping literature review. Biomedical signal processing and control, 73, pp. 103444.

4 Fu, Y., Lei, Y., Wang, T., Curran, W. J., Liu, T., & Yang, X. (2020). Deep learning in medical image registration: A review. Physics in medicine and biology, 65(20), 20TR01. doi: 10.1088/1361-6560/ab843e.

5 Li, M., Jiang, Y., Zhang, Y., & Zhu, H. (2023). Medical image analysis using deep learning algorithms. Frontiers in public health, 11, 1273253. doi: 10.3389/fpubh.2023.1273253.

6 Hossein-Nejad, Z., & Nasri, M. (2017). An adaptive image registration method based on SIFT features and RANSAC transform. Computers & electrical engineering, 62, pp. 524–537.

7 Alzubaidi, L., Zhang, J., & Humaidi, A. J., et al. (2021). Review of deep learning: Concepts, CNN architectures, challenges, applications, future directions. Journal of big data, 8, p. 53. doi: 10.1186/s40537-021-00444-8.

8 Amari, S. (1993). Backpropagation and stochastic gradient descent method. Neurocomputing, 5(4–5), pp. 185–196.

9 Zhang, Z. (2018). "Improved Adam optimizer for deep neural networks." In: 2018 IEEE/ACM 26th International Symposium on Quality Of Service (IWQoS). IEEE.

10 Xiao, H., et al. (2023). Deep learning-based lung image registration: A review. Computers in biology and medicine, 165 (2023): 107434.

11 Yousef, R., et al. (2022). A holistic overview of deep learning approach in medical imaging. Multimedia systems, 28(3), pp. 881–914.

12 Montavon, G., Kauffmann, J., Samek, W., & Müller, K. R. (2022). Explaining the Predictions of Unsupervised Learning Models. In: Holzinger, A., Goebel, R., Fong, R., Moon, T., Müller, K. R., Samek, W. (eds), xxAI – Beyond Explainable AI. xxAI 2020. Lecture Notes in Computer Science, vol. 13200. Springer, Cham. doi: 10.1007/978-3-031-04083-2_7.

13 Jaderberg, M., Simonyan, K., & Zisserman, A. (2015). Spatial transformer networks. Advances in neural information processing systems, 28, pp. 1–13.

14 Mahapatra, D. (2018). GAN based medical image registration. arXiv preprint arXiv:1805.02369.

15 Elmahdy, M. S., et al. (2019). "Adversarial optimization for joint registration and segmentation in prostate CT radiotherapy." In: Medical Image Computing and Computer Assisted Intervention – MICCAI 2019: 22nd International Conference, Shenzhen, China, October 13–17, 2019, Proceedings, Part VI 22. Springer International Publishing.

16 Liu, B., Wang, L., & Wang, J., et al. (2023). Dual discriminator weighted mixture generative adversarial network for image generation. Journal of ambient intelligence and humanized computing, 14, pp. 10013–10025. doi: 10.1007/s12652-021-03667-y.

17 Chen, M., Tustison, N. J., & Jena, R., et al. (2023). Image Registration: Fundamentals and Recent Advances Based on Deep Learning (Chapter 14). In: Colliot O. (ed.), Machine Learning for Brain Disorders [Internet]. Humana, New York, NY. Available from: https://www.ncbi.nlm.nih.gov/books/NBK597490/ doi: 10.1007/978-1-0716-3195-9_14.

18 Haskins, G., et al. (2019). Learning deep similarity metric for 3D MR–TRUS image registration. International journal of computer assisted radiology and surgery, 14, pp. 417–425.

19 Chan, H. P., Samala, R. K., Hadjiiski, L. M., & Zhou, C. (2020). Deep learning in medical image analysis. Advances in experimental medicine and biology, 1213, pp. 3–21. doi: 10.1007/978-3-030-33128-3_1.

20 Elyan, E., Pattaramon V., Pamela J. et al. (2022). Computer vision and machine learning for medical image analysis: recent advances, challenges, and way forward. Artificial Intelligence Surgery 2(1): 24–45.

21 Bouchard, C., Bernatchez, R., & Lavoie-Cardinal, F. (2023). Addressing annotation and data scarcity when designing machine learning strategies for neurophotonics. Neurophotonics, 10(4), 044405. doi: 10.1117/1.NPh.10.4.044405.

22 Guo, Y., et al. (2023). Adversarial deep transfer learning in fault diagnosis: Progress, challenges, and future prospects. Sensors 23(16), p. 7263.

23 Cunningham, P., Cord, M., & Delany, S. J. (2008). Supervised Learning. In: Matthieu Cord, Pádraig Cunningham, Machine Learning Techniques for Multimedia: Case Studies on Organization and Retrieval (pp. 21–49). Springer, Berlin, Heidelberg.

24 Learning, Semi-Supervised. Semi-supervised learning. CSZ2006. html 5 (2006).

25 Krizhevsky, A., Sutskever, I., & Hinton, G. E. (2012). ImageNet classification with deep convolutional neural networks. In: Advances in Neural Information Processing Systems 25 (NIPS 2012, NeuIPS Proceedings) (pp. 1097–1105).

26 Simonyan, K., & Zisserman, A. (2014). Very deep convolutional networks for large-scale image recognition. arXiv preprint arXiv:1409.1556.

27 Szegedy, C., et al. (2015). Going deeper with convolutions. In Proceedings of the IEEE Conference on Computer Vision and Pattern Recognition (CVPR), Boston, MA, USA.

28 He, K., Zhang, X., Ren, S., & Sun, J. (2016). Deep residual learning for image recognition. In Proceedings of the IEEE Conference on Computer Vision and Pattern Recognition (CVPR), Las Vegas, NV, USA.

29 Huang, G., Liu, Z., Van Der Maaten, L., & Weinberger, K. Q. (2017). Densely connected convolutional networks. In Proceedings of the IEEE Conference on Computer Vision and Pattern Recognition (CVPR), Honolulu, HI, USA.

30 Marques, G., Agarwal, D., & De la Torre Díez, I. (2020). Automated medical diagnosis of COVID-19 through EfficientNet convolutional neural network. Applied soft computing, 96, p. 106691.

31 Saifuddin, H. (2018). Evaluating ResNeXt model architecture for image classification. arXiv preprint arXiv:1805.08700.

32 Raza, K., & Singh, N. K. (2021). A tour of unsupervised deep learning for medical image analysis. Current medical imaging, 17(9), pp. 1059–1077.

33 Chen, X., et al. (2022). Recent advances and clinical applications of deep learning in medical image analysis. Medical image analysis, 79, p. 102444.

34 Baur, C., Albarqouni, S., & Navab, N. (2017). "Semi-supervised deep learning for fully convolutional networks." In: Medical Image Computing and Computer Assisted Intervention – MICCAI 2017: 20th International Conference, Quebec City, QC, Canada, September 11–13, 2017, Proceedings, Part III 20. Springer International Publishing.

35 Huynh, T., Nibali, A., & He, Z. (2022). Semi-supervised learning for medical image classification using imbalanced training data. Computer methods and programs in biomedicine, 216, p. 106628.

36 Feng, H., Jia, Y., Xu, R., Prasad, M., Anaissi, A., & Braytee, A. (2024). "Integration of self-supervised BYOL in semi-supervised medical image recognition." In: International Conference on Computational Science (pp. 163–170). Cham: Springer Nature Switzerland.

37 Yu, K., et al. (2020). A consistency regularization based semi-supervised learning approach for intelligent fault diagnosis of rolling bearing. Measurement, 165, p. 107987.

38 Wenzel, M. (2023). Generative Adversarial Networks and Other Generative Models. In: Colliot, O. (eds) Machine Learning for Brain Disorders. Neuromethods, vol 197. Humana, New York, NY. https://doi.org/10.1007/978-1-0716-3195-9_5.

39 Wang, R., Lei, T., Cui, R., Zhang, B., Meng, H., & Nandi, A. K. (2022). Medical image segmentation using deep learning: A survey. IET image processing, 16(5), pp. 1243–1267.

40 Yang, L., et al. (2017). "Suggestive annotation: A deep active learning framework for biomedical image segmentation." In: Medical Image Computing and Computer Assisted Intervention – MICCAI 2017: 20th International Conference, Quebec City, QC, Canada, September 11–13, 2017, Proceedings, Part III 20. Springer International Publishing.

41 Tajbakhsh, N., et al. (2020). Embracing imperfect datasets: A review of deep learning solutions for medical image segmentation. Medical image analysis, 63, 101693.

42 Liu, X., et al. (2021). A review of deep-learning-based medical image segmentation methods. Sustainability, 13(3), p. 1224.

43 Long, J., Shelhamer, E., & Darrell, T. (2015). Fully convolutional networks for semantic segmentation. Proceedings of the IEEE Conference on Computer Vision and Pattern Recognition (pp. 3431–3440).

44 Sony, S., et al. (2021). A systematic review of convolutional neural network-based structural condition assessment techniques. Engineering structures, 226, p. 111347.

45 Lin, C. Y., Chiu, Y. C., Ng, H. F., Shih, T. K., & Lin, K. H. (2020). Global-and-local context network for semantic segmentation of street view images. Sensors (Basel), 20(10), 2907. doi: 10.3390/s20102907.

46 Zhang, J., et al. (2019). Concrete cracks detection based on FCN with dilated convolution. Applied sciences, 9(13), p. 2686.

47 Ronneberger, O., Fischer, P., & Brox, T. (2015). "U-net: Convolutional networks for biomedical image segmentation." In: Medical Image Computing and Computer-Assisted Intervention – MICCAI 2015: 18th International Conference, Munich, Germany, October 5–9, 2015, Proceedings, Part III 18. Springer International Publishing.

48 Yin, X. X., Sun, L., Fu, Y., Lu, R., & Zhang, Y. (2022). U-Net-based medical image segmentation. Journal of healthcare engineering, 4189781. doi:10.1155/2022/4189781.

49 Nahian, S., Paheding, S., Colin, E. et al.(2011). U-Net and its variants for medical image segmentation: Theory and applications. Preprint at arxiv, 1118, v1.

50 Zhou, Z., et al. (2018). "Unet++: A nested u-net architecture for medical image segmentation." In: Deep Learning in Medical Image Analysis and Multimodal Learning for Clinical Decision Support: 4th International Workshop, DLMIA 2018, and 8th International Workshop, ML-CDS 2018, held in conjunction with MICCAI 2018, Granada, Spain, September 20, 2018, Proceedings 4. Springer International Publishing.

51 Chaudhari, S., et al. (2021). An attentive survey of attention models. ACM transactions on intelligent systems and technology (TIST), 12(5), pp. 1–32.

52 Abdi, M., & Nahavandi, S. Multi-residual networks: Improving the speed and accuracy of residual networks. arXiv preprint arXiv:1609.05672 (2016).

53 Niyas, S., et al. (2022). Medical image segmentation with 3D convolutional neural networks: A survey. Neurocomputing 493, pp. 397–413.

54 Alom, M. Z., et al. (2019). Recurrent residual U-Net for medical image segmentation. Journal of medical imaging, 6(1), pp. 014006–014006.

55 Badrinarayanan, V., Kendall, A., & Cipolla, R. (2017). SegNet: A deep convolutional encoder-decoder architecture for image segmentation. IEEE transactions on pattern analysis and machine intelligence, 39(12), pp. 2481–2495.

56 Wang, J., & Liu, X. (2021). Medical image recognition and segmentation of pathological slices of gastric cancer based on Deeplab v3+ neural network. Computer methods and programs in biomedicine, 207, p. 106210.

57 Liu, Z., et al. (2017). Deep learning Markov random field for semantic segmentation. IEEE transactions on pattern analysis and machine intelligence, 40(8), 1814–1828.

58 Wu, J., Ji, W., Liu, Y., Fu, H., Xu, M., Xu, Y., & Jin, Y. (2023). Medical sam adapter: Adapting segment anything model for medical image segmentation. arXiv preprint arXiv:2304.12620.

59 Rayed, M. E., Islam, S. S., Niha, S. I. et al. (2024). Deep learning for medical image segmentation: State-of-the-art advancements and challenges. Informatics in Medicine Unlocked, 47, 101504

60 Chen, H., Dou, Q., Yu, L., Qin, J., & Heng, P. A. (2018). VoxResNet: Deep voxel-wise residual networks for brain segmentation from 3D MR images. NeuroImage, 170, pp. 446–455.

61 Hu, S., Hoffman, E. A., & Reinhardt, J. M. (2001). Automatic lung segmentation for accurate quantitation of volumetric X-ray CT images. IEEE transactions on medical imaging, 20(6), pp. 490–498.

62 Fernandez-Gonzalez, R., Deschamps, T., Idica, A., Malladi, R., & de Solorzano, C. O. (2004). Automatic segmentation of histological structures in mammary gland tissue sections. Journal of biomedical optics, 9(3), pp. 444–453.

63 Painchaud, N., Skandarani, Y., Judge, T., Bernard, O., Lalande, A., & Jodoin, P. M. (2020). Cardiac segmentation with strong anatomical guarantees. IEEE transactions on medical imaging, 39(11), pp. 3703–3713.

64 Jiang, X., Hu, Z., Wang, S., & Zhang, Y. (2023). Deep learning for medical image-based cancer diagnosis. Cancers (Basel), 15(14), p. 3608. doi: 10.3390/cancers15143608.

65 Mall, P. K., Singh, P. K., Srivastav, S. et al. (2023). A comprehensive review of deep neural networks for medical image processing: Recent developments and future opportunities. Healthcare analytics, p. 100216.

66 Wang, G. (2019) High temporal-resolution dynamic PET image reconstruction using a new spatiotemporal kernel method. IEEE transactions on medical imaging, 38(3), pp. 664–674. doi: 10.1109/TMI.2018.2869868.

67 Lin, D. J., Johnson, P. M., Knoll, F., & Lui, Y. W. (2021). Artificial intelligence for MR image reconstruction: An overview for clinicians. Journal of magnetic resonance imaging, 53(4), pp. 1015–1028. doi: 10.1002/jmri.27078.

68 Komolafe, T. E., Sun, Y., Wang, N., Sun, K., Cao, G., & Shen, D. (2022, September). DPDudoNet: Deep-Prior Based Dual-Domain Network for Low-Dose Computed Tomography Reconstruction. In International Workshop on Machine Learning for Medical Image Reconstruction (pp. 123–132). Cham: Springer International Publishing.

69 Zhou, B., Miao, T., Mirian, N., Chen, X., Xie, H., Feng, Z., Guo, X., Li, X., Zhou, S. K., Duncan, J. S., & Liu, C. (2023). Federated transfer learning for low-dose PET denoising: A pilot study with simulated heterogeneous data. IEEE transactions on radiation and plasma medical sciences, 7(3), pp. 284–295. doi: 10.1109/trpms.2022.3194408.

70 Li, X., et al. (2020). One-dimensional convolutional neural network (1D-CNN) image reconstruction for electrical impedance tomography. Review of scientific instruments, 91(12), 124704.

71 Gupta, H., et al. (2018). CNN-based projected gradient descent for consistent CT image reconstruction. IEEE transactions on medical imaging, 37(6), pp. 1440–1453.

72 Perdios, D., et al. (2021). CNN-based image reconstruction method for ultra-fast ultrasound imaging. IEEE transactions on ultrasonics, ferroelectrics, and frequency control, 69(4), pp. 1154–1168.

73 Yang, C., Wang, W., Cui, D., Zhang, J., Liu, L., Wang, Y., & Li, W. (2023). Deep learning image reconstruction algorithms in low-dose radiation abdominal computed tomography: assessment of image quality and lesion diagnostic confidence. Quantitative imaging in medicine and surgery, 13(5), p. 3161.

74 Karl, W. C. (2005). Regularization in Image Restoration and Reconstruction. In Handbook of Image and Video Processing, A. Bovik, ed, Academic Press Limited (pp. 183–185).

75 Sarvamangala, D. R., & Kulkarni, R. V. (2022). Convolutional neural networks in medical image understanding: A survey. Evolutionary intelligence, 15(1), pp. 1–22. doi: 10.1007/s12065-020-00540-3.

76 Lan, H., et al. (2020). Y-Net: Hybrid deep learning image reconstruction for photoacoustic tomography in vivo. Photoacoustics, 20, 100197.

77 Wu, D., Kim, K., Fakhri, G. E, Li, Q. (2017). A cascaded convolutional neural network for x-ray low-dose CT image denoising. arXiv preprint arXiv:1705.04267.

78 Ahmed, S. F., Alam, M. S. B., & Hassan, M., et al. (2023). Deep learning modelling techniques: Current progress, applications, advantages, and challenges. Artificial intelligence review, 56, pp. 13521–13617. doi: 10.1007/s10462-023-10466-8.

79 Pain, C. D., Egan, G. F., & Chen, Z. (2022). Deep learning-based image reconstruction and post-processing methods in positron emission tomography for low-dose imaging and resolution enhancement. European journal of nuclear medicine and molecular imaging. 49(9), pp. 3098–3118. doi: 10.1007/s00259-022-05746-4.

80 Makhlouf, A., Maayah, M., & Abughanam, N. et al. (2023). The use of generative adversarial networks in medical image augmentation. Neural computing & applications, 35, pp. 24055–24068. doi: 10.1007/s00521-023-09100-z.

81 Armanious, K., et al. (2020). MedGAN: Medical image translation using GANs. Computerized medical imaging and graphics, 79, 101684.

82 Bhadra, S., Zhou, W., & Anastasio, M. A. (2020). Medical Image Reconstruction with Image-Adaptive Priors Learned by Use of Generative Adversarial Networks. In: Medical Imaging 2020: Physics of Medical Imaging, vol. 11312. SPIE.

83 Kim, B., Han, I., & Ye, J. C. (2022). "DiffuseMorph: Unsupervised deformable image registration using diffusion model." In: Computer Vision – ECCV 2022: 17th European Conference, Tel Aviv, Israel, October 23–27, 2022, Proceedings, Part XXXI (pp. 347–364). Springer.

84 Wolleb, J., Bieder, F., Sandkühler, R., & Cattin, P. C. (2022). "Diffusion models for medical anomaly detection." In: Medical Image Computing and Computer Assisted Intervention–MICCAI 2022: 25th International Conference, Singapore, September 18–22, 2022, Proceedings, Part VIII (pp. 35–45). Springer.

85 Fernandez, V., Pinaya, W. H. L., Borges, P., Tudosiu, P.-D., Graham, M. S., Vercauteren, T., & Cardoso, M. J. (2022). "Can segmentation models be trained with fully synthetically generated data?" In: International Workshop on Simulation and Synthesis in Medical Imaging (pp. 79–90). Springer.

86 Jalal, A., Arvinte, M., Daras, G., Price, E., Dimakis, A. G., & Tamir, J. (2021). Robust compressed sensing MRI with deep generative priors. Advances in neural information processing systems, 34, pp. 14938–14954.

3

HOW TO INCORPORATE PRIOR KNOWLEDGE FOR EFFECTIVE fMRI DATA ANALYSIS

A Comprehensive Review and Future Direction

Yuhu Shi, Nizhuan Wang, and Weiming Zeng

3.1 Introduction

Functional magnetic resonance imaging (fMRI) is an advanced neuroimaging technique with many advantages. It has been widely used in the study of many fields such as neurocognitive regularity, brain diseases, and mental health detection [1–3]. It can noninvasively enter the brain of a person who is awake and behaving normally. By tracking whole brain signals for various cognitive and behavioral states, mapping differences associated with specific characteristics or clinical conditions advances our understanding of brain function and its connections to normal and atypical behaviors. At the same time, it provides a solid foundation for promoting effective and reproducible open scientific practice by exploring the capacities of human cognitive, emotional, and motor, as well as obtaining corresponding data across species through non-invasive access to spatial and temporal information at the whole brain level. More recently, Finn et al. proposed that fMRI could be a catalyst for integrating neuroscience based on a systematic introduction of applied research in each subfield of neuroscience, providing a roadmap for the future advances needed to achieve this integrated vision and demonstrating how fMRI could help usher in a new era of interdisciplinary coherence in neuroscience [4].

In the process of applying fMRI technology, how to analyze fMRI data accurately and reliably is the key step. There are many methods that can be used for fMRI data analysis, and they are usually divided into model-driven methods [5, 6] and data-driven methods [7–9]. Among them, the model-driven methods need prior knowledge about the experimental paradigm such as the generalized linear model and Pearson correlation analysis, and these

DOI: 10.1201/9781003481959-3

methods usually consider only local brain region data, rather than whole brain data. Therefore, the data-driven methods emerged that do not require any prior knowledge such as independent component analysis (ICA), sparse component analysis, and non-negative matrix factorization, and they have been fruitfully applied for fMRI data analysis which demonstrated a better performance.

However, in the process of using these methods, it was found that there are still some shortcomings that need to be removed by further research. Some studies showed that these issues can be overcome to a certain extent by introducing prior knowledge and their performance of fMRI data analysis can be improved simultaneously [10, 11]. For example, Li et al. proposed a spatiotemporal constrained nonnegative matrix factorization method by incorporating available temporal and spatial prior knowledge from fMRI data of group participants, which was then used to extract large-scale brain networks to identify transdiagnostic changes in neurocognitive networks associated with multiple diseases [12]. Chen et al. proposed to extract the intrinsic prior knowledge hidden in fMRI data, and then them were integrated into the constrained ICA (CICA) method which was used to decompose the corresponding functional independent components under two states to solve the problem of choosing differential features under different emotional states [13].

In addition, adding prior knowledge to the model is also widely used in other fields of related researches [14, 15]. For example, in order to more effectively capture the biological mechanisms involved in association networks in bionomic analysis. Benedetti et al. proposed a strategy to incorporate prior knowledge into correlation network cutoff selection, and the results showed that prior knowledge can effectively assist the reconstruction of association networks, and it is still effective even when the prior knowledge is rough, missing, and wrong [16]. Deng et al. presented a comprehensive multi-genome imaging framework called multidimensional constraint joint non-negative matrix decomposition to identify modules associated with sarcomatous lung metastasis by using sample-matched full-entity images, DNA methylation, and copy number variation features as prior knowledge [17].

Among them, ICA is a data analysis method based on high-order statistics, which has shown good performance in fMRI data analysis on the premise that the source signals are independent and non-Gaussian. By adding prior knowledge to it, its analytical performance can be greatly improved, and it is also widely concerned with, and applied in, many other fields, such as biomedical signal processing, speech signal processing, machine fault diagnosis, and so on [18–20]. Therefore, this chapter mainly focuses on how to improve the analytical ability of fMRI data by incorporating prior knowledge into ICA and details two model frameworks that incorporate prior knowledge into ICA, namely, constraint optimization framework and multi-objective optimization framework. Then, the relevant issues involved in these two frameworks are discussed, and it further looks into the direction of how to better play the role of prior knowledge in the future.

3.2   Methods

3.2.1   Why incorporating prior knowledge into ICA

ICA is a data-driven blind source separation technique which does not require any prior knowledge, but some additional prior knowledge about the desired independent components usually existed in practical applications. A growing number of researchers have proposed that incorporating prior knowledge into the estimation process of ICA can improve its ability to analyze fMRI data, and many algorithms have been proposed to solve the problem of incorporating prior knowledge into the ICA model [21–23]. For example, Lu and Rajapakse proposed a general CICA framework using a constrained optimization model that automatically extracts the required components in a predefined order and reduces computational costs by incorporating additional prior knowledge into ICA, and then they used the augmented Lagrangian multiplier method and Newton-like learning algorithm to solve it [24, 25]. Subsequently, Lin et al. proposed a semi-blind spatial ICA on the framework of CICA by utilizing spatial prior knowledge, and then applying it to estimate the desired independent components from fMRI data by using a fixed-point learning algorithm [26].

When using ICA for the fMRI data analysis, the original fMRI mixing data is decomposed into a mixed matrix containing temporal information and a source signal matrix containing spatial information. Therefore, the prior knowledge that can be utilized by ICA is also divided into two types: temporal prior knowledge and spatial prior knowledge [27, 28]. However, the above CICA methods usually include only one kind of prior knowledge, and spatial prior knowledge is used in most cases, which may increase the dependency of CICA on the accuracy of prior knowledge. Furthermore, the accuracy of the results will be reduced in another domain if only one type of prior knowledge is used. In order to solve these problems, Wang et al. proposed a spatiotemporal CICA method, which simultaneously uses spatiotemporal prior knowledge as the references in CICA to improve its robustness and reduce the impact of the accuracy of prior knowledge on CICA [29]. Shi et al. proposed a constrained spatiotemporal ICA method on the framework of multi-objective optimization that contains temporal and spatial prior knowledge simultaneously, which improved the detection ability of spatial and temporal domains to a certain extent and reduced the dependency on the accuracy of prior knowledge [30]. Figure 3.1 shows the framework of adding different kinds of prior knowledge into ICA for fMRI data analysis on both single-subject and multi-subject levels.

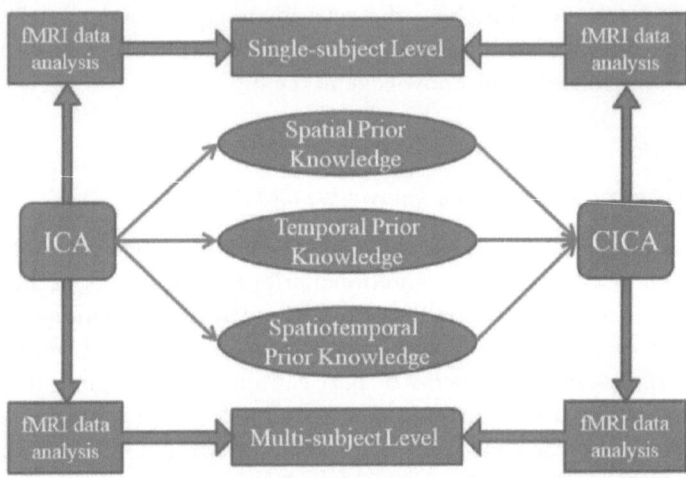

FIGURE 3.1 The framework of adding different kinds of prior knowledge into ICA for fMRI data analysis on both single-subject and multi-subject levels.

3.2.2 How to incorporate prior knowledge into ICA

3.2.2.1 CICA based on constrained optimization framework

In order to integrate prior knowledge into the ICA estimation process, it is necessary to define a distance metric to constrain the similarity between the output signal and prior knowledge. Commonly used distance measures include mean square error and correlation [31]. In classical ICA methods, contrast functions are mainly used to measure the statistical independence of the output signal, where non-Gaussian measures (such as negentropy or kurtosis) and mutual information are often utilized. Similar to most studies, this chapter uses negentropy as a contrast function, which is flexible and reliable because the entropy of the output signal is unknown in practice [32]. Then the traditional CICA model can be formulated as a constraint optimization problem as follows:

$$\text{Maximize } J(y) \approx \left\{ E[G(y)] - E[G(v)] \right\}^2$$

$$\text{Subject to } g(y) = \varepsilon(y, r) - \xi \leq 0 \text{ and } h(y) = E[y^2] - 1 = 0 \quad (3.1)$$

where y is the output signal and $J(y)$ is the contrast function used to measure the statistical independence of $y = wx$ in which w is the unmixing vector and x is the observed fMRI data. $E[\cdot]$ denotes the mathematical expectation. $G(\cdot)$ is a non-quadratic function [33], and v is a Gaussian random variable. r is a reference signal, $\varepsilon(y, r)$ is a distance measure, and ξ is a threshold parameter used to compel the desired output signal to be the only one satisfying

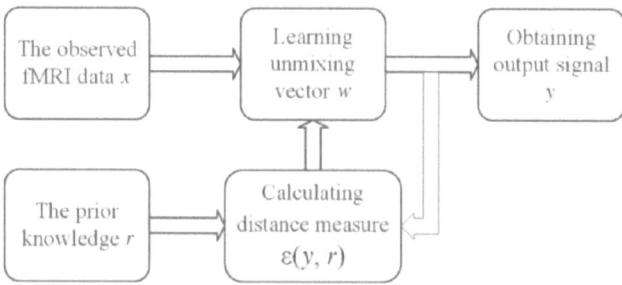

FIGURE 3.2 The schematical diagram of incorporating prior knowledge into ICA.

the inequality constraint. The equality constraint $h(y)$ is used to ensure that the output signal y and the contrast function $J(y)$ are bounded. Through introducing a slack variable c, the inequality constraint can be transformed into an equality constraint, namely, $\hat{g}(y) = g(y) + c = 0$. Then, the augmented Lagrange method combined with a Newton-like learning algorithm or fixed-point learning algorithm is used to solve the constrained optimization problem. Figure 3.2 presents the schematical diagram of incorporating prior knowledge into ICA for fMRI data analysis.

3.2.2.2 CICA based on multi-objective optimization framework

However, it is difficult to predetermine the threshold parameter in the traditional CICA algorithms since the output signals are blind, so the choice of an appropriate threshold depends largely on the experience of applying CICA. An improper parameter usually leads to two possible consequences. When the threshold exceeds the upper bound of the feasible range, the output may produce an unwanted source signal; on the contrary, when it is less than the lower bound of the range, the output cannot produce any source signal, so special efforts must be made to determine the appropriate parameter. In order to solve this problem, the multi-objective optimization framework is used to estimate source signals in the CICA which has circumvented the selection of threshold parameters [34]. Furthermore, in addition to the spatial prior knowledge, there is also some available temporal prior knowledge that can be used in certain situations, such as specific experimental paradigms of cognitive task experiments. According to previous studies, adding spatiotemporal prior knowledge can improve the performance of CICA. Therefore, the CICA model with both temporal and spatial prior knowledge can be established on the multi-objective optimization framework as follows:

$$\textit{Maximize} \begin{cases} J(w_i) \approx \left\{ E\left[G(S_i) \right] - E[G(v)] \right\}^2 \\ \varepsilon_1(w_i) = E\left[S_i R S_i \right] \\ \varepsilon_2(w_i) = E\left[T_i R T_i \right] \end{cases} \tag{3.2}$$

where $J(w_i)$ is the negentropy of the estimated source signal $S_i = w_i^T Y$. $Y = ZX$ denotes the whitening process of X, and Z denotes the whitening matrix. $T_i = Z^{-1}w_i$ denotes the time course corresponding to S_i. $G(\cdot)$ is a non-quadratic function which is the same as in equation (3.1). RS_i denotes a spatial prior knowledge, and $\varepsilon_1(w_i) = E[S_i RS_i]$ is specifically defined as the Pearson correlation to measure the similarity between S_i and RS_i, where both of them have a zero mean and unit variance. RT_i denotes a temporal prior knowledge, and $\varepsilon_2(w_i) = E[T_i RT_i]$ is specifically defined as the Pearson correlation to measure the similarity between T_i and RT_i, where both of them have a zero mean and unit variance. Many methods can be used to solve the multi-objective optimization problem, in which optimizing a linear weighting sum of the contrast functions is an effective method to solve the general multi-objective optimization problem, if the weights are strictly positive and add up to 1 [35], although only one point of the Pareto optimal set is found with one choice of such weights [36]. The process of adding prior knowledge to the CICA algorithm under this framework is consistent with Figure 3.1 and further gives the algorithm steps of this method, as shown in Table 3.1.

TABLE 3.1 The algorithm steps of incorporating prior knowledge into ICA on the framework of multi-objective optimization

---

Step 1: Preprocessing of the observed fMRI data X and prior knowledge RS_i and RT_i.
Step 1.1: The observed fMRI data X was centralized, and then whitened by the whitening matrix Z to obtain Y.
Step 1.2: The prior knowledge RS_i and RT_i are normalized so that they have zero mean and unit variance.
Step 2: The main iterative steps corresponding to each prior knowledge RS_i and RT_i
Step 2.1: Initialize w_i :

$$w_i(0) = \left[\left((RS_i \cdot Y^+)^T + (RT_i \cdot Z^T)^+\right)/2\right] / \left\|\left((RS_i \cdot Y^+)^T + (RT_i \cdot Z^T)^+\right)/2\right\|$$

Step 2.2: Update $\nabla f(w_i(k))$ according to (10) in [28] to get the gradient ascending direction

$$d_i(k) = \nabla f(w_i(k)) / \|\nabla f(w_i(k))\|$$

Step 2.3: Update $w_i(k+1)$ according to (11) in [28] and standardize it, i.e.

$$w_i(k+1) = w_i(k+1) / \|w_i(k+1)\|$$

Step 2.4: Calculate the objective function $f(w_i(k+1))$ according to (5) in [28]. If

$$f(w_i(k+1)) < f(w_i(k)) + \beta \cdot \mu \cdot \nabla f(w_i(k))^T \cdot d_i(k)$$

Then $\mu = \mu \cdot \rho$, return to **Step 2.2**; otherwise, go to **Step 2.5**.
Step 2.5: Check if $\|w_i(k+1) - w_i(k) < \delta\|$, then $w_i = w_i(k+1)$, where δ is an iterative end parameters; otherwise, $k = k+1$, return to **Step 2.2**.
Step 3: Once the source signal $S_i = w_i^T Y$ is obtained, its corresponding time course can be estimated by $T_i = Z^{-1}w_i$.

3.2.3 Evaluation of incorporate prior knowledge into ICA

In order to verify the effectiveness of incorporating prior knowledge into ICA mentioned in this chapter, we conducted an experimental analysis on simulated data, task-related fMRI data, and resting-state fMRI data, respectively, for which the parameter description of simulated data and task-related fMRI data, as well as the pre-processing steps of task-related fMRI data, can be found in [30], while the parameter description and pre-processing steps of resting-state fMRI data can be found in [10].

In the simulated data, CICA with spatiotemporal prior knowledge under the multi-objective framework (denoted as STCICA), CICA with spatial prior knowledge and temporal prior knowledge under the constraint optimization framework (denoted as SCICA and TCICA respectively), and the traditional ICA are involved and compared, in which the corresponding prior knowledge is the simulated spatial region and stimulus mode. In the task-related fMRI data, STCICA, TCICA, and ICA are included, and the corresponding temporal prior knowledge is the BLOCK stimulus mode. In the resting-state fMRI data, STCICA, SCICA, and ICA are included, and the corresponding spatial prior knowledge is obtained by using the method proposed in [37] to carry out group-level data analysis.

The experimental results are shown in Figure 3.3. Among them, Figure 3.3(a) shows the comparison of the correlation coefficient between the real-time course and the time course calculated by STCICA, SCICA, TCICA, and ICA for each subject in the simulated data, respectively. It can be seen from the figure that the correlation coefficients calculated by STCICA, SCICA, and TCICA by adding prior knowledge are all significantly higher than those calculated by ICA, indicating that adding prior knowledge can significantly improve the source signal recovery performance of ICA in the temporal domain. Figure 3.3(b) shows the comparison of the correlation coefficient between the real source signal and the component calculated by STCICA, SCICA, TCICA, and ICA for each subject in the simulated data, respectively. It can be found from the figure that the correlation coefficients calculated by STCICA and SCICA are significantly higher than those calculated by ICA, indicating that the spatial components calculated by STCICA and SCICA are improved to a certain extent compared with those calculated by ICA.

Figure 3.3(c) shows the spatial map corresponding to the visual network calculated by STCICA, TCICA, and ICA in the task-related fMRI data. Meanwhile, Figure 3.3(d) shows the correlation coefficient between the average time courses calculated by the preceding three methods and the prior time course. The results display that the correlation coefficient calculated by STCICA is higher than that calculated by TCICA and ICA, which demonstrate that the method of adding prior knowledge has a better ability of source signal recovery than ICA.

Figure 3.3(e) shows the spatial map corresponding to the default mode network calculated by STCICA, SCICA, and ICA on the group level of

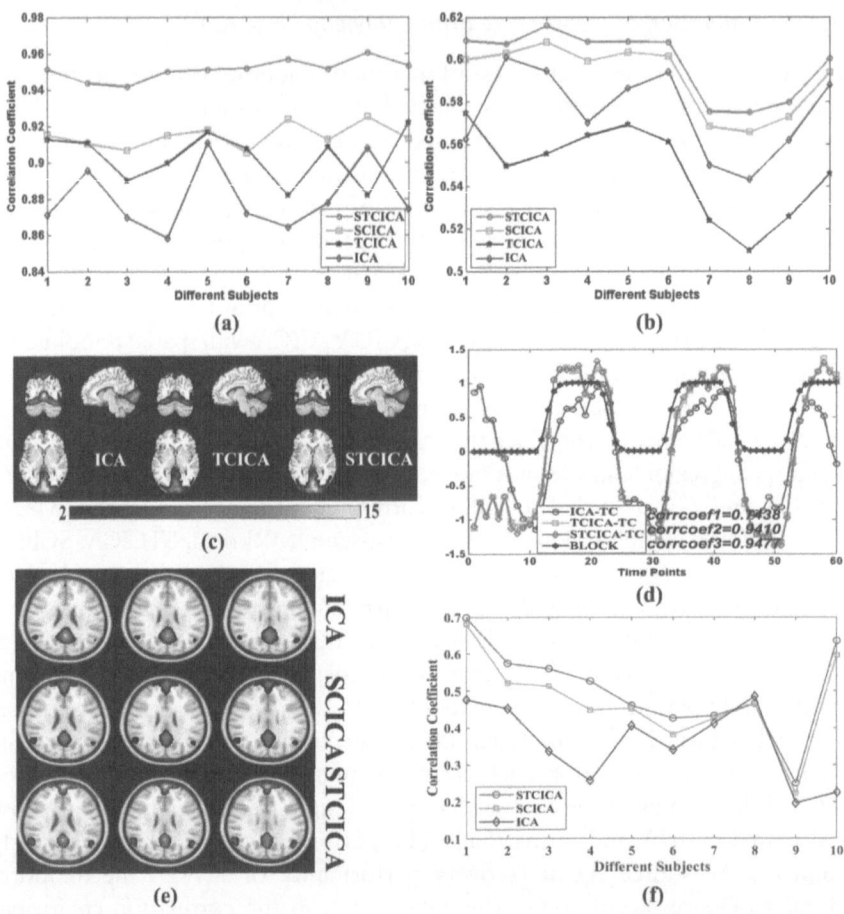

FIGURE 3.3 The results on the simulated data, task-related fMRI data, and resting-state fMRI data.

resting-state fMRI data. It can be seen from the figure that the spatial default network detected by STCICA is improved to some extent compared with those detected by ICA and SCICA. Further, the correlation coefficients between the default mode network of group-level calculated by these three methods and the corresponding default mode network of each subject in the group are given, as shown in Figure 3.3(f). It can be seen from the figure that the correlation coefficients calculated by STCICA and SICA with prior knowledge are higher than those calculated by ICA on most subjects, indicating that the introduction of prior knowledge can significantly improve the universal expression performance of ICA at the group level.

3.3 Discussion

In summary, compared with traditional ICA, CICA has significantly improved the performance for fMRI data analysis to a certain extent, especially for CICA on the framework multi-objective optimization. Therefore, it is expected to be a useful tool for fMRI data analysis. There are many reasons to account for why adding prior knowledge to an ICA model can refine its performance. For example, we can extract only the components of interest without extracting all components compared with classical ICA, thus avoiding the calculation of the components of uninteresting, facilitating subsequent applications, while reducing the computation time and storage requirements required by ICA [38]. Most importantly, incorporating prior knowledge into ICA can improve the quality and accuracy of the separation of components of interest [39].

Of course, it is noted that the performance of CICA is related to the accuracy of prior knowledge. If there is a strong correlation between the given prior knowledge and the target component, the higher is the accuracy of the prior knowledge, which can enable CICA to obtain a better result. On the contrary, if the correlation between the prior knowledge and the target component is weak, the accuracy of the prior knowledge is low, which will cause the algorithm to converge to a poor solution. Therefore, how to reduce the requirement of CICA on the accuracy of prior knowledge, and improve the knowledge of fault-tolerant ability in the calculation process of the algorithm, will be the main contents requiring further investigations.

Moreover, existing methods with prior knowledge usually consider only specific knowledge of the source, such as specific spatial activation templates or specific characteristics of the source. However, this knowledge about the sources is not always known, especially in the case of complex cognitive activity. Therefore, it is important to acquire prior knowledge from the existing data itself. For example, Du and Fan used the group components computed by ICA on a multi-subject level to guide ICA on the single-subject level, which can obtain independent components with subject specificity, stronger independence, better spatial correspondence between different subject, and higher spatiotemporal accuracy [34]. Furthermore, Shi et al. proposed a data-driven method to extract some intrinsic, spatial prior knowledge from data from groups of subjects and then incorporate it into ICA to obtain the group independent component which is more representative of the commonality of the subjects in the group [40].

In practice, ICA is mostly used for multi-subject fMRI data analysis, often referred to as group ICA, and the fMRI data of multiple subjects are typically grouped into three different ways with different hypotheses imposed upon the multi-subject fMRI data, including spatial concatenation, temporal concatenation, and tensor concatenation [41, 42]. The spatial concatenation method assumes that all subjects have common temporal information in each corresponding component and concatenates the multi-subject fMRI data along the spatial dimension. The temporal concatenation method assumes that all subjects have common spatial components and concatenates multi-subject fMRI data along the temporal dimension. The tensor concatenation method assumes that different subjects have common group spatial components and temporal information but a subject-specific magnitude and concatenates the original multi-subject fMRI data along a separate third dimension. For different cascading manners, the way to introduce prior knowledge in ICA will be different due to different dimensions. Therefore, how to introduce different kinds of prior knowledge in multi-subject fMRI data analysis is also a problem that needs to be further studied and solved in the future.

Finally, when the linear weighted summation method is used to solve the CICA model under the multi-objective optimization framework, the summation function will contain the corresponding weight parameters, which are usually determined manually according to manual experience. In other words, the selection of weight parameters is usually subjective, which may introduce certain errors in the results. For the different weight parameter values used in the linear weighted summation objective function, the method can find different solutions to the Pareto front set, which means that the results obtained by the method will contain multiple cases. Therefore, it is necessary to select the best situation through additional post-processing steps according to certain evaluation indicators.

3.4 Future Direction

First, for the problem of introducing prior knowledge into ICA estimation, how to construct and select appropriate prior knowledge is one of the most important factors for their successful application. At present, the prior knowledge that can be embedded into CICA usually is some specific and directly usable prior knowledge, which generally only exists in simple task experiments and does not always exist, or may exist in some cases, but is not easy to obtain. For example, fMRI data in the resting state or complex cognitive task state is difficult to obtain such prior knowledge. It is precisely because of the difficulty in obtaining such prior knowledge that some studies have to abandon the use of the CICA method, and instead use the traditional ICA method to recover all source signals and then make post-selection. From this point of view, mining the prior knowledge implied in data is not only to overcome the problem of difficult acquisition of prior knowledge in CICA but also very beneficial to the wide application of the CICA method. Therefore, how to obtain the available prior knowledge from the existing conditions is particularly important.

Second, the basic idea of CICA is adding prior knowledge into the contrast function of ICA to make sure that the output of the algorithm is the required source signal. Among them, one way is constructing prior knowledge into an inequality constraint by introducing a similarity measure function into the optimization process of the ICA algorithm. Therefore, the solution of CICA becomes a constrained optimization problem, and then the quasi-Newton optimization method or fast fixed-point iteration method is used to solve it. The other way is transforming the inequality constraint containing prior knowledge in the traditional CICA method into an optimization objective function, and forms a multi-objective optimization strategy with the contrast function of traditional ICA, and then use linear weighted summation and genetic algorithm to solve it.

No matter whether the prior knowledge is obtained directly from the experiment or the hidden prior knowledge is mined by data-driven methods, they provide only some rough information about the source signal, which is not 100% correct, while the prior knowledge with different precision has different effects on improving the analytical ability of ICA algorithm. Moreover, it may contain some error information more or less among some available prior knowledge except for the low precision. The basic idea of the CICA method is to guide the algorithm optimization process to converge to the desired output through prior knowledge. If the prior knowledge contains false information, it will inevitably mislead the convergence direction of the algorithm optimization process, so that the output is not the expected result. Therefore, how to improve the fault-tolerant ability of the CICA algorithm to prior knowledge and reduce the adverse impact of false information on the algorithm is a key problem to be solved urgently.

Next, according to the analysis in Section 3.2.1, it can be seen that prior knowledge can be divided into temporal prior knowledge and spatial prior knowledge. Therefore, the use of prior knowledge to construct constraints in the model can be divided into three situations: the use of temporal prior knowledge to construct constraints, the use of spatial prior knowledge to construct constraints, and the use of temporal and spatial prior knowledge to construct constraints. At the same time, the traditional ICA method divides the observation data into a mixed matrix containing temporal information and a source signal matrix containing spatial information. Therefore, according to the different constraints, it can be divided into two ways to constrain the mixed matrix and the source signal matrix in the ICA model by using prior knowledge. Although they all use prior knowledge to constrain the optimization process, the solution methods of the model and the final results are different with different kinds of prior knowledge or different constraints. Therefore, exploration of the specific impacts of different kinds of prior knowledge and different constraints on the CICA algorithm is also the subject that needs to be focused in the future.

Thirdly, as a data-driven method, ICA decomposes the observed fMRI data into several sources without any prior knowledge under the assumption that the sources are mutually statistically independent and non-Gaussian. Based on the assumption whether statistical independence is madding in the temporal or spatial domain, ICA is divided into spatial ICA (SICA) and temporal ICA (TICA). SICA decomposes the observed data into components that are spatially independent to the greatest extent possible, while TICA obtains these components by optimizing the temporal independence between them. Among them, TICA is less robust because the number of spatial voxels is much larger than the number of time points, and TICA is also much more computative because it requires the calculation of a difficult mixed matrix, which becomes unfeasible in practice. Therefore, TICA is generally used to analyze only a few slices of fMRI data, rather than the whole brain fMRI data, which greatly limits the analytical performance of TICA and its ability to be widely used in the analysis of whole brain fMRI data.

Therefore, it is important to develop a feasible version of TICA for whole brain fMRI data analysis. While improving the robustness of TICA, it also helps to expand its application in fMRI data analysis. In order to solve this problem, Shi et al. proposed to adopt a split strategy in ICA to overcome this problem, and the results proved the effectiveness of this strategy, thus making TICA available for whole brain fMRI data analysis [40]. Of course, there are still some limitations to the proposed method. For example, optimization of the packet numbers is a challenge, and different packet numbers may lead to different results. We do not know how other packet number values will affect the results; thus, further studies are needed.

Finally, as neuroimaging data increases in volume and dimension, it becomes increasingly important to improve big data analytics capabilities. Therefore, more and more methods like deep neural networks are being rapidly applied for fMRI data analysis in various fields. However, for end-to-end deep neural networks, although it can automatically learn some distinguishing features, it often fits some non-important features, resulting in the partial collapse of the model to some bad features. In order to solve this problem, some studies can make the model learn some key features by adding artificially designed prior knowledge to the model. Therefore, how to add prior knowledge into the methods including deep neural networks to improve their ability for fMRI data analysis is a problem that needs further research in the future.

3.5 Conclusion

Taking the ICA algorithm as an example, this chapter introduces the role and significance of adding prior knowledge to ICA, elaborates two common CICA frameworks containing prior knowledge, and conducts verification analysis in three experiments of simulation data, task-related fMRI data, and resting-state fMRI data. The results show that adding prior knowledge to ICA can effectively improve its performance of fMRI data analysis. In the end, the existing problems are discussed in detail, and the introduction of prior knowledge into other algorithms for fMRI data analysis is prospected in the future.

References

1 Raichle M E, MacLeod A M, Snyder A Z, et al. A default mode of brain function. Proceedings of the National Academy of Sciences, 2001, 98(2): 676–682.
2 Shi Y, Zeng W, Deng J, et al. The identification of Alzheimer's disease using functional connectivity between activity voxels in resting-state fMRI data. IEEE Journal of Translational Engineering in Health and Medicine, 2020, 8: 1–11.
3 Shi Y, Li Y. The effective connectivity analysis of fMRI based on asymmetric detection of transfer brain entropy. Cerebral Cortex, 2024, 34(3): bhae070.
4 Finn E S, Poldrack R A, Shine J M. Functional neuroimaging as a catalyst for integrated neuroscience. Nature, 2023, 623(7986): 263–273.
5 Friston K J, Holmes A P, Worsley K J, et al. Statistical parametric maps in functional imaging: a general linear approach. Human Brain Mapping, 1994, 2(4): 189–210.
6 Sun F T, Miller L M, D'Esposito M. Measuring interregional functional connectivity using coherence and partial coherence analyses of fMRI data. Neuroimage, 2004, 21(2): 647–658.
7 Cordes D, Haughton V, Carew J, et al. Hierarchical clustering to measure connectivity in fMRI resting-state data. Magnetic Resonance Imaging, 2002, 20(4): 305–317.
8 Calhoun V D, Adali T. Unmixing fMRI with independent component analysis. IEEE Engineering in Medicine and Biology Magazine, 2006, 25(2): 79–90.
9 Wang N, Zeng W, Chen D. A novel sparse dictionary learning separation (SDLS) model with adaptive dictionary mutual incoherence constraint for fMRI data analysis. IEEE Transactions on Biomedical Engineering, 2016, 63(11): 2376–2389.
10 Shi Y, Zeng W, Wang N, et al. A new method for independent component analysis with priori information based on multi-objective optimization. Journal of Neuroscience Methods, 2017, 283: 72–82.
11 Jie B, Liu M, Liu J, et al. Temporally constrained group sparse learning for longitudinal data analysis in Alzheimer's disease. IEEE Transactions on Biomedical Engineering, 2016, 64(1): 238–249.
12 Li Y, Zeng W, Deng J, et al. Exploring dysconnectivity of the large-scale neurocognitive network across psychiatric disorders using spatiotemporal constrained nonnegative matrix factorization method. Cerebral Cortex, 2022, 32(20): 4576–4591.
13 Chen X, Zeng W, Shi Y, et al. Intrinsic prior knowledge driven CICA FMRI data analysis for emotion recognition classification. IEEE Access, 2019, 7: 59944–59950.
14 James C J, Gibson O J. Temporally constrained ICA: an application to artifact rejection in electromagnetic brain signal analysis. IEEE Transactions on Biomedical Engineering, 2003, 50(9): 1108–1116.
15 Deng J, Zeng W, Kong W, et al. Multi-constrained joint non-negative matrix factorization with application to imaging genomic study of lung metastasis in soft tissue sarcomas. IEEE Transactions on Biomedical Engineering, 2019, 67(7): 2110–2118.

16 Benedetti E, Pučić-Baković M, Keser T, et al. A strategy to incorporate prior knowledge into correlation network cutoff selection. Nature Communications, 2020, 11(1): 5153.

17 Deng J, Zeng W, Luo S, et al. Integrating multiple genomic imaging data for the study of lung metastasis in sarcomas using multi-dimensional constrained joint non-negative matrix factorization. Information Sciences, 2021, 576: 24–36.

18 Wang Z, Chen J, Dong G, et al. Constrained independent component analysis and its application to machine fault diagnosis. Mechanical Systems and Signal Processing, 2011, 25(7): 2501–2512.

19 De Vos M, De Lathauwer L, Van Huffel S. Spatially constrained ICA algorithm with an application in EEG processing. Signal Processing, 2011, 91(8): 1963–1972.

20 Shi Y, Zeng W, Tang X, et al. An improved multi-objective optimization-based CICA method with data-driver temporal reference for group fMRI data analysis. Medical & Biological Engineering & Computing, 2018, 56: 683–694.

21 Wang Z. Fixed-point algorithms for constrained ICA and their applications in fMRI data analysis. Magnetic Resonance Imaging, 2011, 29(9): 1288–1303.

22 Ma X, Zhang H, Zhao X, et al. Semi-blind independent component analysis of fMRI based on real-time fMRI system. IEEE Transactions on Neural Systems and Rehabilitation Engineering, 2012, 21(3): 416–426.

23 Mi J X, Xu Y. A comparative study and improvement of two ICA using reference signal methods. Neurocomputing, 2014, 137: 157–164.

24 Lu W, Rajapakse J C. Approach and applications of constrained ICA. IEEE Transactions on Neural Networks, 2005, 16(1): 203–212.

25 Lu W, Rajapakse J C. ICA with reference. Neurocomputing, 2006, 69(16): 2244–2257.

26 Lin Q H, Liu J Y, Zheng Y R, et al. Semiblind spatial ICA of fMRI using spatial constraints. Human Brain Mapping, 2010, 31(7): 1076–1088.

27 Lin Q H, Zheng Y R, Yin F L, et al. A fast algorithm for one-unit ICA-R. Information Sciences, 2007, 177(5): 1265–1275.

28 Calhoun V D, Adali T, Stevens M C, et al. Semi blind ICA of fMRI: a method for utilizing hypothesis derived time courses in a spatial ICA analysis. NeuroImage, 2005, 25(2): 527–538.

29 Wang Z, Xia M G, Jin Z, et al. Temporally and spatially constrained ICA of fMRI data analysis. PloS One, 2014, 9(4): e94211.

30 Shi Y, Zeng W, Wang N, et al. A new constrained spatiotemporal ICA method based on multi-objective optimization for fMRI data analysis. IEEE Transactions on Neural Systems and Rehabilitation Engineering, 2018, 26(9): 1690–1699.

31 Huang D S, Mi J X. A new constrained independent component analysis method. IEEE Transactions on Neural Networks, 2007, 18(5): 1532–1535.

32 Comon P. Independent component analysis, a new concept? Signal Processing, 1994, 36(3): 287–314.

33 Hyvarinen A. Fast and robust fixed-point algorithms for independent component analysis. IEEE Transactions on Neural Networks, 1999, 10(3): 626–634.

34 Du Y H, Fan Y. Group information guided ICA for fMRI data analysis. NeuroImage, 2013, 69: 157–197.

35 Klamroth K, Jørgen T. Constrained optimization using multiple objective programming. Journal of Global Optimization, 2007, 37: 325–355.

36 Marler R T, Arora J S. Survey of multi-objective optimization methods for engineering. Structural and Multidisciplinary Optimization, 2004, 26: 369–395.

37 Shi Y, Zeng W, Wang N, et al. A novel fMRI group data analysis method based on data-driven reference extracting from group subjects. Computer Methods and Programs in Biomedicine, 2015, 122(3): 362–371.

38 Barros A K, Vigário R, Jousmaki V, et al. Extraction of event-related signals from multichannel bioelectrical measurements. IEEE Transactions on Biomedical Engineering, 2000, 47(5): 583–588.

39 Rasheed T, Lee Y K, Kim T S. Constrained spatiotemporal ICA and its application for fMRI data analysis[C]//13th International Conference on Biomedical Engineering: ICBME 2008 3–6 December 2008 Singapore. Springer Berlin Heidelberg, 2009: 555–558.

40 Wu L, Calhoun V D, Jung R E, et al. Connectivity-based whole brain dual parcellation by group ICA reveals tract structures and decreased connectivity in schizophrenia. Human Brain Mapping, 2015, 36(11): 4681–4701.

41 Shi Y, Zeng W, Wang N. SCGICAR: spatial concatenation based group ICA with reference for fMRI data analysis. Computer Methods and Programs in Biomedicine, 2017, 148: 137–151.

42 Shi Y, Zeng W. SCTICA: sub-packet constrained temporal ICA method for fMRI data analysis. Computers in Biology and Medicine, 2018, 102: 75–85.

4

AI APPLICATIONS IN DIAGNOSTICS AND TREATMENT

Yuchi Tian, Temitope Emmanuel Komolafe, and Wenxiu Zhang

4.1 Introduction

Medical imaging technology has become an indispensable part of modern clinical diagnosis and disease research. Doctors cannot do without the assistance of medical imaging information in the diagnosis of diseases. They can quickly and accurately diagnose diseases through imaging data and improve the cure rate and survival rate of patients.

With the continuous development of medical technology, large-scale medical imaging equipment (computed tomography (CT), X-ray (X-radiation), magnetic resonance imaging (MRI), etc.) has been widely popularized and applied, resulting in a continuous and substantial increase in the amount of medical imaging data. Nowadays, the diagnosis of medical imaging is mainly relying on doctors for purely manual diagnosis, but the training speed of professional radiologists cannot keep up with the increase in image data. The two have presented an unbalanced development and a situation of short supply, resulting in low diagnosis efficiency and slow diagnosis results. Moreover, doctors are facing such a huge workload and often have to diagnose medical images in an overloaded state, so the rate of misdiagnosis and missed diagnosis is inevitably increased; at the same time, the generation of massive medical imaging data not only brings huge work pressure to doctors but also leads to a lot of waste of valuable medical information. Doctors do not have extra time and energy to conduct information mining analysis and medical research on the acquired medical images. By using valuable medical images to extract and analyze rich feature information, it becomes possible to address the challenge

DOI: 10.1201/9781003481959-4

of quantitatively evaluating the heterogeneity of certain diseases, such as tumors. This will have important clinical value and significance for disease prediction and efficacy evaluation.

In recent years, artificial intelligence (AI) has developed rapidly, demonstrating its advantages and potential in the medical field. The essence of AI is embodied in the formation of valuable conclusive information and knowledge models by collecting, processing, analyzing, and mining data, simulating human cognition and reaction. At the same time, it can extend the simulated human ability to serve human-specific task requirements. AI-based intelligence algorithms rely on the powerful computing power of computers and have the ability to process massive amounts of data to solve some complex problems, which can far exceed the processing capabilities of human beings. With the gradual maturity of computer vision and cognitive computing in the field of AI, AI technology has begun to become an important factor affecting the development of the medical industry and improving the level of medical services.

The application advantages of AI in medical image analysis can be summarized in the following aspects: (1) Improving diagnostic efficiency: AI can quickly and accurately mark specific abnormal structural areas for the reference of radiologists, help doctors improve the efficiency of film reading and diagnostic decision-making ability, quickly feedback patient diagnosis results, and alleviate the problem of a short supply of radiologists. (2) Reducing misdiagnosis caused by human subjective factors: Because it is a computer diagnosis, there will be no problem with fatigue and low efficiency, and it also reduces the diagnostic errors caused by some subjective biases or mistakes. (3) Mining medical information: Understanding medical images and extracting the key information that has value for treatment decision-making are very important links in the process of curative effect prediction. The computer can analyze massive data, and through feature mining, it can gain insight into the level of information that cannot be obtained by human eyes. This information can be quantified and divided, providing a theoretical basis for the prognosis of diseases and the evaluation of surgical efficacy.

AI-driven techniques have shown remarkable potential in improving the accuracy, efficiency, and accessibility of medical diagnosis and treatment. This review aims to explore the role of AI in medical diagnostics, medical imaging, and the analysis of physiological signals. We will delve into the applications of machine learning algorithms in computer-aided diagnosis (CAD), the use of AI in medical imaging processing, and its impact on the analysis of physiological signals. Figure 4.1 provides an overview of AI applications in medical imaging, specifically in diagnosis and treatment.

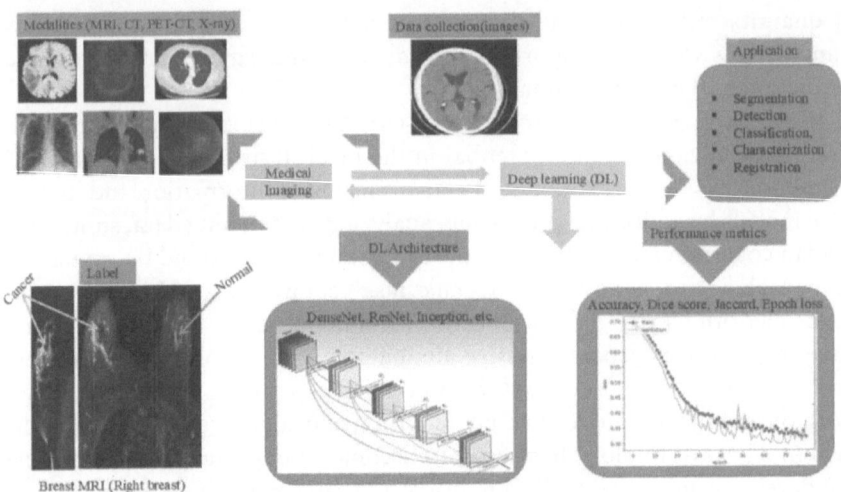

FIGURE 4.1 Deep learning implementation and traits for medical imaging application [1].

4.2 AI in computer-aided diagnosis

CAD systems represent a cornerstone of AI applications in diagnostics and imaging. These systems harness the power of machine learning algorithms to analyze medical images and assist healthcare professionals in making accurate diagnoses. CAD systems are equipped with sophisticated algorithms capable of identifying subtle abnormalities and patterns indicative of various diseases across different imaging modalities. The integration of CAD into clinical practice has significantly enhanced diagnostic accuracy, particularly in fields such as radiology and pathology.

4.2.1 Segmentation

Segmentation is especially important in the development of surgical plans, which can help physicians determine the exact boundaries of the lesion, guide the operation, and provide technical support in the quantitative analysis of some clinical parameters related to shape. The application of AI in medical image segmentation can free doctors from the laborious manual delineation of regions of interest (ROI), and the study of automatic segmentation is the most common topic in medical application papers. The best performance of medical image segmentation using AI is the automatic segmentation method using deep learning convolutional neural network (CNN). Numerous CNN-based deep learning models have been developed for medical image segmentation tasks, such as U-Net, DeepLab, Mask R-CNN, etc. These models have their own characteristics in structural design and training strategies and can be optimized and adjusted for different medical imaging tasks. In addition, some advanced medical image segmentation methods also combine multi-modal image data and prior knowledge to further improve the accuracy and stability of segmentation. The most famous one is the U-Net neural network model proposed by Ronneberger et al. [2] in 2015. The advantage of this model is that it connects a contraction path and an expansion path in equal parts. The contraction path can capture semantic information, and the expansion path is used for accurate positioning. U-Net also uses the idea of short-circuit connection to connect the corresponding convolutional layer and deconvolution layer, so that more low-level feature information can be fused into the feature map, while taking into account the feature information of different scales. In addition, U-Net's training strategy based on data amplification makes more effective use of limited labeled samples so that even with a small number of labeled samples, the model can be trained and excellent segmentation results can be obtained. Later, the U-Net algorithm was extended to 3D medical image segmentation, and many derivatives of U-Net network models were born. For example, Çiçek et al. [3] proposed a 3D-U-Net network model in 2016, which changed 2D operations (convolution, pooling, etc.) in 2D-U-Net into 3D operations. In the same year, Milletari et al. [4] also proposed the V-net network for 3D image segmentation and conducted segmentation experiments on MRI prostate scan sequences, obtaining the Dice coefficient of 0.869. Choi et al. [5] have developed a fast and accurate method for striatum segmentation based on deep CNN architecture in their research on brain summary striatum segmentation. A Dice coefficient of 0.893 ± 0.017 was obtained, and the speed and accuracy of this method make it suitable for application in neuroscience and other clinical fields. The emergence of an AI-based 3D segmentation algorithm is adapted to the current situation and actual needs of most clinical 3D image analysis. Stollenga et al. [6] proposed a 3D network model that rearranged the traditional cuboid computing order in MD-LSTM in a pyramid way and segmented the six directions of brain MRI images, achieving excellent segmentation results in the MRBrainS Competition in 2015. Moeskops et al. [7] constructed an MRI brain image segmentation model composed of three CNN models, and the modified model could automatically segment different tissues (white matter, gray matter, and cerebrospinal fluid) in the three brain images, and the Dice coefficient of about 0.85 was obtained by this algorithm. Singh et al. [8] used a generative adversarial network (GANs) to continuously learn the internal characteristics of breast masses and to segment the masses. They achieved a Jaccard index of 0.89 and a Dice coefficient of 0.94. Andermatt et al. [9] proposed the use of 3D recurrent neural networks (RNNs) with gated units to segment white matter and gray matter in brain images and achieved a good segmentation effect.

As an important branch of medical image processing, medical image segmentation aims to accurately divide and segment structures or tissues in medical images, providing key support for clinical diagnosis, treatment planning, and disease research. Traditional medical image segmentation methods mainly rely on the features and rules of manual design, and there are some problems such as low precision, strong subjectivity, and heavy workload.

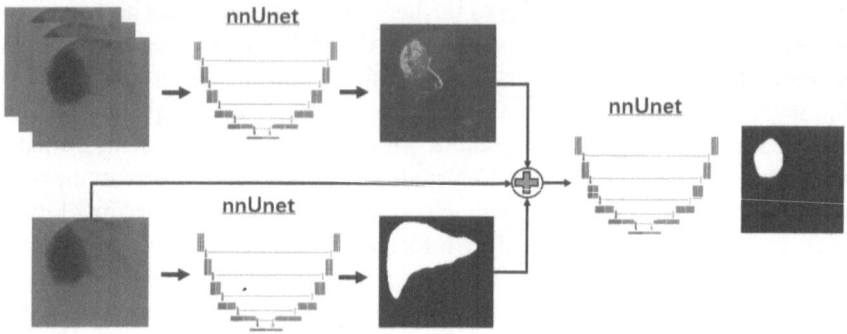

FIGURE 4.2   Liver tumor segmentation using CNN architecture [10].

With the rise of deep learning technology, especially the wide application of CNN, medical image segmentation has made remarkable progress.

The successful application of deep learning in medical image segmentation is mainly due to its ability to automatically learn high-level feature representations without manually designing feature extractors. By training on a large amount of medical image data, CNN can learn features such as structure, texture, and shape in the image and use them for accurate segmentation. At present, medical image segmentation based on deep learning has achieved success in various medical image analysis tasks, including organ segmentation, tumor localization, and blood vessel extraction. Figure 4.2 shows a schematic representation of how a deep-learning model like U-Net can be applied to liver tumor segmentation. For more details, see Ref [10].

Despite the remarkable results of deep learning methods, medical image segmentation still faces some challenges. First, the high cost of annotation and acquisition of medical image data limits the training and application of deep learning models. Second, the deep learning model is poor in interpretation, and it is difficult to understand the reason and basis of its segmentation results. In addition, the diversity and complexity of medical image data also brings challenges to segmentation tasks, requiring more intelligent and robust algorithms to cope with different clinical scenarios and data characteristics.

In summary, medical image segmentation, as an important research direction in the field of medical image processing, has made remarkable progress with the help of AI technologies such as deep learning. With the continuous development of technology and the accumulation of medical image data, medical image segmentation technology will further improve the efficiency and accuracy of medical image analysis and provide more reliable support for clinical diagnosis and treatment.

4.2.2 Classification

With the development of medical imaging technology, the collection of medical images is more convenient, and the storage is almost fully digitized.

Doctors are increasingly relying on medical images for disease diagnosis. However, doctors are highly subjective in the diagnosis of images, and their energy is limited, so it is difficult to improve the amount of film reading every day. In addition, there may be cases of misdiagnosis due to fatigue. Therefore, the construction of intelligent medical-assisted diagnosis, especially the automatic medical image diagnosis system based on an AI algorithm, can improve the clinical diagnosis efficiency and reduce the misdiagnosis rate of human factors. Intelligent image classification is the earliest and most extensive application of AI in medical images. The typical operation in medical examination classification is to take medical image film as the input of the model, and then the model outputs the judgment result of whether there is a disease. In recent years, the development of AI algorithm has brought a series of new breakthroughs in the field of medical image classification.

The evolution of AI in medical classification has witnessed significant advancements in machine learning algorithms, particularly deep learning models such as CNNs and RNNs. These algorithms excel in learning complex patterns and features from large-scale medical datasets, enabling accurate classification and diagnosis of diseases across diverse medical specialties. Intelligent medical image classification is a process of automated analysis and classification of medical image data using AI technology, which aims to help doctors accurately and quickly diagnose diseases, evaluate conditions, and guide treatment. With the rapid growth of medical image data and the continuous development of AI technology, intelligent classification of medical images has become one of the important research directions in the field of medical images.

The core of intelligent medical image classification is to use machine learning and deep learning algorithms to extract features from medical image data and classify them. Traditional machine learning methods include support vector machines (SVM), decision trees, random forests, etc., while deep learning methods have attracted much attention for their excellent performance in image recognition and classification tasks, especially the application of CNN. By training on a large number of medical image data, the intelligent classification system can learn the feature representation in the image and achieve accurate classification and recognition of different diseases and lesions. Figure 4.3 shows

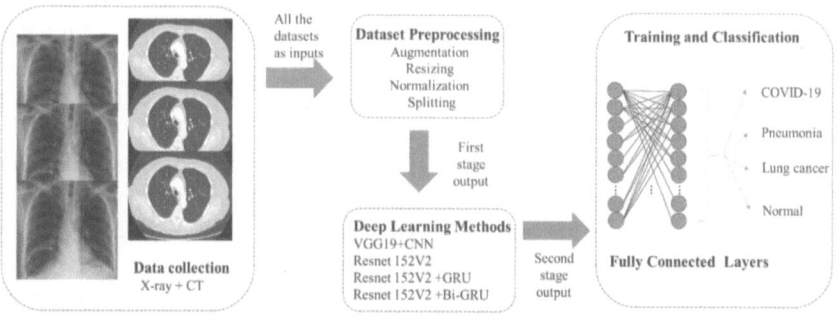

FIGURE 4.3 Classification and predictions of lung diseases from chest X-rays [11].

how different deep-learning models have been applied to classify COVID-19 from lung infections, such as pneumonia. For more details, please see Ref [11].

Sunwoo et al. [12] analyzed MRI of craniocerebral metastases with a CAD system, and the diagnostic sensitivity increased from 77.6% to 81.9%, and the diagnostic time of each patient was reduced by 42 s compared with before. For interns with relatively weak professional knowledge, the sensitivity of diagnosis also increased by about 10%. Masood et al. [13] used an AI algorithm to diagnose lung cancer by analyzing chest CT images and obtained an average lung cancer screening accuracy of 84.58%. Hepsa et al. [14] used the neural network method to diagnose 143 breast cancer patients, and the accuracy rate of diagnosis results (82%) reached the level of professional radiologists (79–87%). Kumar et al. [15] proposed a method for classifying pulmonary nodules using CNN. The accuracy of this method was 0.75, the sensitivity was 0.83, and after ten cross-validations, the false positive of each patient was 0.39. Lakhani and Sundaram used convolutional deep networks to automatically classify X-ray images of tuberculosis. The sensitivity and specificity of the classification results were both over 90%, while the AUC (area under curve) was about 0.98 [16]. The AUC score of the CNN model trained by Becker et al. [17] in the detection of breast cancer was 0.82, which reached the level of experienced breast cancer diagnostic physicians. Shin et al. [18] used GoogLeNet to construct a detection model for CT scanning to detect thoracic and abdominal lymph nodes and interstitial lung disease. An AUC of 0.95 and a sensitivity of 0.85 are obtained. Yan et al. [19] developed a detection algorithm based on 3D information. On DeepLesion dataset [20] (including lung nodules, liver tumors, pancreas, bone, kidney soft tissue, and other lesions), multiple lesions could be detected simultaneously, and the lesion recognition accuracy rate reached 84.37%. It provides the technical possibility for assisting doctors to quickly diagnose various types of lesions in patients. Ciresan et al. [21] used CNNs to identify mitosis through feature learning on breast histological images and obtained a recall rate of 0.70 and a precision of 0.88 in the published histopathological electronic image dataset test. Wang et al. [22] used the CNN model to classify and learn T2-weighted MRI sequences of prostate cancer and obtained an AUC score of 0.84. The above studies show that AI technology can assist doctors in imaging diagnosis in clinical practice. It not only improves the diagnostic accuracy of doctors but also reduces the time of diagnosing medical images, which has an important auxiliary role and clinical value. Another important technology application for medical image classification based on CNN is transfer learning technology. The training of CNN requires the support of massive labeled training data, while medical images require experienced doctors to spend a lot of time on high-quality labeling, so it is often unrealistic to obtain a large number of high-quality labeled training data. The transfer learning technology can solve this problem well. Its core idea is to transfer the models or features learned in a certain domain to another related domain and solve new problems in the target domain based on the prior knowledge of the source domain. Maqsood et al. [23] developed a domain adaptive classifier by transferring the model parameters and prior distribution learned from natural image classification in the source domain to the target domain. They finetuned a natural image classifier containing more than a million images and 1,000 categories, then fed MRI images with Alzheimer's disease (AD) into the model, which had been pre-trained on natural images, and then trained it to get good AD diagnosis results. Transfer learning has also been used in other studies [24]. To solve the expensive problem of acquiring annotated medical images, in addition to the transfer learning method, the CNN multi-example learning algorithm is also proposed, and the CNN multi-example learning algorithm belongs to the semi-supervised learning method. In multi-instance learning, the label knowledge of the training set processed is incomplete; that is, each instance of the training set is considered to be a set with labels, and the elements in the set are unlabeled, and the machine has to learn the labels of the elements in the set by itself. This method is particularly suitable for medical image classification training with only image-level labels (i.e., diseased and disease-free), without marking the focal areas. For example, Shen et al. [25] built a network for patient-grade lung cancer prediction by first training a nodule-grade CNN model and then based on a model of the maximum probability MIL strategy. Han et al. [26] proposed an attention-based deep 3D multi-instance learning for automatic screening of COVID-19. By treating 3D chest CT as a set of instances, the algorithm achieved an overall accuracy of 97.9% and an AUC of 99.0%.

Although intelligent classification of medical images shows great potential in clinical applications, it also faces some challenges. First, the quality and quantity of medical image data have an important impact on the performance of intelligent classification systems, so a large amount of high-quality data is needed for training and verification. Second, the privacy and security of medical image data also need to be fully considered to ensure the security and privacy of patient data. In addition, the interpretability and credibility of intelligent classification systems are also a focus of concern, and doctors need to understand the working principle of the algorithm and the reliability of the results in order to fully trust and accept its auxiliary diagnosis.

In summary, as a cutting-edge technology in the field of medical imaging, intelligent classification of medical images provides important support for improving the efficiency and accuracy of medical image analysis and promoting the personalization and precision of clinical diagnosis and treatment. With the continuous advancement of technology and the continuous evolution of clinical needs, intelligent classification of medical images will continue to play an important role and inject new vitality into further development and innovation in the field of medical imaging.

4.2.3 Lesion detection

Medical image object detection is the process of automatically detecting and locating structures, lesions, or abnormal areas of interest from medical images using computer vision and machine learning techniques. This technology has important application significance in medical image analysis and clinical diagnosis, which can help doctors more accurately diagnose diseases, evaluate conditions, and guide treatment.

The key to medical image target detection is to identify and locate the target of interest in medical images, such as tumors, organs, lesions, etc. Traditional medical image analysis methods often rely on the doctor's experience and intuition, which is subjective and inefficient. The use of machine learning and deep learning technology for medical image target detection can achieve automatic, efficient, and accurate target positioning.

Medical image target detection has a wide application prospect in clinical practice. First of all, it can help doctors quickly and accurately find and locate lesions, tumors, and other targets, providing important auxiliary information for clinical diagnosis. Second, medical image target detection can also be used to assess the severity of the disease, predict the development trend of the disease, and guide the formulation and adjustment of treatment programs. In addition, medical image target detection can also be used for the screening and early detection of diseases, helping to improve treatment outcomes.

In medical image object detection, deep learning technology is particularly prominent, especially the method based on a CNN. By training on a large number of medical image data, CNN can learn the feature representation in the image and achieve accurate detection and positioning of the target. At present, many medical image target detection algorithms based on deep learning have achieved remarkable results, including Faster R-CNN, YOLO, Mask R-CNN, and so on. Girshick [27] et al. proposed the R-CNN model in 2014 for the first time by combining the preselection frame of object detection with CNN technology and realized more accurate image object detection and location. Subsequently, improved or new deep learning object detection algorithms have been successfully proposed, such as Fast-R-CNN [28], Faster-R-CNN [29], and YOLO [30], and some models have also achieved good results in lesion detection and segmentation. Zhang et al. [31] proposed a CNN (Mask R-CNN) method based on multi-scale mask regions, which uses PET imaging to detect lung tumor area. The authors trained three R-CNN models on three images at different scales and then integrated the three R-CNN models using a weighted voting strategy to reduce false positive results. Zhang et al. [32] adopted the improved Faster-R-CNN to introduce multi-scale features and multi-resolution candidate boundary extraction mechanism, and the average accuracy of lesion detection in breast ultrasound images was 91.3%. Montalbo [33] used the YOLO model to train the brain tumor detection model on T1-weighted MRI images labeled with ROI region and adopted transfer learning technology, finally obtaining an average accuracy of 93.14%. Bousabarah et al. [34] manually labeled the liver lesion area weighted by MRI T1, used U-Net to train the tumor detection model, and used the random forest classifier for post-processing. The classifier adopted radiomic features and average neural activation threshold (TR) to reduce the average false positive rate and finally obtained a detection accuracy of 68%. Hasegawa et al. [35] proposed a phase attention Mask R-CNN method for simultaneous detection and segmentation of liver tumors in multiphase CT images. The attention network selectively extracts each feature of a three-phase image for each scale, while preserving information for each single phase. Finally, the detection accuracy of single-phase CT images is about 77%. Frid-Adar et al. [36] adopted a two-channel and multi-scale CNN model to detect lesions in CT and divided lesions into image blocks of different scales to train the lesion detection model. Vivanti et al. [37] proposed a global CNN to automatically detect liver tumor lesions. Kim et al. [38] proposed an optimization network that can automatically select hyper-parameter combinations to realize automatic detection of hepatocellular carcinoma lesions. Shin et al. [18] evaluated five CNN structures for use in CT scans to detect thoracic and abdominal lymph nodes. Detecting lymph nodes is important because they can be markers of infection or cancer. They used GoogLeNet to obtain a mediastinal lymph node detection model with an AUC score of 0.95 and sensitivity of 85%. Becker et al. [17] trained a model to locate breast tumor areas from mammogram images, and the AUC score was 0.82, comparable to that of experienced radiologists. Wang et al. [39] used T2-weighted MR images to train the CNN model to detect prostate lesions, and the AUC score was 0.84, which was significantly higher than that of traditional machine learning methods (such as SVM model based on scale-invariant feature transformation features, with an AUC of 0.70). DeepLesion [40] is the largest multi-category, focus-grade labeled open access clinical image dataset in the world so far, containing 32,735 labeled lesion instances, including key imaging findings from various parts of the body, such as lung nodules, liver tumors, and lymph node swelling. Yan et al. [41] developed a universal lesion detector based on the DeepLesion dataset, providing technical possibilities to help radiologists find all types of lesions in patients. The difficulty of general lesion detection is much higher than that of specific lesion detection. DeepLesion contains various lesions of lung, liver, kidney, lymph, pancreas, bone, soft tissue, etc., with large differences within the lesion category but small differences between the lesion categories (lesions of lung and liver are relatively easy to detect, while some lesions in abdominal cavity have little difference from surrounding normal tissues). In addition, histopathological images are also becoming increasingly digitized. Ciresan et al. [42] used 11–13 layers CNN to detect mitosis in breast histological images from the MITOS dataset. Sirinukunwattana et al. [43] used CNN to detect nuclei in colorectal adenocarcinoma histological images.

Computer-aided detection (CADe) is an important research field because overlooking lesions during examinations can have serious consequences for patients and clinicians. The goal of CADe is to locate abnormal or suspicious areas in images, thereby alerting clinicians. CADe aims to improve the detection rate of diseased areas while reducing the false negative rate. Medical imaging intelligent detection, aided by deep learning and other AI algorithms, can extract rich information and features from medical imaging data, enabling automated diagnosis and analysis. For example, algorithms based on CNNs are capable of effectively identifying and locating abnormal areas in images, such as tumors and lesions, while accurately segmenting and labeling structures within the images. Through extensive training on large volumes of medical imaging data, intelligent detection systems can learn rich feature representations, thereby achieving precise identification and classification of different diseases and abnormalities. Therefore, CADe and medical imaging intelligent detection are both committed to improving the efficiency of medical image analysis and diagnosis, alleviating the workload of clinicians, and ensuring the early detection and treatment of diseases, thus maximizing patient health and safety. Figure 4.4 shows how deep learning models can be applied to disease detection, such as chest lesions. For details, see Ref. [44].

Although medical image target detection shows great potential in clinical applications, it also faces some challenges. These problems include the quality and quantity limitation of medical image data, the robustness and

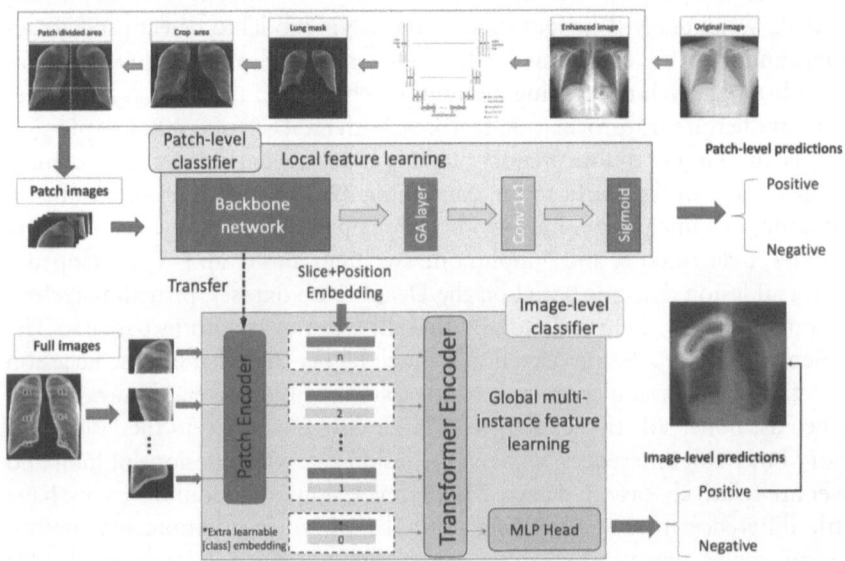

FIGURE 4.4 A deep learning model of chest lesion detection for X-ray images [44].

generalization ability of the model, and the interpretation of the algorithm. Addressing these challenges requires interdisciplinary collaboration and sustained research efforts.

In summary, as an important technology in the field of medical image analysis, medical image target detection provides important support for improving the efficiency and accuracy of medical image analysis and promoting the personalization and precision of clinical diagnosis and treatment. With the continuous advancement of technology and the continuous evolution of clinical needs, medical image target detection will continue to play an important role and inject new vitality into the further development and innovation in the field of medical imaging.

4.2.4 Aiding in treatment and prognosis

The application of AI in predicting therapeutic outcomes and assessing prognosis involves utilizing advanced AI technologies to analyze and interpret clinical data from patients. This approach enables the prediction of treatment efficacy and the evaluation of potential outcomes following therapy. Such technology holds significant promise in clinical medicine, as it supports healthcare professionals in devising more precise treatment strategies, evaluating the effectiveness of interventions, and making informed clinical decisions.

The key to the efficacy prediction and prognosis evaluation of AI treatment is to use machine learning and deep learning technologies to learn potential treatment patterns and prognostic rules from a large number of clinical data. These clinical data include clinical characteristics, biochemical indicators, medical image data, and other information about patients, which can comprehensively reflect the disease condition and treatment process of patients. By analyzing this data, AI systems can build predictive models and evaluation metrics to predict treatment effects and assess patient outcomes.

In terms of efficacy prediction of AI treatment modalities, machine learning and deep learning algorithms can use information such as clinical characteristics and biochemical indicators of patients to predict the response and efficacy of patients to different treatment modalities. For example, for tumor treatment, AI systems can predict a patient's response to chemotherapy, radiotherapy, or targeted therapy by analyzing tumor gene expression data, image characteristics, etc. and help doctors choose the best treatment plan. In terms of prognosis assessment of AI treatment methods, machine learning and deep learning algorithms can analyze patients' clinical data and dynamic changes during treatment and predict patients' post-treatment survival, recurrence risk, complication rate, and other prognostic indicators, providing an important reference for clinical decision-making. For details on deep learning the prediction of treatment response to liver cancer (Figure 4.5).

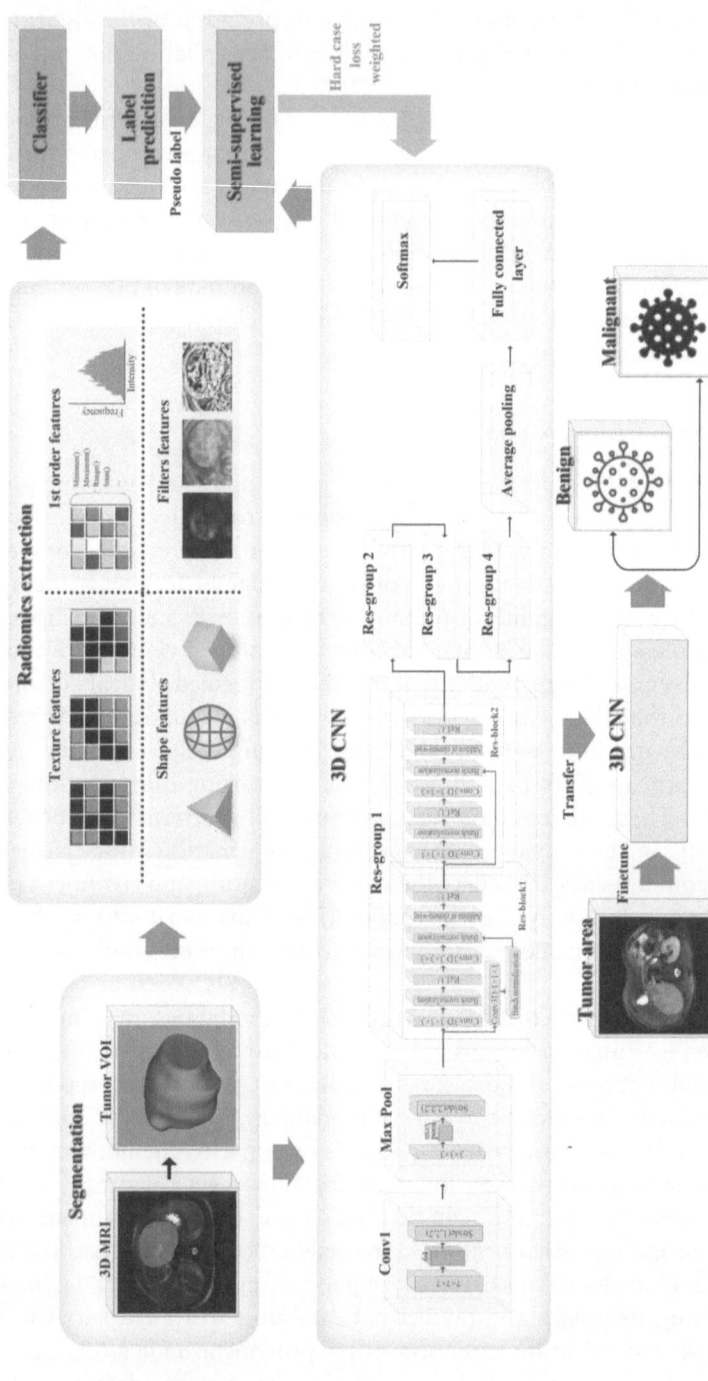

FIGURE 4.5 Prediction of prognosis and treatment response in liver cancer patients from MRI images using deep learning and radiomics [45].

The technology of therapeutic effect prediction and prognosis evaluation of AI therapy has a wide application prospect in clinical practice. First of all, it can help doctors more accurately develop individualized treatment plans, according to the patient's individual characteristics and disease conditions for precise treatment, improving the treatment effect and survival rate. Second, AI prognosis assessment technology can help doctors find risk factors and complications in the treatment process as early as possible, adjust treatment plans in time, and improve the treatment safety and prognosis quality of patients. In addition, AI therapeutic efficacy prediction and prognosis assessment technology can also be used in clinical trial design, drug development, and medical resource allocation, providing important support for medical research and practice.

Imaging examination is not only the main means of diagnosis of diseases but also a very important basis for operation, diagnosis, and treatment plan formulation and prognosis prediction. A large number of studies have shown that the macroscopic image features of tumors are closely related to the microscopic gene, protein, and molecular changes. Changes in gene or protein patterns at the microscopic level can be expressed in macroscopic imaging features [46]. In recent years, medical image analysis technology to obtain tumor microscopic information through medical images has become a research hotspot. With the development of AI, advanced image analysis technology has been successively applied to the research of predicting tumor biomarkers [47]. The main representative techniques are deep learning and radiomics. However, the construction of tumor therapeutic efficacy prediction models generally requires the results of pathological examination or long-term postoperative follow-up as the gold standard for data labeling, which leads to the high cost of data acquisition and data labeling. Therefore, studies on tumor therapeutic efficacy prediction are usually based on small samples. Since it is difficult for data-driven methods represented by deep learning to construct effective prediction models on small sample sets, most research works adopt the method of image omics. As a new research method in the field of medical imaging, radiomics [48] technology has achieved particularly remarkable results. Through advanced mathematical statistical analysis algorithms, a large amount of image information can be extracted from images (CT, MRI, PET, etc.) in high throughput, and rich information about tumor phenotype and microenvironment can be obtained based on quantitative image features such as image density, shape, volume, and texture [49]. Through in-depth mining and analysis of this massive image data information, clinical information analysis, tumor efficacy evaluation and prognosis analysis, and other applications can be realized [50–52]. For example, it has been found that Ct-based radiomics analysis can predict Kirsten rat sarcoma viral oncogene homolog (KRAS) mutations in colorectal cancer patients [53], and there are other studies that can also predict preoperative KRAS mutation status in colorectal cancer patients through imaging texture analysis based on magnetic resonance T2-weighted imaging [54]. Feng et al. [55] analyzed the microvascular invasion (MVI) of HCC patients before the surgical operation to predict the effect of surgical treatment, built a prediction model based on the preoperative intratumoral and peritumoral MRI image characteristics, and included 160 HCC patients as research objects. The resulting AUC is 0.83, sensitivity is 0.90, and specificity is 0.75. Hectors et al. [56] combined quantitative and qualitative image-tomic features to predict PD-L1 expression before operation, and they found specific texture features that are related to PD-L1 expression. Liao et al. [57] predicted CD-8+ T cell tumor invasion in HCC patients based on enhanced CT imaging features and studied the correlation between tumor immune features and radiomics scores. 142 HCC patients were taken as samples in the experiment, 100 of which were used as the training set and 42 as the validation set. The result is an AUC of 0.705. Kong et al. [58] developed an MRI-based image-omics nomograph model, which can provide a pre-assessment of personalized immunotherapy response to HCC. 99 HCC patients receiving immunotherapy were included in the study, and a total of 396 image-omics features were extracted from T2-weighted pre-immunotherapy MRI images. The LASSO regression analysis method was applied to feature selection and model construction, and the AUC value of 0.866 was obtained. Zhang et al. [59] used radiomics to build a prediction model of immunotherapy efficacy, included 98 liver cancer patients receiving immunotherapy, quantified the MRI imaging features of liver cancer patients before surgery into radiomics scores to analyze the expression of immunotherapy biomarker PD-L1 and obtained an AUC of 0.750. Chen et al. [60] analyzed the imaging features of preoperative enhanced MRI images to predict the concentrations of CD-3+ and CD-8+T cells and then evaluated the efficacy of HCC immunotherapy. 207 HCC patients were included in the study, and 1044 imaging features were extracted from the MRI sequences of each patient. The extraction regions included the intra- and peri-tumor regions, and the prediction model was constructed using the random forest method, and the AUC was 0.926.

These case studies and clinical trials demonstrate the profound impact of AI on personalized medicine and treatment planning. Through analysis based on image features and genomic markers, AI models can predict tumor response to chemotherapy, immunotherapy, and targeted therapy. The advent of industrial intelligence has brought about the era of personalized medicine, where treatment decisions can be tailored to a patient's individual characteristics and disease conditions. By combining imaging data with clinical and genomic information, AI enables the identification of patient-specific biomarkers, treatment response predictors, and prognostic indicators to support clinical decision-making.

Although AI therapeutic efficacy prediction and prognosis assessment technology has shown great potential in clinical application, it also faces some challenges. These include issues such as the quality and integrity of clinical data, the interpretability and credibility of models, and the robustness and generalization ability of algorithms. Addressing these challenges will require the collaboration of the medical community, the computer science community, and government regulators to drive the innovation and application of technology to ultimately providing patients with more accurate, safe, and effective treatment.

4.3 Challenges and opportunities

While the integration of AI into diagnostics and imaging holds immense promise, it also poses several challenges and opportunities. Ethical considerations, regulatory constraints, and data privacy concerns must be carefully addressed to ensure the responsible and ethical use of AI technologies in healthcare. Moreover, the heterogeneity and complexity of medical data present challenges in algorithm development, validation, and deployment. Collaborative efforts between clinicians, data scientists, and policymakers are essential to overcome these challenges and unlock the full potential of AI in diagnostics and imaging.

4.3.1 *Ethical considerations and regulatory challenges*

The ethical implications of AI in healthcare, particularly in diagnostics and imaging, are multifaceted and require careful consideration. Issues such as algorithmic bias, transparency, accountability, and patient consent must be addressed to ensure the ethical use of AI technologies [61, 62]. Moreover, regulatory frameworks and standards for AI-driven medical devices and software are still evolving, posing challenges for healthcare providers and technology developers. Robust governance mechanisms and regulatory oversight are essential to mitigate risks and safeguard patient safety and privacy.

4.3.2 *Data privacy and security issues*

The proliferation of medical data generated from imaging modalities, electronic health records, and wearable devices raises concerns about data privacy and security. Healthcare organizations must implement robust data protection measures, such as encryption, anonymization, and access controls, to safeguard patient information from unauthorized access or misuse. Moreover, AI algorithms trained on sensitive medical data must adhere to strict privacy regulations, such as the Health Insurance Portability and Accountability Act (HIPAA) in the United States, to ensure compliance and accountability [63]. Figure 4.6 shows challenges and opportunities of AI.

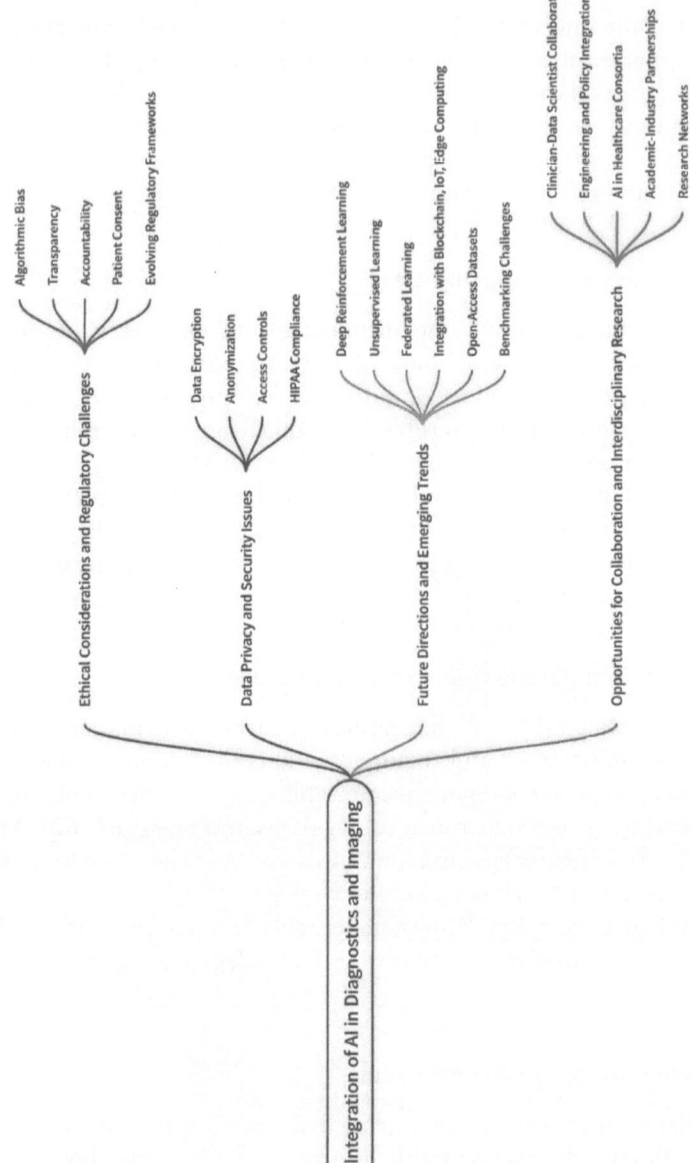

FIGURE 4.6 The schematic diagram of challenges and opportunities of AI.

4.3.3   Future directions and emerging trends in AI diagnostics and imaging

Looking ahead, several emerging trends and future directions are poised to shape the landscape of AI in diagnostics and imaging. Advancements in AI algorithms, such as deep reinforcement learning, unsupervised learning, and federated learning, hold the promise of more robust, interpretable, and generalizable models. Moreover, the integration of AI with other emerging technologies, such as blockchain, Internet of Things (IoT), and edge computing, offers new opportunities for data sharing, interoperability, and real-time decision support. Collaborative initiatives, such as open-access datasets, benchmarking challenges, and interdisciplinary research consortia, are essential to accelerate innovation and translation of AI into clinical practice [64].

4.3.4   Opportunities for collaboration and interdisciplinary research

The complex challenges and opportunities in AI diagnostics and imaging require collaborative efforts and interdisciplinary research collaborations. Clinicians, data scientists, engineers, and policymakers must work together to address the unmet needs and challenges in healthcare delivery. By fostering a culture of collaboration, knowledge sharing, and innovation, stakeholders can harness the full potential of AI to improve patient outcomes, reduce healthcare disparities, and advance medical research and innovation. Initiatives such as AI in Healthcare Consortia, research networks, and academic-industry partnerships play a crucial role in driving interdisciplinary research [65].

4.4   Conclusion

In conclusion, the integration of AI into diagnostics and imaging represents a transformative shift in healthcare delivery, offering unprecedented opportunities to enhance diagnostic accuracy, efficiency, and patient care. From computer-aided diagnosis systems to advanced image analysis techniques and personalized medicine approaches, AI-driven solutions are revolutionizing the practice of medicine. While challenges such as ethical considerations, regulatory constraints, and data privacy concerns persist, collaborative efforts and interdisciplinary research collaborations hold the key to unlocking the full potential of AI in diagnostics and imaging. By harnessing the power of AI technologies responsibly and ethically, healthcare providers can usher in a new era of precision medicine, tailored to the individual needs and preferences of each patient. The future of healthcare lies at the intersection of AI, diagnostics, and imaging, paving the way for more accurate, efficient, and personalized healthcare delivery.

References

1 Yousef R, Gupta G, Yousef N, et al. A holistic overview of deep learning approach in medical imaging. Multimedia systems, 2022, 28(3): 881–914.

2 Ronneberger O, Fischer P, Brox T. U-Net: Convolutional networks for biomedical image segmentation. International conference on medical image computing and computer-assisted intervention. Springer, Cham, 2015: 234–241.

3 Çiçek Ö, Abdulkadir A, Lienkamp S S, et al. 3D U-Net: learning dense volumetric segmentation from sparse annotation. International conference on medical image computing and computer-assisted intervention. Springer, Cham, 2016: 424–432.

4 Milletari F, Navab N, Ahmadi S A. V-net: Fully convolutional neural networks for volumetric medical image segmentation. 2016 fourth international conference on 3D vision (3DV). IEEE, 2016: 565–571.

5 Choi H, Jin K H. Fast and robust segmentation of the striatum using deep convolutional neural networks. Journal of neuroscience methods, 2016, 274: 146–153.

6 Stollenga M F, Byeon W, Liwicki M, et al. Parallel multi-dimensional LSTM, with application to fast biomedical volumetric image segmentation. Advances in neural information processing systems, 2015, 28: 2998–3006.

7 Moeskops P, Viergever M A, Mendrik A M, et al. Automatic segmentation of MR brain images with a convolutional neural network. IEEE transactions on medical imaging, 2016, 35(5): 1252–1261.

8 Singh V K, Romani S, Rashwan H A, et al. Conditional generative adversarial and convolutional networks for X-ray breast mass segmentation and shape classification. International conference on medical image computing and computer-assisted intervention. Springer, Cham, 2018: 833–840.

9 Andermatt S, Pezold S, Cattin P. Multi-dimensional gated recurrent units for the segmentation of biomedical 3D-data. Deep learning and data labeling for medical applications. Springer, Cham, 2016: 142–151.

10 Zhang L, Jiang Y, Jin Z, et al. Real-time automatic prediction of treatment response to transcatheter arterial chemoembolization in patients with hepatocellular carcinoma using deep learning based on digital subtraction angiography videos. Cancer imaging, 2022, 22(1): 23.

11 Ibrahim D M, Elshennawy N M, Sarhan A M. Deep-chest: Multi-classification deep learning model for diagnosing COVID-19, pneumonia, and lung cancer chest diseases. Computers in biology and medicine, 2021, 132: 104348.

12 Sunwoo L, Kim Y J, Choi S H, et al. Computer-aided detection of brain metastasis on 3D MR imaging: Observer performance study. PLoS One, 2017, 12(6): e0178265.

13 Masood A, Sheng B, Li P, et al. Computer-assisted decision support system in pulmonary cancer detection and stage classification on CT images. Journal of biomedical informatics, 2018, 79: 117–128.

14 Hepsağ P U, Özel S A, Yazıcı A. Using deep learning for mammography classification. 2017 International conference on computer science and engineering (UBMK). IEEE, 2017: 418–423.

15 Kumar D, Wong A, Clausi D A. Lung nodule classification using deep features in CT images. 2015 12th conference on computer and robot vision. IEEE, 2015: 133–138.

16 Lakhani P, Sundaram B. Deep learning at chest radiography: automated classification of pulmonary tuberculosis by using convolutional neural networks. Radiology, 2017, 284(2): 574–582.

17 Becker A S, Marcon M, Ghafoor S, et al. Deep learning in mammography: diagnostic accuracy of a multipurpose image analysis software in the detection of breast cancer. Investigative radiology, 2017, 52(7): 434–440.

18 Shin H C, Roth H R, Gao M, et al. Deep convolutional neural networks for computer-aided detection: CNN architectures, dataset characteristics and transfer learning. IEEE transactions on medical imaging, 2016, 35(5): 1285–1298.

19 Yan K, Bagheri M, Summers R M. 3D context enhanced region-based convolutional neural network for end-to-end lesion detection. International conference on medical image computing and computer-assisted intervention. Springer, Cham, 2018: 511–519.

20 Yan K, Wang X, Lu L, et al. DeepLesion: automated mining of large-scale lesion annotations and universal lesion detection with deep learning. Journal of medical imaging, 2018, 5(3): 036501.

21 Cireşan D C, Giusti A, Gambardella L M, et al. Mitosis detection in breast cancer histology images with deep neural networks. International conference on medical image computing and computer-assisted intervention. Springer, Berlin, Heidelberg, 2013: 411–418.

22 Wang X, Yang W, Weinreb J, et al. Searching for prostate cancer by fully automated magnetic resonance imaging classification: deep learning versus non-deep learning. Scientific reports, 2017, 7(1): 1–8.

23 Maqsood M, Nazir F, Khan U, et al. Transfer learning assisted classification and detection of Alzheimer's disease stages using 3D MRI scans. Sensors, 2019, 19(11): 2645.

24 Raina R, Battle A, Lee H, et al. Self-taught learning: transfer learning from unlabeled data. Proceedings of the 24th international conference on machine learning. 2007: 759–766.

25 Shen W, Zhou M, Yang F, et al. Learning from experts: Developing transferable deep features for patient-level lung cancer prediction. International conference on medical image computing and computer-assisted intervention. Springer, Cham, 2016: 124–131.

26 Han Z, Wei B, Hong Y, et al. Accurate screening of COVID-19 using attention-based deep 3D multiple instance learning. IEEE transactions on medical imaging, 2020, 39(8): 2584–2594.

27 Girshick R, Donahue J, Darrell T, et al. Rich feature hierarchies for accurate object detection and semantic segmentation. Proceedings of the IEEE conference on computer vision and pattern recognition. 2014: 580–587.

28 Girshick R. Fast r-cnn. Proceedings of the IEEE international conference on computer vision. 2015: 1440–1448.

29 Ren S, He K, Girshick R, et al. Towards real-time object detection with region proposal networks, 2015. ArXiv. Available online: https://arxiv.org/abs/1506.01497 (accessed on June 2021), 2019.

30 Redmon J, Divvala S, Girshick R, et al. You only look once: Unified, real-time object detection. Proceedings of the IEEE conference on computer vision and pattern recognition. 2016: 779–788.

31 Zhang R, Cheng C, Zhao X, et al. Multiscale mask R-CNN–based lung tumor detection using PET imaging. Molecular imaging, 2019, 18: 1536012119863531.

32 Zhang Z, Zhang X, Lin X, et al. Ultrasonic diagnosis of breast nodules using modified faster R-CNN. Ultrasonic imaging, 2019, 41(6): 353–367.

33 Montalbo F J P. A computer-aided diagnosis of brain tumors using a fine-tuned YOLO-based model with transfer learning. KSII transactions on internet and information systems (TIIS), 2020, 14(12): 4816–4834.

34 Bousabarah K, Letzen B, Tefera J, et al. Automated detection and delineation of hepatocellular carcinoma on multiphasic contrast-enhanced MRI using deep learning. Abdominal radiology, 2021, 46(1): 216–225.

35 Hasegawa R, Iwamoto Y, Lin L, et al. Automatic segmentation of liver tumor in multiphase CT images by mask R-CNN. 2020 IEEE 2nd global conference on life sciences and technologies (LifeTech). IEEE, 2020: 231–234.

36 Frid-Adar M, Diamant I, Klang E, et al. Modeling the intra-class variability for liver lesion detection using a multi-class patch-based CNN. International workshop on patch-based techniques in medical imaging. Springer, Cham, 2017: 129–137.

37 Vivanti R, Szeskin A, Lev-Cohain N, et al. Automatic detection of new tumors and tumor burden evaluation in longitudinal liver CT scan studies. International journal of computer assisted radiology and surgery, 2017, 12(11): 1945–1957.

38 Kim J, Min J H, Kim S K, et al. Detection of hepatocellular carcinoma in contrast-enhanced magnetic resonance imaging using deep learning classifier: a multi-center retrospective study. Scientific reports, 2020, 10(1): 1–11.

39 Wang X, Yang W, Weinreb J, et al. Searching for prostate cancer by fully automated magnetic resonance imaging classification: deep learning versus non-deep learning. Scientific reports, 2017, 7: 15415.

40 Yan K, Wang X, Lu L, et al. DeepLesion: automated mining of large-scale lesion annotations and universal lesion detection with deep learning. Journal of medical imaging, 2018, 5(3): 036501–036501.

41 Yan K, Bagheri M, Summers R, et al. 3D context enhanced region-based convolutional neural network for end-to-end lesion detection. International conference on medical image computing and computer-assisted Intervention, September 16–20, 2018, Granada, Spain. Heidelberger: Springer, 2018: 511–519.

42 Ciresan D C, Giusti A, Gambardella L M, et al. Mitosis detection in breast cancer histology images with deep neural networks. Medical image computing and computer assisted intervention, 2013,16(Pt 2): 411–418.

43 Sirinukunwattana K, Raza S, Tasng Y W, et al. Locality sensitive deep learning for detection and classification of nuclei in routine colon cancer histology images. IEEE Transactions on medical imaging, 2016, 35(5): 1196–1206.

44 Tian Y, Wang J, Yang W, et al. Deep multi-instance transfer learning for pneumothorax classification in chest X-ray images. Medical physics, 2022, 49(1): 231–243.

45 Tian Y, Komolafe T E, Chen T, et al. Prediction of TACE treatment response in a preoperative MRI via analysis of integrating deep learning and radiomics features. Journal of medical and biological engineering, 2022, 42(2): 169–178.

46 Moon S H, Kim J, Joung J G, et al. Correlations between metabolic texture features, genetic heterogeneity, and mutation burden in patients with lung cancer. European journal of nuclear medicine and molecular imaging, 2019, 46(2): 446–454.

47 Bi W L, Hosny A, Schabath M B, et al. Artificial intelligence in cancer imaging: clinical challenges and applications. CA: A cancer journal for clinicians, 2019, 69(2): 127–157.

48 Mayerhoefer M E, Materka A, Langs G, et al. Introduction to radiomics. Journal of nuclear medicine, 2020, 61(4): 488–495.

49 Tomaszewski M R, Gillies R J. The biological meaning of radiomic features. Radiology, 2021, 298(3): 505–516.

50 Lambin P, Leijenaar R T H, Deist T M, et al. Radiomics: the bridge between medical imaging and personalized medicine. Nature reviews Clinical oncology, 2017, 14(12): 749–762.

51 Liu Z, Wang S, Dong D. et al. The applications of radiomics in precision diagnosis and treatment of oncology: opportunities and challenges. Theranostics, 2019, 9(5): 1303.

52 Starmans M P A, van der Voort S R, Tovar J M C, et al. Radiomics: data mining using quantitative medical image features. Handbook of medical image computing and computer assisted intervention. Academic Press, 2020: 429–456.

53 Yang L, Dong D, Fang M, et al. Can CT-based radiomics signature predict KRAS/ NRAS/BRAF mutations in colorectal cancer? European radiology, 2018, 28(5): 2058–2067.

54 Oh J E, Kim M J, Lee J, et al. Magnetic resonance-based texture analysis differentiating KRAS mutation status in rectal cancer. Cancer research and treatment: official journal of Korean Cancer Association, 2020, 52(1): 51–59.

55 Feng S T, Jia Y, Liao B, et al. Preoperative prediction of microvascular invasion in hepatocellular cancer: a radiomics model using Gd-EOB-DTPA-enhanced MRI. European radiology, 2019, 29(9): 4648–4659.

56 Hectors S J, Lewis S, Besa C, et al. MRI radiomics features predict immuno-oncological characteristics of hepatocellular carcinoma. European radiology, 2020, 30(7): 3759–3769.

57 Liao H, Zhang Z, Chen J, et al. Preoperative radiomic approach to evaluate tumor-infiltrating CD8+ T cells in hepatocellular carcinoma patients using contrast-enhanced computed tomography. Annals of surgical oncology, 2019, 26(13): 4537–4547.

58 Kong C, Zhao Z, Chen W, et al. Prediction of tumor response via a pretreatment MRI radiomics-based nomogram in HCC treated with TACE. European radiology, 2021, 31(10): 7500–7511.

59 Zhang J, Wu Z, Zhang X, et al. Machine learning: an approach to preoperatively predict PD-1/PD-L1 expression and outcome in intrahepatic cholangiocarcinoma using MRI biomarkers. ESMO open, 2020, 5(6): e000910.

60 Chen S, Feng S, Wei J, et al. Pretreatment prediction of immunoscore in hepatocellular cancer: a radiomics-based clinical model based on Gd-EOB-DTPA-enhanced MRI imaging. European radiology, 2019, 29(8): 4177–4187.

61 Naik N, Hameed B M, Shetty D K, et al. Legal and ethical consideration in artificial intelligence in healthcare: who takes responsibility? Frontiers in surgery, 2022, 9: 266.

62 Farhud D D, Zokaei S. Ethical issues of artificial intelligence in medicine and healthcare. Iranian journal of public health, 2021, 50(11): i.

63 Roy S. Privacy prevention of health care data using AI. Journal of data acquisition and processing, 2022, 37(3): 769.

64 Romagnoli A, Ferrara F, Langella R, et al. Healthcare systems and artificial intelligence: focus on challenges and the international regulatory framework. Pharmaceutical research, 2024, 41(4): 721–730.

65 Sunarti S, Rahman F F, Naufal M, et al. Artificial intelligence in healthcare: opportunities and risk for future. Gaceta sanitaria, 2021, 35: S67–S70.

5

eHEALTH PLATFORMS FACILITATE BREAST CANCER

A Systematic Review

Arpit Kumar Sharma, Arvind Dhaka, and Amita Nandal

5.1 Introduction

For women, breast cancer is one of the most prevalent cancers that are diagnosed and the primary cause of cancer-related fatalities. The World Health Organization (WHO) estimates that 2.1 million of the women population worldwide get breast cancer annually. An estimated number of about 627,000 women passed away in 2018 due to this, accounting for almost 15% of all female cancer deaths around the world. With a rate of up to 30%, it is one of the most frequent cancers in the United States of America and was estimated to be diagnosed in women in 2019. Breast tissue can be classified as normal, benign, in-situ cancer, or invasive carcinoma [1]. Benign refers to a tissue that is used to describe a slight alteration in the breast's structure. it is not considered cancer and is usually not damaging to health. In-situ cancer does not spread to the other organs of the body; it usually stays within the mammary duct of the lobule system. In-situ carcinoma is curable if it is diagnosed at an early stage. On the other hand, invasive carcinoma is a cancerous growth that often spreads to other organs. X-ray mammography, 3-D, CT-Scan, PET, MRI, and breast temperature assessment are only a few of the methods available for detecting breast cancer. Nonetheless, pathological diagnosis is sometimes thought of as the "golden standard" [2].

5.1.1 Broad development of current AI analysis disorders

AI is the umbrella term including all the ways for the machine to emulate and surpass human intelligence, particularly in cognitive capabilities. The primary topics of AI study include machine learning (ML), pattern recognition,

DOI: 10.1201/9781003481959-5

natural language processing, etc. [3]. In particular, ML has made a substantial impact on medical advancements. It is employed in the pathological diagnosis of various cancer types, including breast, stomach, colon, lung, and cervical cancers. The application's scope is centered on early tumor screening, staining analysis, disease grading, and benign and malignant diagnosis. A weakly supervised multi-layer hidden conditional random field model, for instance, is proposed in this work to classify cervical histopathology images into well-differentiated, moderately differentiated, and poorly differentiated stages. The study evaluates the efficacy and potential of the proposed method using six cervical IHC datasets. The maximum classification accuracy of the six datasets, at 88%, is obtained with an overall classification accuracy of 77.32%. A deep learning (DL)-based framework, called GastricNet, is proposed for automatic gastric cancer identification in the field of gastric cancer. This DL framework outperforms cutting-edge networks such as DenseNet and ResNet, as demonstrated by the experimental findings, which also show that it can attain 100% accuracy in slice-based classification. The rectum or inner linings of the colon are the primary sites of growth, known as polyps, that precede colorectal cancer, a malignant tumor [4].

The work of [1] proposes an automated supervised DL strategy to maintain the original image size in this publication, which uses a 31-layer deep convolutional neural network (DCNN) to perform five-grade cancer classification. For two-class grading and five-class cancer grading, the suggested model yields classification accuracy of 96.97% and 93.24%, respectively. Regarding lung cancer histology, the two most common subtypes of the disease are LUSC: Lung Squamous Cell Carcinoma and LUAD: Lung Adenocarcinoma. In [2], a DCNN (inception-v3) is trained on whole slide images (WSIs) from The Cancer Genome Atlas to classify them automatically and reliably into normal lung tissue, LUAD, and LUSC, with an average area under the curve (AUC) of 0.9.

It is noteworthy that artificial neural networks (ANNs), a subfield of ML, are crucial for pathological diagnosis. An approach to mathematical modeling or computation that mimics the structure and operation of a biological neural network is the ANN method, which includes both deep and conventional neural networks. ANNs are now often utilized for image segmentation, feature extraction, and classification in Breast Histopathological Image Analysis (BHIA), which illustrates the development path of BHIA utilizing ANNs.

5.1.2 Motivation

A thorough review of methods for using deep neural networks (DNNs) and traditional neural networks for image processing of breast histopathology is provided. Clarifying the history of ANN development, comprehending popular technology and ANN application trends, and identifying ANNs' potential in the BHIA area going forward are the driving forces behind this effort. To the best of our knowledge, some survey papers have been written summarizing studies about the BHIA study (see, for example, the reviews). We examine the survey studies that are associated with the BHIA effort in the section that follows [4].

This provides an overview of ML techniques used in histopathology image processing, including feature extraction, segmentation, supervised learning, and unsupervised learning. Out of the summarized more than 130 studies on histological image processing, only five discuss BHIA using ANNs. The research survey published focuses on recent advancements in digital image processing as well as the application of AI and DL to the diagnosis of breast disease images. Of these, our focus is solely on providing an overview of the advancements made in DL as it relates to pathological breast diagnostics from an application standpoint.

The outcomes that have been obtained for each research approach are not discussed in the chapter, though. The review provides an overview of recent developments in breast histology and mammography DL methods. This chapter solely focuses on DL methods applied to photos of breast his- topathology. Sixteen publications are summarized based on BHIA accord- ing to various tasks, namely, nuclei analysis, tubular analysis, epithelial and stromal region analysis, mitotic activity analysis, and other tasks in the breast digital histopathology image process. The DL applications in breast cancer image processing in the US, MRI, DBT, screen-film mammography (SFM), digital mammography (DM), and US imaging modalities are compiled in the survey. Six papers of our interest are found at the same time. A summary containing 106 linked works on "recent trends in computer assisted diag- nosis system for breast cancer diagnosis using histopathological images" is given in ref. [3]. Four technological steps—image preprocessing, segmenta- tion, feature extraction and selection, and classification—are used to sum- marize that research in this review. Nevertheless, this paper includes just 20 relevant publications about BHIA with ANNs.

According to data on cancer worldwide, lung cancer is the deadliest type of cancer globally, with breast cancer coming at second. In 2018, 2 billion new cases of breast cancer were reported globally, with 627,000 deaths from the disease [4]. According to research conducted in Australia, the likelihood of a patient surviving breast cancer is 98% if the tumor's size at the time of discovery is less than 10 mm. According to a cohort study, 30% of cases of breast cancer are discovered when the tumor is 30 mm in size. During screen- ing, breast cancer is often identified when the tumor is at least 20 mm in size [5]. Thus, it is essential to detect breast cancer early to start treatment. Fol- lowing identification by screening exams like the clinical breast examination (CBE) and breast self-examination (BSE), early therapy can be advantageous.

While BSE is carried out by an individual to examine physical changes and changes in the appearance of breasts, CBE is a routine medical examination carried out by healthcare professionals to detect lesions in the breasts. BSE gives women the confidence to take charge of their health. So, the WHO advises BSE to increase awareness among vulnerable women. Medical pictures of breasts are produced via screening techniques. Radiologists and physicians, among other human professionals, typically interpret these images [6]. Research reveals that a lack of technical proficiency and experience in analyzing thermograms is the reason for their poor diagnostic accuracy. Researchers and medical professionals are using computer-assisted technology to reduce errors in breast thermography-based diagnosis due to the rise of various diseases and the scarcity of human labor. Thus, it is necessary to have a computer system that can automatically categorize thermograms into normal and abnormal groups. This requirement has led to an ongoing increase in research into computer-based methods for classifying medical images. To help clinicians analyze medical images, a number of computer-assisted diagnosis techniques have been created. DL model development has received a lot of attention during the past ten years [7].

DL models are simply implemented using pre-trained networks because they are publicly available. Numerous investigations on the identification of breast cancer rely on DL employing mammograms, histological pictures, tomosyntheses, and ultrasound images, all of which have demonstrated adequate accuracy. Conversely, only a small number of studies have used the DNN approach to do non-invasive thermal imaging of the breasts. Given the limited resources available at the moment, this problem is still in its early phases of investigation. Therefore, a great deal of work needs to go into creating trustworthy non-invasive computer-assisted technology that will help in the early identification of breast cancer. The significance of reviewing pertinent past, present, and upcoming studies on thermal imaging and DL for breast cancer diagnosis cannot be overstated.

On the significant unresolved concerns found in this study, further research could be done. In this work, we examine recent developments in the non-invasive use of thermography and DL for breast cancer screening. In addition, we indicate future research directions that are critical to enhancing the precision of thermal imaging and DL in the identification of breast cancer.

This chapter's contributions and state-of-the-art can be summed up as follows [8]:

- A summary of the potential applications of breast thermography, including the dataset of breast thermograms that is available for cancer diagnosis.
- A detailed description of the convolutional neural networks (CNN) idea.
- Breast cancer thermograms: a basic feature learning visualization.

- A summary of the most recent developments in DL techniques and thermal imaging for early detection of breast cancer.
- To outline the possible research obstacles in creating a quick and precise CNN-thermal imaging system for the diagnosis of breast cancer.

5.2 Related work

This section provides an overview of the key conclusions, techniques, and strategies for deep learning (DL) model-based breast MRI segmentation. It highlights prominent research from the literature that uses CNN-based models to classify individual pixels using a sliding window technique for segmentation.

The primary procedures for segmenting images are as follows:

a   preprocessing MRI data;
b   developing and training models;
c   evaluating models;
d   inference; and
e   post-processing.

Single-modal models employ only one kind of input modality, but multi-modal models combine data from several input MRI modalities, such as T1, T1 contrasted, and T2.

5.2.1 Multi-models

The limited morphology of breast cancers and the difficulty in differentiating between the tumors and the normal blood arteries make it difficult to segment breast tumors in single-modal pictures. Nevertheless, because cancers differ from other tissues in terms of shape or grayscale, multi-modal images provide a richer picture of the tumor. Piantadosi et al. [9] integrated the three time points (3TP) technique into the U-Net architecture in order to achieve multi-modality in lesion segmentation in magnetic resonance imaging slices. With temporal acquisitions ($T = 0$, 2, and 6 min) entered before and after the contrast agent injection, they were able to obtain a median dice similarity coefficient of 61.24%.

By utilizing the three U-Net models with the distinct inputs as 3TP acquisitions, an entire series of images, and the pre, the last, and the standard deviation images of the entire series—Khaled et al. [10] it is investigated that the ensemble and the U-Net framework for the lesion segmentation. Additionally, they included a breast mask in every model and used residual basic blocks in place of U-Net convolutional blocks. Hirsch [11] used a very large training set of data of about the 60,108 benign breast and **that of**

2,455 units of the malignant breast pictures to achieve radiologist-level performance with a 3D U-Net. The initial postcontrast picture, T1 postcontrast minus pre-contrast image (DCE-in), washout (DCE-out), and a radiologists' reference were all included in the input MRI. The way DL models use labeled and/or unlabeled data for training allows them to be categorized as supervised, semi-supervised, or unsupervised.

5.3 Breast cancer prediction using ML algorithm

ML is an automatic learning technique. The algorithms are built to learn from historical datasets. We provide a lot of data, the ML model analyzes it, and we may forecast the future using the train model [12]. The following are the main ML algorithms for breast cancer prediction. Figure 5.1 shows the implementation of breast cancer detection.

5.3.1 Artificial neural network (ANN)

One popular technique for the data mining process is the ANN. The input layer, hidden layer, and output layer make up a neural network. The overly complex pattern is extracted using this method. Parallel processing, distributed memory, collaborative solutions, and network architecture are the foundations of algorithms [12].

5.3.2 Logistics regression (LR)

There are more dependent variables in this supervised learning approach. The binary form represents the algorithm's response. The continuous result of a given set of data can be obtained by logistics regression. The statistical model used in this technique uses binary variables [12].

5.3.3 K-nearest neighbor (KNN)

Pattern recognition uses this algorithm. It's a useful method for predicting breast cancer. To identify the pattern, equal weight is assigned to every class. From a big dataset, K-nearest neighbor extracts the featured data that are related. We classify a large dataset based on feature similarity [13].

5.3.4 Decision tree (DT)

Regression modeling and categorization are the foundations of the decision trees algorithms. The dataset used is further segmented into fewer subsets of the data. The best degree for the precision in the prediction may be achieved with the help of these smaller sets of data that are segmented. CART, C4.5, C5.0, and conditional trees are examples of decision tree methods [13].

5.3.5 Naive Bayes algorithm (NB)

The huge training dataset assumption is made using this model. The Bayesian approach is included in the procedure to compute the probability. When determining the probability of the noisy data that is used as the input, it offers the maximum accuracy. The training dataset and training tuple are compared using this analogy classifier.

5.3.6 Support vector machine (SVM)

It is one of the supervised learning methods that can also be used to solve problems with the classification and the regression approach. In order to solve the regression problems, it makes use of theoretical and mathematical functions. It provides the highest accuracy rate for predicting large-scale datasets. It is one of the most powerful ML techniques based on both 2D and 3D modeling approaches [14].

5.3.7 Random forest (RF)

The supervised learning foundation of the random forest algorithm allows it to handle both regression and classification issues. It is one of the fundamental components of ML that is employed in this in order to forecast new data based on historical datasets [14].

5.3.8 K mean algorithm

The K mean clustering algorithm allows data to be divided into smaller clusters. To determine the degree of similarity between several data points, algorithms are utilized. The data points are precisely made up of one or more clusters that are best suited for large-scale dataset evaluation [15].

5.3.9 C mean algorithm

The similarity criterion is used to identify clusters. A cluster made up of comparable data points is a member of a single family. Every data entry pointed in the C mean algorithm is a member of a single cluster. Its primary applications are in illness prediction and medical image segmentation.

5.3.10 Hierarchical algorithm

Most of the time, a hierarchical algorithm offers an evaluation of raw data as a matrix. A hierarchy is used to keep each cluster apart from the others. Each and every cluster is made up of comparable data points. Each cluster's distance is calculated using a probabilistic approach.

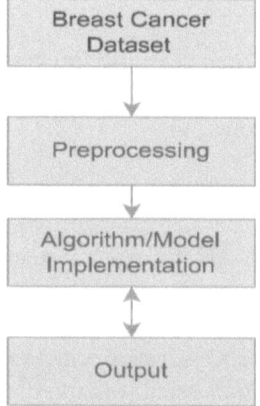

FIGURE 5.1   Basic methodology for implementing breast cancer detection.

5.3.11   Gaussian mixture algorithm

It is the most often used unsupervised learning method. The method used to calculate the likelihood of various forms of clustered data is referred to as the soft clustering methodology. This algorithm's implementation is predicated on maximizing expectations [15].

5.4   Particular techniques for breast cancer

There are two types of ensemble techniques: the homogeneous (as described in), which combines one of the base methods with two or more configuration methods (e.g., bagging and boosting technique); the heterogeneous is for a combination of two or more base methods. Ensemble techniques are based on supervised learning and also yield good predictions based on certain hypotheses [16].

5.4.1   Bagging

Bootstrap aggregation is another term for the bagging approach, which is used to predict any of the disease. It is built on several models, each of which is then trained independently before being integrated for prediction.

5.4.2   Boosting

Boosting is a technique that combines multiple weak classifiers to create a single strong classifier, using a homogeneous weak learner. It is predicated on methodical approaches to gradually construct the model from a small amount of training data.

5.4.3 Stacking

A heterogeneous weak learner, stacking integrates various ML methods to make predictions using the same dataset. It combines the predictions of two or more basic models into one.

5.5 Breast cancer prediction using DL techniques

An expanded version of an ANN (artificial neural network) is termed deep learning. DL algorithms are made up of an architecture with several layers. These algorithms are capable of recognizing all of the data from the various categories and are used to process a significant amount of natural data. When we have a large amount of unlabeled training data, we typically use unsupervised DL algorithms [16].

5.5.1 Autoencoder

In essence, an autoencoder is a decoder followed by an encoder. The encoder often transfers data in the form of variables, such as x and y, while the decoder uses that same input and attempts to recover the complete original input. Autoencoders are primarily used to learn from large datasets by training their networks to disregard the noise and other irrelevant signals.

5.5.2 Sparse autoencoders

The sparse autoencoder effectively manages sparsity and regularization, ensuring that the hidden layer of the neural network produces a sparse output. Sparse autoencoders are automatically able to learn from the unlabeled data. The sparse autoencoder is essentially used with a feed forward and backpropagation algorithm with regular autoencoders.

5.5.3 Stacked sparse autoencoder

Each stacked layer consists of hidden layers that function as classifiers, ultimately generating the output. The basic layers of the stacked-sparse autoencoder (SSAE) are then combined to create the stretched sparse. The output of the first layer is then merged into the output of the second layer for further processes.

5.5.4 Convolutional neural network CNN

This can analyze the image-based cancer dataset. During the preprocessing stage, CovNet is used to analyze various datasets, and various filters are applied to enable CovNet to collect various picture dimensions. The pooling layer, convolutional layer, classification layer, and completely contacted layer are the different types of layers. All of these layers come together to form CNN.

5.5.5   Recurrent neural network (RNN)

It is a type of neural network that uses the output of a previous state as input for the next state and consists of multiple hidden states. It is less accurate than other neural networks in reducing parameter complexity when processing a series of inputs that use the same parameters at each layer. However, it is unable to process a large number of sequences of inputs using Tanh and ReLU (rectified linear unit) activation functions [17].

5.6   MRI data as breast cancer

Three important MRI modalities are used in the diagnosis of breast cancer: DWI, T1-/T2-weighted imaging, and DCE-MRI. Even with multiple slices in each modality, there is frequently insufficient information to distinguish between tumors and breast nodules, which have comparable sizes and forms. In order to access a larger dataset for abnormality identification, the use of multi-modal images becomes essential. As such, the utilization of image processing methods becomes imperative.

5.6.1   Input MRI data

Models with multi-modal inputs are more effective than those with single-modal inputs, and the DL method uses multi-modal MRIs and mask labels as input data [18]. Anatomical information was obtained by using the pre-contrast picture as input, which excluded enhancements from the chest region of the heart. Parallel to this, using the contralateral subtraction image as input reduced the number of false positives from parenchymal enhancements—a crucial step for DL models and radiologists' interpretation. To evaluate the accuracy of segmentation, specialists manually create ground truth labels using graphical tools. The smallest box containing proximal peritumor tissue demonstrated the highest accuracy when assessing the impact of the tumor alone plus various annotation boxes. To improve result reliability, researchers have used a variety of strategies on raw data.

5.6.2   Processing techniques

5.6.2.1   Preprocessing

In order to eliminate labels, markers, non-breast tissues, and black areas from the image, this crucial stage in image segmentation must be completed. The following are commonly used methods: motion correction through 3D rigid and non-rigid image registration [19], data augmentation using geometric transformations such as rotations, flips, and translations, and normalization.

5.6.2.2 During processing

The substantial disparity between voxels depicting damaged and healthy tissues makes data balancing essential in medical imaging. In order to address this issue, Galli et al. [19] implemented an eras/epochs training schema that makes sure that the same amount of lesions and healthy slices are sampled at each training step. Yue et al. [20] used a random selection technique for patch cropping in order to balance the data. With equal probability, the patches' centers were selected from either the background or the foreground. Before feeding the input data into the model for assessment, they further applied different degrees of rotation (augmentation) to the data during inference. Among these strategies are patch extraction, transfer learning, and attention processes.

5.6.2.3 Post-processing

Segmentation results can be improved by applying morphological procedures (such as erosion and dilation), thresholding, and linked component analysis. To improve the segmentation results, various techniques have been used, such as removing skin folds to improve fibroglandular tissue segmentation, keeping only the largest continuous regions of segmentation, removing outliers within connected regions [20], and applying a threshold of 0.35 with hole filling.

5.7 Key aspects of CNN

This section delves into the fundamental features and diverse basic architectures of CNNs, providing valuable insights into the key components that enable them to successfully segment breast MRI images.

5.7.1 CNN components

Depending on the particular segmentation task requirements and dataset characteristics, many CNN architectures can be created by modifying the component parameters as listed below.

5.7.1.1 Convolutional layers

They use the convolution operation to extract features from the input data, which entails sliding a tiny matrix known as a filter.

5.7.1.2 Activation functions

After every convolutional layer, they inject non-linearity, which helps the network understand intricate patterns and produce precise predictions. Hidden layers frequently employ ReLU. By adding a tiny hyperparameter for negative input values, the leaky ReLU activation function helps the network sustain the gradient flow and overcomes a restriction known as the "dying ReLU" problem in standard ReLU. Furthermore, at the ultimate classifier layers, SoftMax or Sigmoid have been employed.

5.7.1.3 Batch normalization

End-to-end training using the same optimal solver may be made possible as a result. Prior to each ReLU, this strategy was used to decrease the internal covariate shift [21] and improve gradient flow, which led to faster convergence. It was also used after every ReLU block in order to decrease internal covariate shift [21], increase training speed, strengthen the model's resistance to changes in input [19], and lessen the model's susceptibility to weight initialization.

5.7.1.4 Pooling layers

Through techniques like max-pooling and average pooling, they lower the spatial dimensions of the feature maps, which lowers the number of parameters in later layers. As a result, the training pace is increased and overfitting is avoided.

5.7.1.5 Optimizers

Through gradient computation and application, they determine parameter adjustments during training; typically utilized alternatives include stochastic gradient descent (SGD), adaptive moment (Adam), and Adadelta, which is an AdaGrad [10] extension.

5.7.1.6 Skip connections

Skip connections work by concatenating feature maps from the encoder with those in the decoder, creating additional pathways for backpropagation between network layers. By bypassing certain layers, these connections help preserve and reuse low-level features during upsampling, enhancing the model's ability to retain important spatial information.

5.7.1.7 Dropout

During training, a fraction of the neurons is randomly "dropped out" as part of a regularization process designed to reduce overfitting and enhance generalization. To improve network performance, Hazirbas et al. [21], for example, used dropout in both the encoder and the decoder.

5.7.2 Architectures

5.7.2.1 SegNet

SegNet is encoder-decoder architecture, in which the encoder layers match the VGG16 architecture's convolutional layers. In order to store pooling indices for usage in the relevant decoder levels for upsampling, the encoder uses max-pooling layers. A multi-class softmax classifier receives the decoder output as input and produces independent class probabilities for every pixel. SegNet measures the dissimilarity between the projected segmentation map and ground truth labels using a variation of cross-entropy loss, and it optimizes using SGD with backpropagation. Advantages include precise tumor localization and breast boundary delineation made possible by SegNet's use of max-pooling indices during downsampling [21]. Figure 5.2 shows architecture of SegNet.

For medical photos with varying resolutions and aspect ratios, SegNet's capacity to accept input images of diverse sizes is especially helpful. However, compared to U-Net, SegNet did not produce as effective results for breast tumor segmentation in 2D slices. Its sole dependence on stored pooling indices during convolution was blamed for this. SegNet may not adequately capture the broader contextual information because it primarily concentrates on local spatial data [22].

5.7.2.2 FuseNet

The encoder in FuseNet is a two-branch network that uses the VGG 16-layer model to fine-tune its encoder parameters. It simultaneously extracts features

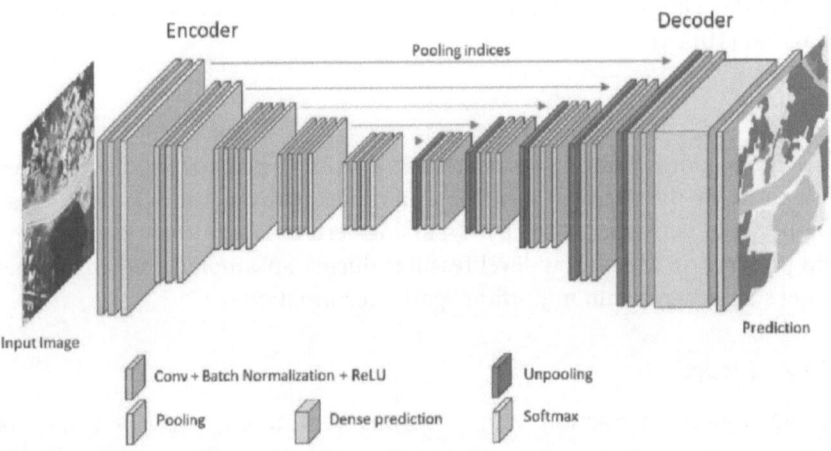

FIGURE 5.2 The SegNet architecture [21].

from complimentary depth input and fuses them into primary feature maps [21]. T1C MRI was the primary modality utilized by Li et al. [18] because it can highlight breast masses and irrelevant regions. T2W was used as an auxiliary modality to help distinguish actual breast masses from other enhanced areas. FuseNet enhances segmentation accuracy by capturing complementary features from multiple imaging modalities and integrating data from various MRI sequences.

5.7.2.3 U-Net

The U-Net design consists of an expanding channel (decoder) that symmetrically supports accurate localization and a contracting pathway (encoder) that gathers contextual information. In order to enable the model to capture both local and global contextual information, U-Net includes skip links between the encoder and the decoder. One benefit of U-Net is that it does not require patch division because it may use entire images of any size [23]. Despite having a very small quantity of training data, the architecture has proven to be resilient and robust. Figure 5.3 presents the U-Net architecture for breast segmentation.

The architecture of U-Net makes it possible to combine detailed spatial information from the decoder with high-level information from the encoder. However, because of issues such as fuzzy borders between the FGT and surrounding organs, false-positive segmentation of the pectoral muscle area and fat in cases of low breast density, and under-segmentation in

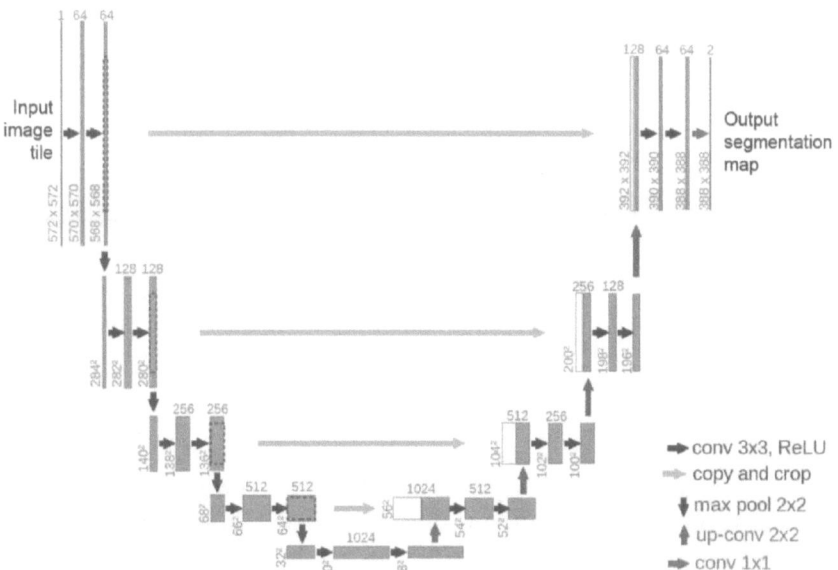

FIGURE 5.3 The U-Net and GAN architecture for breast segmentation [23].

cases of high breast density, U-Net was unable to reliably segment the FGT. Careful regularization strategies, including dropout or data augmentation, should be used when training data is scarce in order to reduce the likelihood of overfitting.

5.7.2.4 GAN

A generator and a discriminator in a GAN are trained adversarially until convergence. The discriminator separates genuine segmentations from artificial ones, whereas the generator creates realistic segmentations. Realistic synthetic images are produced by GANs, which can supplement the scarce training data. This is especially helpful when there is a lack of labeled data. Consequently, unsupervised learning—that is, learning from unannotated images—can be facilitated by GANs. However, differences in breast sizes, shapes, and imaging techniques may affect how well GANs segment breast MRI data.

5.8 Gaps and challenges

5.8.1 Well-annotated big data

For precise segmentation model training, well-annotated huge data is essential; nonetheless, human annotation is labor-intensive and requires specialized knowledge. The lack of sizable public datasets containing thorough and precise ground facts is a major impediment to developing new DL models for breast MRI segmentation. The "Cancer Imaging Archive" webpage offers datasets as part of efforts to close this gap, although more work is required. On the other hand, creating segmentation methods that are not dependent on annotated data is becoming more and more popular. DL and globally optimal inference in a continuous space were merged by Maicas et al. [22]. Additional endeavors in this regard are documented in the publications of Meng et al. [24] and Parekh et al. [25]. Inter-observer variability in annotation and 3D annotation challenges arise when creating huge public datasets with thorough and accurate annotations. Uncertainty can be introduced into the ground truth annotations used for model training by radiologists' differences in how they segment regions of interest in breast MRIs. For example, Hirsch [11] employed threshold tweaking and testing after 266 cancerous breasts were segmented by four radiologists. Neighboring slices in 3D annotations frequently depend on one another. Accurate segmentation presents challenges, including maintaining consistency and seamless slice transitions during annotations. For this reason, Li et al. [18], for instance, exclusively designated the core slices with the biggest cross-sections for masses.

5.8.2 Inter/intra variations

Due to a variety of imaging methods, patient variables, including race, ethnicity, and illness symptoms, as well as breast morphology, there can be significant variation in the shape, size, position, and appearance of breast MRIs [24]. To address such variabilities, there is a need for robust DL models that have been trained on vast, heterogeneous datasets. To name a few initiatives, Hirsch [11] used a sizable dataset that included difficult situations with patients who had breast implants and minor tumors. A fairly small dataset with varying MRI acquisition procedures and breast kinds was used by Dalmış et al. [23]. Applying pre-trained DL models to a variety of datasets is difficult because of this unpredictability, and additional generalization strategies might be needed.

5.8.3 Generalization techniques

It is difficult to generalize DL models that were trained on a particular dataset to brand-new, sizable, and varied datasets [19]. Many researchers have developed different DL approaches, largely trained on tiny private databases, in an attempt to automate breast MRI segmentation. However, model generality is still lacking and their use may be restricted to their inputs. Some researchers exclusively utilize 2D slices as inputs to learning algorithms, while others exclude patients who have breast implants. For clinical applications, it is imperative to enhance the generalization capabilities of algorithms via transfer learning, domain adaptation, or cross-dataset validation. As single-modal pictures cannot fully capture the tumor morphology without supplementary information from other modalities, multiple MRI modalities have been integrated into the training algorithms.

Inaccurate tumor borders and false positive/negative candidates result from the single-modal segmentation of breast cancers. Moreover, in order to accurately represent the intra- and inter-slice characteristics of the tumor, 3D models are recommended over 2D models. The performance and generalization of models can only be enhanced with the availability of big annotated datasets.

5.8.4 Complex anatomy

Complex anatomical features of the breast include ducts, blood arteries, tissue kinds, and lesions. Precise division of these formations continues to be difficult, particularly when boundaries are hazy or overlap. For example, U-Net was able to segment the whole FGT region in high-density breasts but failed to separate the pectoral muscle and breast fat in low-density breasts. Moreover, class imbalance affects breast MRI segmentation, with a much smaller number of pixels associated with the lesion or anomaly than with the non-target class. The model's capacity to learn and generalize may be impacted by this. Thus, the integration of multiscale and contextual information is necessary to bridge the gap in advanced systems for managing anatomical structures.

References

1 M. Dabass, R. Vig and S. Vashisth, "Five-grade cancer classification of colon histology images via deep learning," in Proc. 2nd Int. Conf. Commun. Comput. Syst. (ICCCS), Taylor and Francis, 2018, p. 18.

2 N. Coudray, A. L. Moreira, T. Sakellaropoulos, D. Fenyö, N. Razavian and A. Tsirigos, "Classification and mutation prediction from non–small cell lung cancer histopathology images using deep learning," Nature Med, vol. 24, no. 10, pp. 1559–1567, 2018.

3 C. Kaushal, S. Bhat, D. Koundal and A. Singla, "Recent trends in computer assisted diagnosis (CAD) system for breast cancer diagnosis using histopathological images," IRBM, vol. 40, no. 4, pp. 211–227, 2019.

4 A. K. Sharma, A. Nandal, T. Ganchev and A. Dhaka, "Breast cancer classification using CNN extracted features: A comprehensive review," in Application of Deep Learning Methods in Healthcare and Medical Science (ADLMHMS-2020). Taylor and Francis, 2022.

5 A. K. Sharma, et al., "HOG transformation based feature extraction framework in modified Resnet50 model for brain tumor detection," Biomedical Signal Processing and Control, vol 84, p. 104737, 2023.

6 M. Rana and M. Bhushan, "Classifying breast cancer using transfer learning models based on histopathological images," Neural Comput. Appl., vol. 35, pp. 14243–14257, 2023.

7 K. Taksali, A. K. Sharma and M. Rai, "Bioinspired genetic algorithm in medical applications," in Bio-Inspired Optimization for Medical Data Mining. Hoboken, NJ: Wiley, 2024.

8 A. K. Sharma, A. Nandal, A. Dhaka and R. Dixit, "Medical image classification techniques and analysis using deep learning networks: A review," in: Patgiri, R., Biswas, A. and Roy, P. (eds) Health Informatics: A Computational Perspective in Healthcare. Singapore: Springer, 2021, vol. 932, pp. 233–258.

9 G. Piantadosi, S. Marrone, A. Galli, M. Sansone and C. Sansone, "DCEMRI breast lesions segmentation with a 3TP U-Net deep convolutional neural network," in Proc. IEEE 32nd Int. Symp. Comput.-Based Med. Syst. (CBMS), Jun. 2019, pp. 628–633.

10 R. Khaled, J. Vidal, J. C. Vilanova and R. Martí, "A U-Net Ensemble for breast lesion segmentation in DCE MRI," Comput. Biol. Med, vol. 140, Jan. 2022, Art. no. 105093.

11 L. Hirsch, "Radiologist-level performance by using deep learning for segmentation of breast cancers on MRI scans," Radiol., Artif. Intell., vol. 4, no. 1, Jan. 2022, Art. no. e200231.

12 N. Aggarwal, P. Samant, S. Bansal, M. Bhushan and S. Kohli, "Methods to Detect Breast Cancer Using Traditional Machine Learning Technique," 2023 International Conference on Computational Intelligence and Sustainable Engineering Solutions (CISES), Greater Noida, India, 2023, pp. 547–552.

13 A. K. Sharma, A. Nandal, L. Zhou, A. Dhaka and T. Wu. Brain Tumor Classification Using Modified VGG Model-Based Transfer Learning Approach, vol. 337, pp. 538–550. IOS Press Ebooks. 2021.

14 A. K. Sharma, A. Nandal, A. Dhaka and R. Dixit, "A survey on machine learning based brain retrieval algorithms in medical image analysis," Health Technol, vol. 10, pp. 1359–1373, 2020.

15 S. N. Singh and M. Bhushan, "Smart ECG Monitoring and Analysis System Using Machine Learning," 2022 IEEE VLSI Device Circuit and System (VLSI DCS), Kolkata, India, 2022, pp. 304–309, doi: 10.1109/VLSIDCS53788.2022.9811433.

16 A. K. Sharma, et al., "Brain tumor classification using the modified ResNet50 model based on transfer learning," Biomed. Signal Process. Control, vol. 86, Part C, 2023.

17 R. Arya, A. Kumar and M. Bhushan, "Affect recognition using brain signals: A survey," in: Singh, V., Asari, V.K., Kumar, S., Patel, R.B. (eds) Computational Methods and Data Engineering. Advances in Intelligent Systems and Computing, vol 1257. Singapore: Springer, 2021.

18 C. Li, H. Sun, Z. Liu and M. Wang, "Learning cross-modal deep representations for multi-modal MR image segmentation," in Proc. MICCAI, Shenzhen, China, 2019, pp. 57–65.

19 A. Galli, S. Marrone, G. Piantadosi, M. Sansone, and C. Sansone, "A pipelined tracer-aware approach for lesion segmentation in breast DCEMRI." J. Imaging, vol. 7, no. 12. https://doi.org/10.3390/jimaging7120276

20 W. Yue, H. Zhang, J. Zhou, G. Li, Z. Tang, Z. Sun, J. Cai, N. Tian, S. Gao, J. Dong, Y. Liu, X. Bai and F. Sheng, "Deep learning-based automatic segmentation for size and volumetric measurement of breast cancer on magnetic resonance imaging," Frontiers Oncol., vol. 12, Aug. 2022, Art. no. 984626.

21 C. Hazirbas, L. Ma, C. Domokos and D. Cremers, "Fusenet: Incorporating depth into semantic segmentation via fusion-based CNN architecture," in Proc. Asian Conf. Comput. Vis., Taipei, Taiwan, 2017, pp. 213–228.

22 G. Maicas, G. Carneiro and A. P. Bradley, "Globally optimal breast mass segmentation from DCE-MRI using deep semantic segmentation as shape prior," in Proc. IEEE 14th Int. Symp. Biomed. Imag. (ISBI), Apr. 2017, pp. 305–309.

23 M. U. Dalmış, G. Litjens, K. Holland and A. Setio, "Using deep learning to segment breast and fibroglandular tissue in MRI volumes," Med. Phys, vol. 44, no. 2, pp. 533–546, 2017.

24 X. Meng, J. Fan, H. Yu, J. Mu, Z. Li, A. Yang, B. Liu, K. Lv, D. Ai, Y. Lin, H. Song, T. Fu, D. Xiao, G. Ma, J. Yang and Y. Gu, "Volume-awareness and outlier-suppression co-training for weakly-supervised MRI breast mass segmentation with partial annotations," Knowl.-Based Syst., vol. 258, Dec. 2022, Art. no. 109988.

25 V. S. Parekh, K. J. Macura, S. C. Harvey, I. R. Kamel, R. EI-Khouli, D. A. Bluemke and M. A. Jacobs, "Multiparametric deep learning tissue signatures for a radiological biomarker of breast cancer: Preliminary results," Med. Phys, vol. 47, no. 1, pp. 75–88, 2020.

6

REHABILITATION AND ASSISTIVE ROBOTICS FOR THE ELDERLY AND PHYSICALLY CHALLENGED

Marwa Mohammed

6.1 Introduction

The number of older adults is anticipated to increase rapidly in the next few years due to the improvements in healthcare management and the decrease in the incidence of death. According to the World Health Organization (WHO), one in six people globally will be aged 60 years or more by 2030, and by 2050, their number will double, and the majority of them will be in developing countries [1]. While the number of older people, at 80 years or more, is expected to triple by 2050 [2]. The shift in a country's population distribution toward population aging started in developed countries; developing countries will experience this tremendous alternation. The increasing number of older people globally and the lack of expenses to aid strain healthcare societies.

In older adults, disability is more significant [3]. Aging is accompanied by different diseases that contribute to movement disability as musculoskeletal disorders (e.g., arthritis and back and hip pain), cardiovascular challenges (e.g., myocardial infarction and peripheral arterial diseases), and neurological disorders (stroke and Parkinson's disease) [4]. The number of years of life with a disability (YLDs) associated with health conditions has increased significantly [5]. The presence of a higher incidence of chronic, noncommunicable diseases, in addition to an increased number of elderly with disability and a decline in function for substantially larger periods of their lives, requires an urgent need for effective elderly care solutions to improve healthy aging, increase independence, and quality of life (QOL).

Assistive technology (AT) includes devices or systems that enhance function and self-care and forbid limitations and co-morbidity [6]. The WHO declared that AT is necessary for older people and patients with physical

DOI: 10.1201/9781003481959-6

disabilities. AT improves independence and QOL [6]. It effectively saves time and the level of assistance healthcare providers need and decreases anxiety and fear with easy task achievement [7]. Those devices extend from comparatively low-technical appliances, such as traditional walk canes, to much more complicated, high-technical ones, such as robotic exoskeletons [8, 9]. Wearable, overground exoskeletons are a wide group of powered orthoses that vary from inflexible multi-joint activating robots that can enable patients with paralysis to stand and locomote at restricted speed to stiff single-joint activating exoskeletons to aid in motion to single- and multi-joint flexible exoskeleton that tailored the patients to move freely to reduce metabolic demand required during their locomotion [10].

Robotics continues to develop rapidly and has shown innovative outcomes in elderly care, a hot topic in the robotics society [11]. They were initially developed to replace humans for repetitive and risky functions; today, they are integrated into various aspects of daily life. They assist individuals in ADLs to shower, cook, and clean the house [12]. Recently, assistive robotics in healthcare has been considered a fruitful market opportunity and a superior and attractive robotic aspect to spend in [13]. So, today, the critical challenge is that technology could improve independence and QOL and reduce family and community expenses to care for, prevent, and address disability and frailty of older individuals [14].

Rehabilitation should be integrated as a core strategy in the long-term care of older people or healthcare conditions to improve the activity of daily living (ADLs) [5]. According to the Global Burden of Disease, about 2.41 billion individuals could benefit from rehabilitation services, and at least one in every three individuals globally requires rehabilitation during their disease or life [5]. Over the past three decades, the need for rehabilitation increased by 63%. This induced staff shortages and increased waiting lists for rehabilitation services [5, 15, 16]. There is an urgent need for facilities that help rehabilitate older people to compensate for the rehabilitation staff shortage.

Rehabilitation robots assist physical therapists in improving the functional motor recovery of people with physical limitations [17]. They were identically developed to relearn therapeutic exercise and reactive residual motor function and prevent further complications such as muscle wasting [17, 18]. These technologies have been able to overwhelm the lack of conventional therapeutic modalities and capabilities of the rehabilitation therapist and caregivers, such as a limited number of exercise repetitions and difficulties applying high-intensity exercise training [19]. The potential usefulness of these technologies to support the care of older patients could reduce costs on healthcare systems in individuals with disability [20]. Fundamentally, their ethical design will ensure that they are developed and used responsibly to benefit older people and are trusted to augment human care [21]. In this chapter, we will discuss the usage of rehabilitation robotics in different diseases contributing to disability in the elderly, impacting their social life and cognitive function, smart homes in the elderly, and rehabilitation advantages and disadvantages of robotics and recommendations to improve them.

6.2 Robotics rehabilitation in stroke patients

Post-stroke, the motor impairments are frequently persistent. The impairment in the upper limb (UL) seems to be more severely affected than the lower limb, and various robotic devices for UL rehabilitation have been improved [22, 23]. They have been categorized generally into end effectors or exoskeletons. Its effectiveness for acute, sub-acute, and chronic stroke patients in a rehabilitation program has been reported [24–26].The joints of end-effector robots do not assemble that of the human limb [27]. They hold the patient's hand or forearm at a single point and make forces at the interface [28]. Exercise with end-effector robots did not substantially enhance arm function compared with exoskeleton robots [28]. At the same time, exoskeleton robots have a structure that assembles human UL, as robot joint axes fit the UL joint axes of human beings [28]. The newly developed single-joint HAL (HAL-SJ) is a new exoskeleton rehabilitation robot. Its action is activated by the participant's voluntary muscular activity as measured by electromyography (EMG), and it can influence the patient's active movements [29]. Recent studies showed that exercise training using HAL-SJ and occupational therapy improves clinical outcomes, ADL parameters, and the function of the UL in acute stroke patients with moderate to severe muscle paralysis [30].

Spastic movement is the dominant feature of functional impairment of the motor system in stroke patients, characterized by alteration in reflex excitability, muscle tone, and range of motion (ROM) restriction, all resulting in difficulty in performing active movement and abilities to perform ADLs [31]. Studies showed positive effects of robotic-assisted training to induce short-term improvement of motor function in post-stroke patients as it provided the affected UL with weight support during exercises, and the tasks performed became the most accurate [32]. A previous study showed that UL kinematics post-robotic training demonstrated significant improvement in functional recovery, reduced muscle tone, improved UL ROMs, hand dexterity, handgrip strength, and visual abilities (e.g., attention, memory, and visuospatial function) [33]. Recently, various planar robots have been utilized in UL rehabilitation, such as the Quanser rehabilitation robot [34], 2-DOF CASIA-ARM robot [35], the In Motion Arm robot [36], 2-DOF planar robot [37], 8-DOF kinematic model [32].

Rehabilitation using exoskeletons with and without body weight support (BWS) systems has shown efficient gait training and better mobility in stroke and Parkinson's disease (PD) patients. It also efficiently improves balance, spasticity, and pain [38]. Balance affection is frequent post-stroke, resulting in poor mobility and inability to do ADL independently. These impairments represent a dominant risk factor for falling, which can induce injury or death [39]. Studies showed that robot-assisted gait training (RAGT) positively affects balance in stroke patients [40]. It is used to regain and improve locomotion [41]. During RAGT, the patient is placed in a supportive harness, and a robotic exoskeleton is attached to the patient's lower extremities. The exoskeleton enables the utilization of guidance force provided by the robotic orthosis during locomotion, thus helping the participants to move in the repeated movement of multiple gait cycles at a near-normal velocity over a more extended period [41]. Studies illustrated that the RAGT combined with conventional physical therapy (CPT) showed significant improvements in static and dynamic balance and lower extremity movement in stroke patients with infratentorial lesion [42]. Other studies have shown that wearable robotic knee orthosis enhances stroke patients' balance, a six-minute walk test (6MWT), and functional ambulation profile [43].

Studies reported that Lokomat improved gait training in stroke patients by improving the single limb stance phase of the paretic lower extremity, increased body muscle mass and cardiovascular fitness, and reduced body fat mass in the exercise training protocol for 30 minutes for four weeks [44]. Earlier studies showed that early application of Lokomat training combined with CPT in hemiparetic patients within three months post-stroke results showed that application of Lokomat training execute automated gait training and improve walking on seven scales of function than during the CPT within each three-week interval. Please note the protocol of the study was that patients were randomized into two treatment groups, ABA or BAB (A) = three weeks of Lokomat training, (B) = three weeks of CPT for whole study duration of nine weeks of exercise. It further means that in group 1 patients perform 3 weeks of Lokomat and then 3 weeks of CPT then 3 weeks of Lokomat, and the whole study duration was 9 weeks [45]. This improvement may refer to the fact that Lokomat stabilized the trunk and pelvis during exercise, supporting the patient's body weight to prevent knee buckling and aid foot clearance and, in turn, executing an automatic and even more natural gait cycle under spatiotemporal control [46]. Applying Lokomat at the onset of the motor learning process more effectively assists the patient in obtaining whole walking coordination. Thus, it may create an essential basis for more individualized and varied training for stroke patients [46]. Still, assistive devices cannot replace CPT, but may serve as an adjunct, particularly early post-stroke and in persistently physically disabled persons. Optimal exercise training protocols with tailored training programs for neurological conditions must be further developed. Additionally, large randomized clinical trials are needed to establish the effectiveness of assistive training over traditional or manually assisted treadmill strategies for locomotion in stroke patients.

6.3   Robotics rehabilitation in Parkinson

PD is among the most significant neurodegenerative diseases, and its prevalence increases steadily with aging. Worldwide, its prevalence is estimated to be doubled to more than 12 million people by 2050 [47]. People with PD are characterized by motor symptoms such as rigidity, bradykinesia, hypokinesia, resting tremor, and postural instability. Motor symptoms progression may lead to complications such as malnutrition and decline in physical function, inducing adverse outcomes and hospital admission [48].

Postural instability is a cardinal feature of PD; it is an extremely disabling symptom that becomes more significant with disease progression and represents a relevant cause of attenuated QOL. A recent systematic review showed high levels of evidence about the efficacy of RAGT on different postural instability patterns such as dynamic and static balance, gait freezing, falls, self-assurance in ADLs, and gait parameters related to balance ability in PD patients compared to CPT-trained at low intensity [49]. Studies reported better improvements in postural instability in PD due to RAGT than treadmill training [50, 51]. In this study, the patients use exoskeleton robotics for 12 sessions (30-minute session; 3 times a week, for 4 consecutive weeks) and they started robotic training at an initial speed of 1.5 km/h, and the speed was gradually increased to between 2.0 km/h and 2.2km/h depending on the participant's condition; no BWS was more effective than equal intensity treadmill training on freezing of gait, especially in individuals with greater walking disability [51].

Studies showed that RAGT using stationary treadmill-based robotic systems provides a method to facilitate gait training in PD patients. This study included patients with PD who were randomly assigned to 45-minute treatment sessions (12 in all), 3 days a week, for 4 consecutive weeks of either robotic stepper training using the Gait Trainer each training session consisted of 3 parts (each one lasting 10 minutes), with a 5-minute rest after each of them. The patients exercised at 20% BWS with a velocity of 1 km/h for 10 minutes, then at 10% BWS with a velocity of 1.3 km/h for 10 minutes, and finally at 0% BWS with a velocity of 1.6 km/h for 10 minutes compared to CPT; results showed significant improvement in gait velocity, walking capability, the number of steps, and resistance to fatigue than the control group [52]. Furthermore, recent systematic reviews showed that RAGT significantly improves motor dysfunction in PD, balance, stride length, and gait speed, 6 MWT, with no adverse events [53]. This significant improvement using RAGT referred to the fact that multiple repetitions of gait motion act as an external proprioceptive input to relearn the neuronal activity circuits to induce a normal gait cycle [54]. Moreover, the patients were instructed to participate in gait training, which made them focus on executing more autonomous gait [52]. Still, there is a lack of sufficient evidence to suggest that RAGT exercise can improve all aspects of lower motor function in addition to results of follow-ups more than three months [52, 53]. Future studies should determine the frequency, duration, speed, and need for BWS that might be most effective and compare RAGT with the treadmill or another active gait intervention to improve walking ability in patients with PD [52].

Studies reported that exercise using bilateral exoskeleton (active, resisted, and functional) with the Keeogo Rehab™ exoskeleton for eight weeks with two sessions/week results showed positive changes in memory, mood, balance, gait, and health-related QOL in adults with PD with substantial enhancement in the cognition SCOPA-COG scale and 6MWT compared to exercise without an exoskeleton [55].

Despite high-intensity exercise, it is particularly effective in treating PD patients [56]. The large difficulties in delivering high-intensity exercise training to them are due to poor health conditions, concern of falling, low self-confidence, low expectations, and attenuated motivation [57]. Overground exoskeleton improved rehabilitation outcomes, as memory and gait provided enough stability to build confidence and self-efficacy, which enabled them to participate in high-intensity exercise [55]. A recent study showed that PD patients with moderate levels of disability trained with overground lower-extremity exoskeletons compared to CPT twice weekly for eight weeks. They can practicably achieve high-intensity exercise in their activity counts per minute (exceed 1354 ACPM) after four weeks of exercise progress and can proceed to increase their intensity for a further four weeks, while in PD patients with CPT, they achieve plateau at moderate-intensity of exercise [55]. The non-BWS overground exoskeleton stresses the biological system, which may evoke neurophysiological consequences that are more appropriate to trigger a series of mechanisms that can lead to improved muscle and brain function [58]. Still, overground exoskeletons are a highly inaccessible technology whose application is an immediate barrier to translating research into practice that impacts practice guidelines that need to be scientifically proven in evidence-based studies [55]. Future studies must include metabolic, blood biomarkers, functional activity, and brain imaging post-rehabilitation [55].

Rehabilitation is still the core treatment modality for PD patients in the smart homeward. A physical therapist guides patients distantly to apply different forms of internet-based rehabilitation exercise training, such as relaxation techniques, joint ROM, breathing exercises, gait, balance, and mental training. During rehabilitation training, the individual vital signs as a smartwatch can monitor pulse rate to forbid exaggerated exercise intensity. In the case of PD patients, a smart lunch box is given to patients to monitor the number and severity of hand tremors on a daily basis while eating to evaluate the efficacy of the exercise training program [59].

6.4 Robotics rehabilitation and cognitive impairment

Studies have illustrated that loneliness is a significant factor in older adults and leads to mental impairments, depression, and frailty [60]. The majority of persons with dementia suffer from behavioral and psychological problems with different levels during the disease course, resulting in more expenses. More than two-thirds of people with dementia suffer from depression [61]. Additionally, the majority complain of anxiety [62]. These challenges may induce prolonged hospitalization, drug use, and decreased QOL for caregivers and patients. Studies showed that AT could enhance the quality of care and security of the elderly with Alzheimer's (AD) by monitoring the time they spend resting in bed and during activity, drug use, surrounding environmental conditions, and emergency communication [63]. In wearable robotics, a cognitive human-robot interface (CHRI) is designed to improve the mental connection between the robot and the human. The CHRI in the human-robot direction is based on information gathered by sensors to measure bio-electrical and bio-mechanical signals, and the information gathered is the result of processing, manipulating, and organizing data [64].

Recent systematic review showed that wide range of technologies (such as GPS, monitoring systems, tablets, touch-screen computers with calendar, clock and task reminders, verbal instruction technology, and robot technology) support people with mild cognitive impairment and dementia (MCI/D) and their seems optimistic, and a wide range of technologies has been evaluated in homes with people with MCI/D and their family carers [65]. A recent study showed that using robotic pet therapy (PARO robotics) day after day for 20 minutes for three months provided a viable alternative to traditional pet therapy to control anxiety and depression symptoms in elderly patients with mild to moderate dementia. Furthermore, heart rate, pain severity, and psychological medication were substantially attenuated while pulse oximetry and galvanic skin response (GSV) were increased compared to the control group [66]. It is critically important to conclude that patients with cognitive deterioration and dementia in research should learn about the required design characteristics to enhance robotics acceptance and usage [65]. Still, there is a lack of research on the impact of technology on QOL, occupational function, or human dignity [65]. Future studies are required regarding provider awareness of evidence-based research using untraditional ways to treat depression, like biofeedback therapy with robotic pets, and the participant's desire to stop or decrease medication use post-therapy when depression declines [66].

Additionally, an earlier study showed that patients trained with human-robotic interactive gait training (HIT) using Walkbot robotics compared CPT in individuals with post-stroke dementia (PSD) [67]. All patients underwent rehabilitation protocols, which consisted of training for 1 hour/sessions day after day for six weeks; the walking velocity was set at 1.00–1.20 km/h and slightly raised by 0.1 km/h every 5 minute, based on patient tolerance with maximum adjustable to 3.00 km/h, results showed that in HIT group enhance mental variables including (sense of orientation, registration, focus, and measurement), furthermore sensorimotor recovery functions, trunk balance, and coordination compared to the group treated with CPT [67]. This improvement occurred as exercise enhanced blood flow to the brain and enhanced neuroplastic alternations in the cognitive part of the brain of older people, with increased hippocampus volume as measured through functional magnetic resonance imaging (fMRI) with improvement in both spatial and verbal memory areas [68]. Still, the efficacy of robotic-induced cognitive neuroplasticity has not been measured yet despite the development of neuroimaging techniques such as fMRI and functional near-infrared spectroscopy (NIRS), which have superior spatial resolutions. Still, its imaging signals are influenced by locomotor movement and robotic machine electromagnetic artifacts that limit its use [69]. Furthermore, a more comprehensive cognitive intervention is required with long-term follow-up.

Studies reported enthusiastic reactions from older people involved in several studies that used assistive robots; results showed their effectiveness in elevated mood, reduced loneliness, and improved mental health conditions [70]. Real-time robotic platforms can accurately anticipate falling risk by sending warning signals and revealing falls and emergencies [70] despite most existing exoskeletons being developed to help rehabilitate patients with neurological conditions or augment human function in the industrial field. Therefore, the exoskeleton industry, physical therapists, and clinicians must collaborate to evolve advanced exoskeleton robotics, which could effectively support independence and enhance the overall well-being of older adults.

6.5 Socially assistive robots (SAR) in elderly care

Healthcare and social policies have recently promoted the "aging in place" concept, where older people stay in their houses and societies. It is the best way to enhance health, QOL, and social connections and decline economic costs for older people [20]. Domestic social robots are a form of robotics that is common in personal lives such as homes and healthcare settings. Those robots are automatic devices that are developed for household environments to interact and communicate with humans socially [71]. They are ordinarily developed to be friendly and show human-like characteristics to listen and answer questions to facilitate users' acceptance and natural interaction. Also, they can help with daily tasks and provide social interaction to relieve loneliness and isolation in older people.

Robotics acceptance and perceptions are evaluated to preserve social interaction between robots and humans [72]. Studies have shown that healthcare providers have a positive attitude toward the long-term application of robotics; they have shown that it is beneficial and practical in psychological and social conditions [73]. Awareness of the elderly toward domestic social robots is classified into four types: (1)"Cautious Optimists" are predominantly aware of technology as they are typically mobile phone users and utilize mobile applications and the internet. They generally have a positive attitude toward innovative technology, particularly social robots. They expect to have the chance to test and learn, but they have important concerns about privacy and safety by using these robots [74]. (2) "Skeptical Traditionalists" or Laggards are the primary mobile phone users; they are slightly friendly with technology. Their attitude regarding social robots tends to be more reserved, with the bulk of them having a negative attitude. Most of them perceive the limited usefulness of social robots in that they are less affected by trends and pressure for social robotic spreads and adhere to conventional values [74]. (3) "Positive Optimists" are basic mobile phone users but showed considerable positivity regarding social robots. They are enthusiastic about the potential benefits and reservations about interacting with humans with social robots. (4) "Technophiles" are generally regular mobile phone users who are aware and satisfied with technology. They showed a positive attitude toward technological advances and social robots. They had sheer confidence: none expressed anxieties about using or interacting with robots [74].

In rehabilitation and healthcare settings, social robots are considered training assistants, coaches, or motivator modalities that enhance the performance or participation of participants through rehabilitation. Social robots have been used for stroke rehabilitation; they showed positive attitudes toward the patients, such as increased willingness to perform prescribed exercises and enthusiastic responses toward the robot [75]. Social interaction is critical during rehabilitation; environmental factors can motivate the patients to achieve their goals. A recent study showed that a human-robot coupled system for the walking posture of older people illustrated that this model can be effectively used as an outdoor walking aid that settles older adults and does not experience resonance and, hence, can be safely used by the elderly as it does not resonate during walking [76].

6.6 Smart homes and rehabilitation for the elderly

Innovative home technologies with artificial intelligence (AI) algorithms can identify abnormalities in normal behavior patterns and provide emergency alerts at an accurate time [77]. AI analyzes data collected from wearable devices and electronic health records, and performs data analysis to detect early warning signs of diseases and to provide individualized treatment protocols [77]. AI-powered systems can help older adults perform ADL activities, such as drug usage, fall detection, and navigation, to enable them to live longer independently [78]. AI may also provide a more sophisticated level of decision-making in the home, such as the ability to respond to emergencies on time for older adults living independently or the desire to automate home safety risk management [77]. The system can send a real-time emergency alarm to their family or healthcare setting without human assistance if it identifies something wrong with the user's health practices or medical recommendations [77].

Smart home technology is rapidly developing, focusing on medical AT to keep older people secure and healthy within their homes [79]. In-home cameras, sensors, and wearable sensors monitor individuals' external activity, gait performance, falls, and overall health, providing alerts to carers when abnormal activity patterns or falls are detected. Smart home technology also allows the operation of numerous household appliances and systems (e.g., lights, heating/cooling) through voice activation or touch screens, thereby supporting older adults with functional limitations in maintaining independent living. Smart refrigerators can monitor contents and usage more efficiently to enhance the nutritional condition of older adults with sarcopenia [79]. Robots also assist older adults in ADLs such as cooking, showering, and cleaning [80]. AI-driven wearable devices also may monitor vital signs and activity levels to promote a healthy and independent lifestyle [77]. AI technology enhances the potential for home hospitalization to enable distant patient monitoring and real-time interaction between healthcare workers and patients. Hospital-at-home attempts to provide necessary medical healthcare services as a practicable method for at-home older adult care [81, 82]. Home hospitalization tracks digital biomarkers (e.g., pulse and respiratory rate, sleep patterns, activity performance, and dietary statues) to provide healthcare workers with a more comprehensive knowledge of a patient's health condition [83].

The new innovative Smart Home Ward (SHW) recently desires to extend healthcare facilities to the home setting. The SHW is a coherent hospital unit controlled by hospital specialists. It was developed to supply patients with the same hospital-medical care level services at home, including clinical monitoring and medical consultation [84]. It also provides early hospital discharge, avoids admission, and provides integrated healthcare follow-up, medical care, and rehabilitation settings in patients' homes [84].

An interdisciplinary care team handles the management of patients in the SHW. Patients receive a primary medical evaluation by their professional clinicians to determine their eligibility for distant home care. If the patient is eligible based on the evaluation and gives consent to participate, the SHW team performs a home environment evaluation. The essential modifications are done, and equipment or devices used for monitoring are installed to safely support care at home with remote expert supervision [84]. The SHW monitors patients' digital biomarkers, ADLs, treatment compliance, and risk hazards through contact or wireless devices. This information can be provided to adapt treatments or inform team workers about deviations from anticipated values [84].

A pre-training ward has been developed in the hospital to adjust the transition of patients from hospital to home care. Patients are exercised to use smart home devices and obtain guidelines on distant rehabilitation intervention [84]. For stroke patients, much effort can contribute to increased mobility and enhanced patient confidence as properly accessible elements are implemented within their home to launch as barrier-free surroundings for easy motion achievement. Physical therapists perform regular assessments in both home visits in addition to performing hospital evaluations [84].

6.7 Tools to assess assistive device validity

Pytheia is a valid and reliable scale assessing rehabilitation, assistive robotics, and other technology-assisted devices. It can also measure end users' satisfaction, individual characteristics, and functionality through rehabilitation and assistive technologies. Its reliability was 0.793, its ICC was 0.992, and its validity was strong to excellent [85].

This scale is composed of two primary domains. The first one, comprised of 15 items, is related to the general evaluation of assistive technology. In comparison, the second one (items 16 to 20) is used to evaluate any individual characteristic of the assistive technology, such as independent motion, oral commands, etc.). In the first domain, the subsequent first nine questions (items 1 to 9) were answered by using the 5-point Likert scale: 0-N/A, 1-Not at all satisfied, 2-Slightly satisfied, 3-Moderately satisfied, 4-Very satisfied, and 5-Extremely satisfied. While the subsequent six questions (items 10 to 15) were answered using the 5-point Likert scale: 0-N/A, 1-Not at all (0% of the time), 2-Sometimes (around 25% of the time), 3-Half the time, neutral (about 50% of the time), 4-Often (around 75% of the time), and 5-All the time (100% of the time). Finally, the questions of the second domain of the scale (items from 16 to 20) use the initially presented Likert scale [85].

6.8 Application and limitations of robotics

6.8.1 Applications of robotics in elderly care

The ethical design of AI systems incorporates human beliefs like the well-being of older people, self-esteem, and the need for independence [86]. Robots are not designed to be tired, distracted, or irritable, and they limit the availability that human careers may demonstrate [87]. Even though care robots are improbable to replace highly skilled medical providers, they may have a role in supplementing lower-skilled work and providing a new chance for patients to engage [88]. Rehabilitation robots have the advantages of being repeatable, accurate, and reliable; they can provide an effective means to improve rehabilitation outcomes and reduce healthcare costs [89]. A recent study showed that the perception and expectation of clinicians and patients involved in rehabilitation procedures toward a social robot showed positive perception among different constructs such as physiological factors, social perception, performance expectations, and entertainment level [90].

6.8.2   Limitations of robotics in elderly care

Robots are human-manufacturer and can perform within the delimited constructs. Robotics lack emotional engagement and human values, challenging the appropriate use of robotic technology in health and social care [87]. The difficulties facing AI researchers and developers include designing algorithms that can distinguish between ethical and unethical values and then transform human belief into technical form [86]. Robot carers can encourage older people to live independently in their homes, but at the cost of personal surveillance and an expected reduction in human interaction [86].

As a robot is used in an older adult's home, there is a conflict concerning privacy; some robots have cameras that see the user inside the home and monitor, collect, and store data on how the older person moves at home, which may trigger intervention and capture their visitors [91]. The user's independence may be inhibited as the robot provides medications to a timetable or even a fall can be prevented, but at the cost of autonomous action and the self-esteem of the individual [91]. When dealing with individuals, robots should be able to interact without expectation. However, classical robots still lack control with uncertainty as they cannot predict the individual's behavior and fall occurrence [32].

The existing literature on social influence in technology adaptation emphasizes that its impact differs for all geriatrics [74]. Not all elderly can deal with robotics; findings suggest that the age and severity of patients' cognitive impairment, as well as their caregivers' age and educational level, could significantly influence the efficacy of technologies in improving the at-home management of patients [63]. Stigma, fear of security, and lack of self-efficacy concerning technology usage could lead to poverty or hedonic motivation for older people, creating barriers to AI usage [92].

Most rehabilitation exoskeletons are aimed toward patients with neurological disorders with less emphasis on musculoskeletal disorders [64]. The significant challenges of robotics in the rehabilitation area are the incompetence of the current system to achieve modulation of the neuromuscular activity while promoting voluntary robotic control and limited understanding of the disability-induced musculoskeletal changes that impede the understanding of how the patient's motor function can be best formulated in a control strategy for robotic device [93]. Other challenges to access robotic devices include compact actuators, long-term power supplies, improved ergonomics and safety, and the use of light materials in structure [64].

A recent study showed that the perception and expectations of therapists and patients participating in rehabilitation intervention toward a social robot showed negative perceptions toward the robot in some concepts. In the case of effort expectation and facility conditions, most patients and clinicians think robot usage can be complex, suggesting that an introduction phase is needed to implement the robot in the future [90]. Furthermore, efforts have been made to enhance the human-robot interaction using EMG. However, the use of EMG has several limitations. It is expected that EMG must be introduced in the whole cycle of robot control, which is only possible by hybrid control strategies [64].

6.9 Recommendations

Studies recommend that policymakers should work with technologists to investigate, prevent, and lessen possible unethical use of AI [94]. They suggest that AI engineers should proceed with the dual-use nature of their work significantly, allowing misuse-related considerations to influence research priorities and models and targeting to reach out to appropriate performers when harmful applications are predictable [94]. Reassurance and robust measures are required to assure the safety and privacy of individual data [74]. They stress the need to identify best practices in research areas with more advanced methods to address dual-use concerns, such as computer security, directing the system of a robotic device that is tailored to the individual's needs and abilities [95], and ensuring participant safety and comfort during robotic use [96, 97].

Understanding and rationalizing these issues is essential for wider acceptance and integration of social robots into the lives of older adults [74]. Their focus is to provide a user-friendly design with clear instructions for easy use of robotics [75]. Developing options for older adults to increase digital skills to enable intelligent assisted technology (IAT) adoption is recommended [74]. It may be necessary for device companies to know that support and training play a role in clinicians' decisions about which IAT to prescribe to older people [93]. Tailored educational initiatives are essential for older adults to promote familiarity and competence with technology [74]. In addition to encouraging individualized, adjustable technology accommodates a patient's home surroundings [92].

Furthermore, clinical standards must be considered when designing robotic rehabilitation strategies to retain compatibility with traditional therapies while involving a minimum amount of robot programming and adjustments [98]. The robot must be adaptable to the human limb segment lengths, ROM, forces, and velocity. The manufacturers should refine the individual's motion and reduce the effects of tremors and spasms [98]. Older people require support from rehabilitation professionals and manufacturers to continue using these technologies independently [92]. Rehabilitation specialists should emphasize their role in motivating older people to consider IAT by persuading them that the technology will help them [93]. Family caregivers may encourage older people to use IAT for rehabilitation and to engage with others socially [92].

Awareness to increase public knowledge about disability and to reduce the stigma around IAT use as a signal of dependence would contribute to increased IAT use [99]. To recreate this function, rehabilitation professionals need knowledge regarding current best practices and the ability to translate them into their clinical practice [99]. Multi-component learning interventions have been used to support this, wherein rehabilitation professionals' self-perceived knowledge and self-perceived practice behavior are observed [100]. This knowledge will become even more critical as IAT is increasingly developed to support older adults and awareness about physical aspects of a patient's home, including narrow passageways, stairs, or weak internet signal [101]. The results did not demonstrate culture or ethnicity as a moderating factor in older people's IAT use for rehabilitation [92]. Gender, age, and experience are recognized as critical constructs in the acceptance of technology and play a pivotal role in modifying a patient's use of an IAT device [102]. Future research should investigate the intersection of age, ethnicity, and gender in the prescription, acquisition, implementation, and adoption of IAT in older adults undergoing rehabilitation [92].

6.10   Conclusion

AT and rehabilitation robotics emerge to alleviate the strain on healthcare and aged care systems. These technologies are not just tools to improve physical abilities but also improve social and mental health. As the skills of such robotics advance, their potential to assist with a broader range of activities of daily living and complex healthcare needs grows, making them indispensable in modern care. However, the process of using assistive robotics technology is challenging. It is urgent to promote multidisciplinary interventions that ensure these innovations are developed and implemented in a manner that is ethical, equitable, and effective. It is imperative to continue research and development in this field to ensure that rehabilitation and assistive robotics technologies become more accessible, affordable, and tailored to the needs of the elderly and physically challenged.

References

1 https://www.who.int/news-room/fact-sheets/detail/ageing-and-health
2 Rudnicka, E., et al., *The World Health Organization (WHO) approach to healthy ageing*. Maturitas, 2020. **139**: p. 6–11.

3 Kraus, L.L., Coleman, E., and Houtenville, R., A., *2017 Disability Statistics Annual Report. A Publication of the Rehabilitation Research and Training Center on Disability Statistics and Demographics.* Institute on Disability, University of New Hampshire, 2018.

4 Kujala, U.M., et al., *Chronic diseases and objectively monitored physical activity profile among aged individuals – a cross-sectional twin cohort study.* Annals of Medicine, 2019. 51(1): p. 78–87.

5 Cieza, A., et al., *Global estimates of the need for rehabilitation based on the Global Burden of Disease Study 2019: A systematic analysis for the Global Burden of Disease Study 2019.* Lancet (London, England), 2021. 396(10267): p. 2006–2017.

6 Scherer, M.J., *Outcomes of assistive technology use on quality of life.* Disability and Rehabilitation, 1996. 18(9): p. 439–448.

7 Madara Marasinghe, K., *Assistive technologies in reducing caregiver burden among informal caregivers of older adults: A systematic review.* Disability and Rehabilitation: Assistive Technology, 2016. 11(5): p. 353–360.

8 Sehgal, M., Jacobs, J., and Biggs, W.S., *Mobility assistive device use in older adults.* American Family Physician, 2021. 103(12): p. 737–744.

9 Molteni, F., et al., *Exoskeleton and end-effector robots for upper and lower limbs rehabilitation*: Narrative review. Physical Medicine and Rehabilitation, 2018. 10(9S2). doi: 10.1016/j.pmrj.2018.06.005.

10 Martini, E., et al., *Gait training using a robotic hip exoskeleton improves metabolic gait efficiency in the elderly.* Scientific Reports, 2019. 9(1): p. 7157.

11 Pearce, A.J., et al., *Robotics to enable older adults to remain living at home.* Journal of Aging Research, 2012. 2012: p. 538169.

12 Bilyea, A., et al., *Robotic assistants in personal care: A scoping review.* Medical Engineering & Physics, 2017. 49: p. 1–6.

13 Riek, L.D., *Healthcare robotics.* Communications of the ACM, 2017. 60(11): p. 68–78.

14 Vancea, M., and Solé-Casals, J., *Population aging in the European information societies: Towards a comprehensive research agenda in eHealth innovations for elderly.* Aging and Disease, 2016. 7(4): p. 526–539.

15 Sheehy, L., et al., *Home-based virtual reality training after discharge from hospital-based stroke rehabilitation: A parallel randomized feasibility trial.* Trials, 2019. 20(1): p. 333.

16 Krishnaswami, A., et al., *Gerotechnology for older adults with cardiovascular diseases: JACC state-of-the-art review.* Journal of the American College of Cardiology, 2020. 76(22): p. 2650–2670.

17 Mohammadi, E., Zohoor, H., and Khadem, S.M., *Design and prototype of an active assistive exoskeletal robot for rehabilitation of elbow and wrist.* Scientia Iranica, 2016. 23(3): p. 998–1005.

18 Najafi, M., et al., *Robotic assistance for children with cerebral palsy based on learning from tele-cooperative demonstration.* International Journal of Intelligent Robotics and Applications, 2017. 1(1): p. 43–54.

19 Huo, W., et al., *Lower limb wearable robots for assistance and rehabilitation: A state of the art.* IEEE Systems Journal, 2016. 10(3): p. 1068–1081.

20 Schulz, R., et al., *Advancing the aging and technology agenda in gerontology.* Gerontologist, 2015. 55(5): p. 724–734.

21 Johnston, C., *Ethical design and use of robotic care of the elderly.* Journal of Bioethical Inquiry, 2022. 19(1): p. 11–14.

22 Germanotta, M., et al., *Reliability, validity and discriminant ability of the instrumental indices provided by a novel planar robotic device for upper limb rehabilitation.* Journal of NeuroEngineering and Rehabilitation, 2018. 15(1): p. 39.

23 Cho, K.H., Hong, M.R., and Song, W.K., *Upper limb robotic rehabilitation for chronic stroke survivors: A single-group preliminary study.* Journal of Physical Therapy Science, 2018. 30(4): p. 580–583.

24 Fukuda, H., et al., *Tailor-made rehabilitation approach using multiple types of hybrid assistive limb robots for acute stroke patients: A pilot study.* Assistive Technology, 2016. 28(1): p. 53–56.

25 Miyasaka, H., et al., *Robot-aided training for upper limbs of sub-acute stroke patients.* Japanese Journal of Comprehensive Rehabilitation Science, 2015. 6: p. 27–32.

26 Volpe, B.T., et al., *Intensive sensorimotor arm training mediated by therapist or robot improves hemiparesis in patients with chronic stroke.* Neurorehabilitation and Neural Repair, 2008. 22(3): p. 305–310.

27 Seidler, R.D., *Neural correlates of motor learning, transfer of learning, and learning to learn.* Exercise and Sport Sciences Reviews, 2010. 38(1): p. 3–9.

28 Bertani, R., et al., *Effects of robot-assisted upper limb rehabilitation in stroke patients: A systematic review with meta-analysis.* Neurological Sciences, 2017. 38(9): p. 1561–1569.

29 Wall, A., Borg, J., and Palmcrantz, S., *Clinical application of the Hybrid Assistive Limb (HAL) for gait training-a systematic review.* Frontiers in Systems Neuroscience, 2015. 9: p. 48.

30 Iwamoto, Y., et al., *Combination of exoskeletal upper limb robot and occupational therapy improve activities of daily living function in acute stroke patients.* Journal of Stroke and Cerebrovascular Diseases, 2019. 28(7): p. 2018–2025.

31 van der Ploeg, H.P., et al., *Physical activity for people with a disability.* Sports Medicine, 2004. 34(10): p. 639–649.

32 Rossa, C., et al., *Robotic rehabilitation and assistance for individuals with movement disorders based on a kinematic model of the upper limb.* IEEE Transactions on Medical Robotics and Bionics, 2021. 3(1): p. 190–203.

33 Adomavičienė, A., et al., *Influence of new technologies on post-stroke rehabilitation: A comparison of Armeo spring to the kinect system.* Medicina (Kaunas), 2019. 55(4): p. 98.

34 Atashzar, S.F., et al., *A computational-model-based study of supervised haptics-enabled therapist-in-the-loop training for upper-limb poststroke robotic rehabilitation.* IEEE/ASME Transactions on Mechatronics, 2018. 23(2): p. 563–574.

35 Luo, L., et al., *A greedy assist-as-needed controller for upper limb rehabilitation.* IEEE Transactions on Neural Networks and Learning Systems, 2019. 30(11): p. 3433–3443.

36 Koeppel, T., and Pila, O., *Test-retest reliability of kinematic assessments for upper limb robotic rehabilitation.* IEEE Transactions on Neural Systems and Rehabilitation Engineering, 2020. 28(9): p. 2035–2042.

37 Zhang, J., and Cheah, C.C., *Passivity and stability of human–robot interaction control for upper-limb rehabilitation robots.* IEEE Transactions on Robotics, 2015. 31(2): p. 233–245.

38 Khan, A.S., et al., *Retraining walking over ground in a powered exoskeleton after spinal cord injury: A prospective cohort study to examine functional gains and neuroplasticity.* Journal of Neuroengineering and Rehabilitation, 2019. 16(1): p. 145.

39 Harris, J.E., et al., *Relationship of balance and mobility to fall incidence in people with chronic stroke.* Physical Therapy, 2005. 85(2): p. 150–158.

40 Kim, S.Y., et al., *Effects of innovative WALKBOT robotic-assisted locomotor training on balance and gait recovery in hemiparetic stroke: A prospective, randomized, experimenter blinded case control study with a four-week follow-up.* IEEE Transactions on Neural Systems and Rehabilitation Engineering, 2015. 23(4): p. 636–642.

41 Sale, P., et al., *Use of the robot assisted gait therapy in rehabilitation of patients with stroke and spinal cord injury.* European Journal of Physical and Rehabilitation Medicine, 2012. **48**(1): p. 111–121.

42 Kim, H.Y., et al., *Robot-assisted gait training for balance and lower extremity function in patients with infratentorial stroke: A single-blinded randomized controlled trial.* Journal of Neuroengineering and Rehabilitation, 2019. **16**(1): p. 99.

43 Wong, C.K., Bishop, L., and Stein, J., *A wearable robotic knee orthosis for gait training: A case-series of hemiparetic stroke survivors.* Prosthetics and Orthotics International, 2012. **36**(1): p. 113–120.

44 Husemann, B., et al., *Effects of locomotion training with assistance of a robot-driven gait orthosis in hemiparetic patients after stroke.* Stroke, 2007. **38**(2): p. 349–354.

45 Mayr, A., et al., *Prospective, blinded, randomized crossover study of gait rehabilitation in stroke patients using the Lokomat gait orthosis.* Neurorehabilitation and Neural Repair, 2007. **21**(4): p. 307–314.

46 Schmidt, R.A., and Wrisberg, C.A., *Motor learning and performance: A situation-based learning approach, 4th ed.* 2008, Champaign, IL, US: Human Kinetics.

47 GBD 2016 Parkinson's Disease Collaborators. *Global, regional, and national burden of Parkinson's disease, 1990-2016: A systematic analysis for the Global Burden of Disease Study 2016.* Lancet Neurology, 2018. **17**(11): p. 939–953. doi: 10.1016/S1474-4422(18)30295-3.

48 Okunoye, O., et al., *Factors associated with hospitalisation among people with Parkinson's disease – A systematic review and meta-analysis.* Parkinsonism & Related Disorders, 2020. **71**: p. 66–72.

49 Picelli, A., et al., *Effects of robot-assisted gait training on postural instability in Parkinson's disease: A systematic review.* European Journal of Physical and Rehabilitation Medicine, 2021. **57**(3): p. 472–477.

50 Picelli, A., et al., *Robot-assisted gait training versus equal intensity treadmill training in patients with mild to moderate Parkinson's disease: A randomized controlled trial.* Parkinsonism & Related Disorders, 2013. **19**(6): p. 605–610.

51 Capecci, M., et al., *Clinical effects of robot-assisted gait training and treadmill training for Parkinson's disease. A randomized controlled trial.* Annals of Physical and Rehabilitation Medicine, 2019. **62**(5): p. 303–312.

52 Picelli, A., et al., *Robot-assisted gait training in patients with Parkinson disease.* Neurorehabilitation and Neural Repair, 2012. **26**(4): p. 353–361.

53 Jiang, X., et al., *Effect of robot-assisted gait training on motor dysfunction in Parkinson's patients: A systematic review and meta-analysis.* Journal of Back and Musculoskeletal Rehabilitation, 2024. **37**(2): p. 253–268.

54 Frenkel-Toledo, S., et al., *Treadmill walking as an external pacemaker to improve gait rhythm and stability in Parkinson's disease.* Movement Disorders, 2005. **20**(9): p. 1109–1114.

55 McGibbon, C.A., Sexton, A., and Gryfe, P., *Exercising with a robotic exoskeleton can improve memory and gait in people with Parkinson's disease by facilitating progressive exercise intensity.* Scientific Reports, 2024. **14**(1): p. 4417.

56 Goodwin, V.A., et al., *The effectiveness of exercise interventions for people with Parkinson's disease: A systematic review and meta-analysis.* Movement Disorders, 2008. **23**(5): p. 631–640.

57 Shulman, L.M., et al., *Randomized clinical trial of 3 types of physical exercise for patients with Parkinson disease.* JAMA Neurology, 2013. **70**(2): p. 183–190.

58 Ben-Zeev, T., and Okun, E., *High-intensity functional training: Molecular mechanisms and benefits.* NeuroMolecular Medicine, 2021. **23**(3): p. 335–338.

59 Chandrabhatla, A.S., Pomeraniec, I.J., and Ksendzovsky, A., *Co-evolution of machine learning and digital technologies to improve monitoring of Parkinson's disease motor symptoms.* NPJ Digital Medicine, 2022. 5(1): p. 32.

60 Haleem, A., et al., *Telemedicine for healthcare: Capabilities, features, barriers, and applications.* Sensors International, 2021. 2: p. 100117.

61 Byers, A.L., and Yaffe, K., *Depression and risk of developing dementia.* Nature Reviews Neurology, 2011. 7(6): p. 323–331.

62 Yu, R., et al., *Use of a therapeutic, socially assistive pet robot (PARO) in improving mood and stimulating social interaction and communication for people with dementia: Study protocol for a randomized controlled trial.* JMIR Research Protocols, 2015. 4(2): p. e45.

63 Pilotto, A., et al., *Information and communication technology systems to improve quality of life and safety of Alzheimer's disease patients: A multicenter international survey.* Journal of Alzheimer's Disease, 2011. 23(1): p. 131–141.

64 Bhardwaj, S., Khan, A.A., and Muzammil, M., *Lower limb rehabilitation robotics: The current understanding and technology.* Work, 2021. 69(3): p. 775–793.

65 Holthe, T., et al., *Usability and acceptability of technology for community-dwelling older adults with mild cognitive impairment and dementia: A systematic literature review.* Clinical Interventions in Aging, 2018. 13: p. 863–886.

66 Petersen, S., et al., *The utilization of robotic pets in dementia care.* Journal of Alzheimer's Disease, 2017. 55(2): p. 569–574.

67 Kim, Y., et al., *Bolstering cognitive and locomotor function in post-stroke dementia using human-robotic interactive gait training.* Journal of Clinical Medicine, 2023. 12(17): p. 5661. doi: 10.3390/jcm12175661.

68 Erickson, K.I., et al., *Exercise training increases size of hippocampus and improves memory.* Proceedings of the National Academy of Sciences of the United States of America, 2011. 108(7): p. 3017–3022.

69 Kim, H., et al., *Neuroplastic effects of end-effector robotic gait training for hemiparetic stroke: A randomised controlled trial.* Scientific Reports, 2020. 10(1): p. 12461.

70 Rajagopalan, R., Litvan, I., and Jung, T.P., *Fall prediction and prevention systems: Recent trends, challenges, and future research directions.* Sensors (Basel), 2017. 17(11): p. 2509. doi: 10.3390/s17112509.

71 Fong, T., Nourbakhsh, I., and Dautenhahn, K., *A survey of socially interactive robots.* Robotics and Autonomous Systems, 2003. 42(3): p. 143–166.

72 Cifuentes, C.A., et al., *Social robots in therapy and care.* Current Robotics Reports, 2020. 1(3): p. 59–74.

73 Chen, S.-C., Jones, C., and Moyle, W., *Health professional and workers attitudes towards the use of social robots for older adults in long-term care.* International Journal of Social Robotics, 2019. 12(5): p. 1135–1147.

74 Žvanut, B., and Mihelič, A., *Qualitative study on domestic social robot adoption and associated security concerns among older adults in Slovenia.* Frontiers in Psychology, 2024. 15: p. 1343077.

75 Matarić, M.J., et al., *Socially assistive robotics for post-stroke rehabilitation.* Journal of Neuroengineering and Rehabilitation, 2007. 4: p. 5.

76 Vitanza, A., et al., Assistive robots for the elderly: Innovative tools to gather health relevant data. In: Consoli, S., Reforgiato Recupero, D., Petković, M. (eds), *Data science for healthcare.* 2019, Springer International Publishing. p. 195–215. doi: 10.1007/978-3-030-05249-2_7.

77 Padhan, S., et al., *Artificial intelligence (AI) and robotics in elderly healthcare: Enabling independence and quality of life.* Cureus, 2023. 15(8): p. e42905.

78 Zhao, M., et al., *Relationship between loneliness and frailty among older adults in nursing homes: The mediating role of activity engagement.* Journal of the American Medical Directors Association, 2019. 20(6): p. 759–764.

79 Muse, E.D., et al., *Towards a smart medical home.* Lancet, 2017. **389**(10067): p. 358.

80 Bilyea, A., et al., *Robotic assistants in personal care: A scoping review.* Medical Engineering & Physics, 2017. **49**: p. 1–6.

81 Ritchie, C., and Leff, B., *Home-based care reimagined: A full-fledged health care delivery ecosystem without walls.* Health Affairs (Millwood), 2022. **41**(5): p. 689–695.

82 Knight, T., and Lasserson, D., *Hospital at home for acute medical illness: The 21st century acute medical unit for a changing population.* Journal of Internal Medicine, 2022. **291**(4): p. 438–457.

83 Qiu, S., et al., *Body sensor network-based robust gait analysis: Toward clinical and at home use.* IEEE Sensors Journal, 2019. **19**(19): p. 8393–8401.

84 Cheng, W., et al., *An introduction to smart home ward-based hospital-at-home care in China.* Journal of Medical Internet Research mHealth and uHealth, 2024. **12**: p. e44422.

85 Koumpouros, Y., et al., *PYTHEIA: A scale for assessing rehabilitation and assistive robotics.* International Journal of Medical, Health, Biomedical, Bioengineering and Pharmaceutical Engineering, 2016. **10**: p. 522–526.

86 Johnston, C., *Ethical design and use of robotic care of the elderly.* Journal of Bioethical Inquiry, 2022. **19**(1): p. 11–14.

87 Moyle, W., *The promise of technology in the future of dementia care.* Nature Reviews Neurology, 2019. **15**(6): p. 353–359.

88 Sharkey, A., and Sharkey, N., *Granny and the robots: Ethical issues in robot care for the elderly.* Ethics and Information Technology, 2012. **14**(1): p. 27–40.

89 Oña, E.D., et al., *Robotics in health care: Perspectives of robot-aided interventions in clinical practice for rehabilitation of upper limbs.* Applied Sciences, 2019. **9**(13): p. 2586.

90 Raigoso, D., et al., *A survey on socially assistive robotics: Clinicians' and patients' perception of a social robot within gait rehabilitation therapies.* Brain Sciences, 2021. **11**(6) :p. 738. doi: 10.3390/brainsci11060738.

91 Houses of Parliament, Parliamentary Office of Science and Technology. 2018. Robotics in social care. POSTNOTE 591(December): 1–7. https://researchbriefings.files.parliament.uk/documents/POST-PN-0591/POST-PN-0591.pdf

92 MacNeil, M., et al., *A scoping review of the use of intelligent assistive technologies in rehabilitation practice with older adults.* Disability and Rehabilitation: Assistive Technology, 2024. **19**(5): p. 1817–1848. doi: 10.1080/17483107.2023.2239277.

93 Durandau, G., et al., *Voluntary control of wearable robotic exoskeletons by patients with paresis via neuromechanical modeling.* Journal of Neuroengineering and Rehabilitation, 2019. **16**(1): p. 91.

94 Brundage, M., et al., *The malicious use of artificial intelligence: Forecasting, prevention, and mitigation.* 2018. ArXiv./abs/1802.07228.

95 Veneman, J.F., et al., *Design and evaluation of the LOPES exoskeleton robot for interactive gait rehabilitation.* IEEE Transactions on Neural Systems and Rehabilitation Engineering, 2007. **15**(3): p. 379–386.

96 Vicentini, F., et al., *SafeNet: A methodology for integrating general-purpose unsafe devices in safe-robot rehabilitation systems.* Computer Methods and Programs in Biomedicine, 2014. **116**(2): p. 156–168.

97 Veneman, J.F., et al., *Design and evaluation of the LOPES exoskeleton robot for interactive gait rehabilitation.* IEEE Transactions on Neural Systems and Rehabilitation Engineering, 2007. **15**(3): p. 379–386.

98 Rossa, C., et al., *Robotic rehabilitation and assistance for individuals with movement disorders based on a kinematic model of the upper limb.* IEEE Transactions on Medical Robotics and Bionics, 2021. **3**(1): p.190–203. doi: 10.1109/TMRB.2021.3050512.

99 Hattink, B., et al., *The electronic, personalizable Rosetta system for dementia care: Exploring the user-friendliness, usefulness and impact.* Disability and Rehabilitation. Assistive Technology, 2014. **11**: p. 1–11.

100 Menon, A., et al., *Strategies for rehabilitation professionals to move evidence-based knowledge into practice: A systematic review.* Journal of Rehabilitation Medicine, 2009. **41**(13): p. 1024–1032.

101 Etingen, B., et al., *Patient perceptions of environmental control units: Experiences of veterans with spinal cord injuries and disorders receiving inpatient VA healthcare.* Disability and Rehabilitation: Assistive Technology, 2018. **13**(4): p. 325–332.

102 Venkatesh, V., Thong, J., and Xu, X., *Consumer acceptance and use of information technology: Extending the unified theory of acceptance and use of technology.* MIS Quarterly, 2012. **36**: p. 157–178.

7

SURGICAL ROBOTS FOR MINIMALLY INVASIVE SURGERY

Li Liu and Yizhao Qian

7.1 Introduction

7.1.1 Minimally invasive surgery robots and their advantages

Surgical procedures have transitioned from traditional open surgery to minimally invasive surgery (MIS). Given the decreased risks and additional advantages associated with MIS, the medical community has increasingly embraced this approach. MIS involves performing procedures through small incisions or even without incisions, aiming to minimize tissue trauma. The advantages of this surgical approach include reduced pain, shorter recovery times, and decreased risks of complications [1]. For example, patients undergoing laparoscopic cholecystectomy through MIS typically discharge within 24–48 hours post-operation, whereas traditional open surgery may require a week of hospitalization.

However, MIS also presents new challenges, such as limited operational space and restricted visibility. This is where minimally invasive surgical robots come into play [2, 3]. Minimally invasive surgical robots can provide a three-dimensional perspective, precise surgical maneuvers, and eliminate tremors in the surgeon's hands, thereby enhancing the accuracy and safety of the procedure [4, 5]. For instance, the da Vinci Surgical System is a widely used minimally invasive surgical robot. Since its FDA approval in 2000, over 5114 systems have been installed and deployed globally, performing millions of surgeries worldwide [6, 7]. In summary, minimally invasive surgical robots offer powerful tools for surgeons to better execute these complex procedures. Thus, the significance of minimally invasive surgical robots in modern healthcare is self-evident.

DOI: 10.1201/9781003481959-7

7.1.2 The evolution of surgical robots

The concept of minimally invasive diagnosis and treatment can be traced back to the orthodox methods of the 1600s [8], involving entry into internal organs through large openings to enhance the safe operation of specific instruments and visualize procedures. Research on minimally invasive diagnosis and treatment and its assistance can be traced back to the 1970s, when traditional methods of medical intervention, such as open surgery, began to be gradually phased out [9, 10]. Subsequently, MIS experienced a period of clinical evaluation and technological advancement in the 1970s and 1980s, followed by vigorous development and establishment in most surgical disciplines. This is considered the foundation of the development of minimally invasive surgical robots.

Over time, patients and surgeons increasingly prefer laparoscopic surgery over traditional open surgery. In addition to reducing postoperative morbidity and improving cosmetic outcomes, the advantages of MIS became the driving force for robot-assisted surgery in the 1980s when the Arthrobot [11] was used for surgeries such as prostatectomy and heart valve repair. A major motivation for robot-assisted MIS interventions was to overcome the limitations of traditional MIS methods and enhance surgeons' capabilities during surgery. Therefore, the concept of minimally invasive flexible surgery (MIFS) was designed to involve procedures of proximal winding surgery devices connected to laparoscopes for human surgical diagnosis and treatment.

In recent years, many innovations in robot-assisted minimally invasive surgery (RAMIS) have emerged, including the da Vinci Surgical System (Figure 7.1) (Intuitive Surgical Inc., Sunnyvale, CA, USA), the Senhance

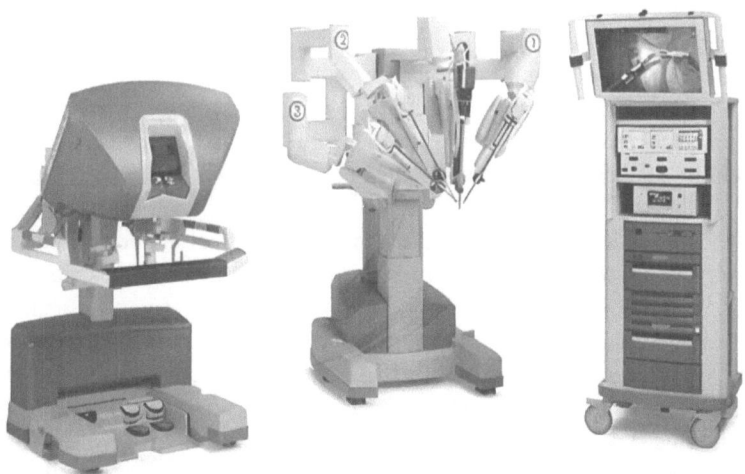

FIGURE 7.1 The da Vinci Surgical Robot, comprising the main console, slave manipulators, and monitors.

Surgical System (Asensus Surgical US, Inc.), the Versius Surgical Robot System (Cambridge Medical Robotics, Cambridge, UK), or the Hugo Surgical System (Medtronic, Minneapolis, MN, USA). The emergence of a large number of minimally invasive surgical robots has enabled the realization of robotic minimally invasive techniques and further changed the operational mode of clinical surgery.

7.2 Characteristics and types of minimally invasive surgical robots

7.2.1 Characteristics and evaluation metrics of minimally invasive surgical robots

In recent years, the continual emergence of minimally invasive surgical robot systems has revolutionized the field of medical technology. The development of these systems aims to strengthen minimally invasive interventions in the body's confined areas, navigating through single-port access routes such as natural orifice or minimal incisions, and intracavity interventions. Compared to traditional surgical methods, minimally invasive surgical robots offer unprecedented technological advantages in terms of higher precision, spatial flexibility, dexterity, and autonomous surgical capabilities. Traditional surgeries often require larger or multiple incisions to access the surgical site, which increases patient pain and recovery time. However, the introduction of minimally invasive surgical robots has made minimally invasive flexible pathways a faster, safer, and more convenient method of intracorporeal intervention, without the need for multiple or wide incisions, reducing patient pain and shortening recovery time. The distinctive attributes of minimally invasive surgical robots are evident in their range of motion, spatial controllability, surgical precision, and level of autonomy. In the following sections, we will provide a detailed exploration of the evaluation metrics for minimally invasive surgical robots from the following four perspectives, while also examining the impact of these characteristics on both the medical industry and patients.

1 Range of Motion of Minimally Invasive Surgical Robots: Traditional robotic arms often face joint limitations that restrict their access during MIS. In contrast, flexible surgical robots prioritize expanding the range of motion. These robots utilize serial chains with closely spaced actuators, enhancing motion flexibility. Their interconnected joints allow for minimal deviation and extension, accommodating acute to blunt angles. While this design sacrifices modular drive, the cumulative effect of each joint significantly improves the robot's posture. With an extended reachable space and agile spatial range, minimally invasive surgical robots can explore more features and perform additional procedures during surgery.

2 Spatial Controllability of Minimally Invasive Surgical Robots: Unlike traditional surgeries constrained by limited operating space, minimally invasive surgical robots excel in precise three-dimensional movements. They accurately control the position and orientation of surgical instruments. Single-port procedures necessitate unique linking modules that enable spatial movement. These modules smoothly traverse curved paths and operate along distinct motion axes. Modular structures, tailored for single-port intracavity surgery, are essential for achieving spatial flexibility and stable navigation in minimally invasive surgical robots.

3 Surgical Precision of Minimally Invasive Surgical Robots: Precision is paramount for safety and reliability in robotic surgery. Flexible robots designed for MIS prioritize surgical precision. This index quantifies and analyzes the stability of flexible poses in additional surgical tool mechanisms—whether static or moving along anatomical paths. Objective analysis considers robot navigation and dynamic stability during minimally invasive procedures. Precise robotic operations maximize patient safety and physical well-being.

4 Autonomy of Minimally Invasive Surgical Robots: Through pre-set programs and intelligent algorithms, robot arms autonomously adjust posture and force, adapting to diverse surgical contexts. This autonomy allows surgeons to focus on critical steps without excessive attention to instrument control, thereby enhancing surgical efficiency and safety. The significance of autonomy lies in improving surgical outcomes, reducing risks, maintaining consistency, expanding applications, and alleviating the burden on surgical teams.

7.2.2 Typical minimally invasive surgical robots

As of today, robotic technology has been widely utilized in clinical medicine, with an increasing number of mature commercialized minimally invasive robotic systems emerging. These intelligent robots play a crucial role in surgical procedures, assisting surgeons in completing complex operations while minimizing patient trauma and recovery time. In this section, we will focus on five leading minimally invasive surgical robot systems.

First, the da Vinci® Robotic Surgical System (DVRSS), one of the most renowned and commonly used minimally invasive surgical systems worldwide, was developed by Intuitive Surgical in the United States in 1995 (Figure 7.2). Even today, DVRSS remains one of the top choices for such surgeries, benefiting over 10 million patients globally. The system comprises three main components: the surgeon's console, a component consisting of four robotic arms (patient cart), and a vision cart (including the console display, recording devices, etc.). DVRSS represents a master-slave remote operation architecture. Surgeons remotely operate the robotic arms from the surgeon's console using two master arms. Currently, DVRSS is widely applied in various fields such as general surgery, urology, cardiovascular surgery, thoracic surgery, gynecology, otolaryngology, pediatric surgery, etc., making it the most widely used minimally invasive surgical robot system.

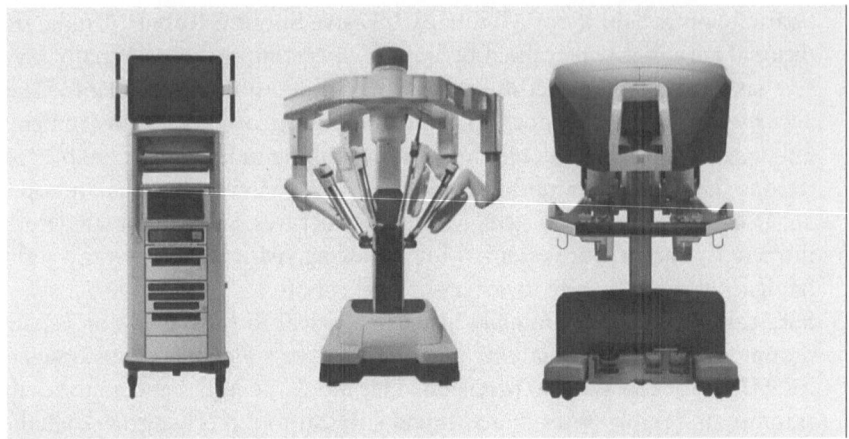

FIGURE 7.2 da Vinci Surgical Robot System.

The emerging "Symani® Surgical System" (Medical Microinstruments, Pisa, Italy) is considered at the forefront of surgical robotics, adopting similar pioneering robotic technology aimed at addressing the scale and complexity issues of microsurgery and ultra-microsurgery (Figure 7.3). Symani is a flexible minimally

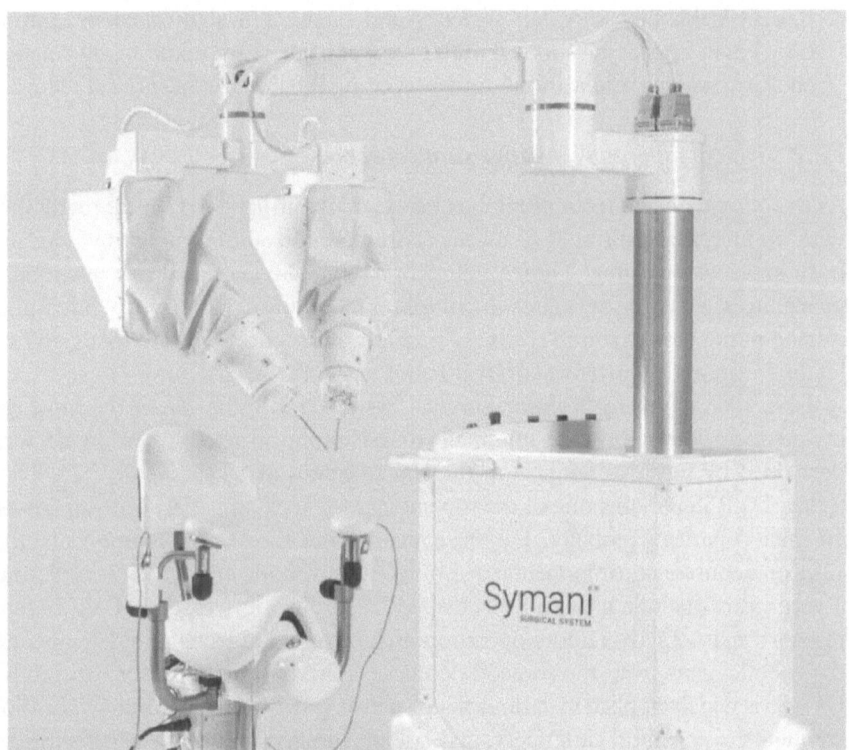

FIGURE 7.3 Symani Surgical Robot System.

invasive surgical robot system composed of two robotic arms capable of performing surgery in any anatomical area. Key features of Symani include micro-wrist instruments, console control, and motion scaling and tremor filtering functions. These features make it suitable for patients requiring soft tissue open surgery, including free flap reconstruction, lymphatic surgery, trauma reconstruction, and peripheral nerve repair surgery. Symani provides better treatment options for patients requiring soft tissue open surgery. Since completing its first human case in October 2020, the system has been used in over 500 surgeries.

The Senhance Surgical Robotic System is a robot-assisted surgical platform featuring 3D high-definition views and three independent remote-controlled robotic arms. The system also integrates tactile force feedback, allowing surgeons to feel tissue stiffness. Additionally, the platform offers advanced camera control with eye-gaze camera control. This feature simplifies camera control for surgeons through eye movements and forward/backward head movements for zooming. The manufacturer conducted two clinical studies. One study involved 150 patients undergoing various gynecological surgeries, and the other involved 45 patients undergoing colorectal surgeries. Senhance has been approved for routine laparoscopic surgery, minimally invasive gynecological surgery, colorectal surgery, cholecystectomy, and inguinal hernia repair surgery (Figure 7.4).

The Hugo RAS System (Medtronic, Minneapolis, USA) was developed as a modular robotic platform featuring four independent arm carts, capable of adjusting surgical strategies for highly customized surgeries. Hugo's introduction aims to provide an alternative robotic platform offering a more ergonomic and personalized working environment. Its significant technological

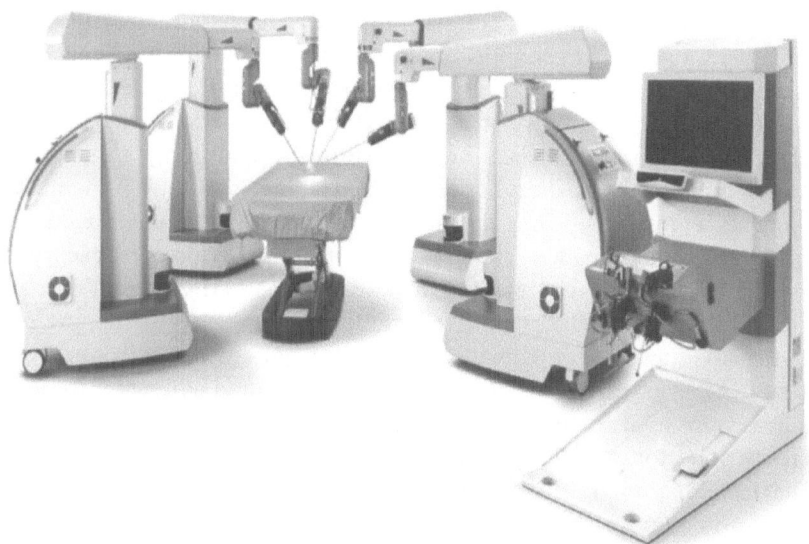

FIGURE 7.4 Senhance Surgical Robot System.

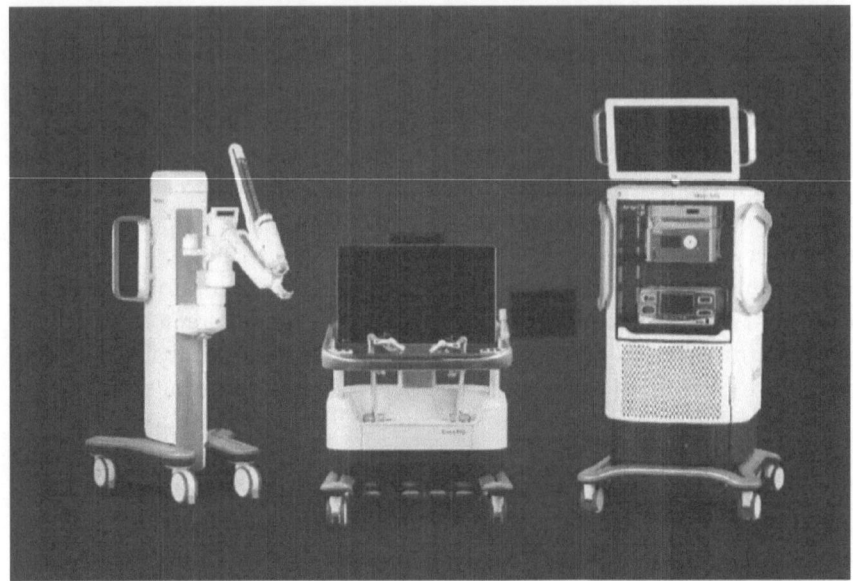

FIGURE 7.5 Hugo RAS Surgical Robotic System.

advantages include more ergonomic trocar positions, a larger workspace for bedside assistants, and cost-effectiveness of individual procedures. It consists of a console, a system tower, and four independent robotic arm carts. The system aims to enable surgeons to perform complex surgeries with higher precision and controllability while reducing patient trauma, pain, and recovery time and providing several key functionalities. Currently, the main application areas of the Hugo RAS system are general surgery, such as cholecystectomy, inguinal hernia repair surgery, low anterior resection, and gastric bypass surgery, as well as urological surgeries such as prostatectomy (Figure 7.5).

The CMR Versius is a robotic system for next-generation general MIS developed by Cambridge Medical Robotics company, consisting of a surgeon's console, modular lightweight robotic arms, and a range of wristed 5-millimeter instruments (Figure 7.6). The system utilizes state-of-the-art 3D high-definition images, significantly enhancing flexibility, and incorporates force feedback, providing surgeons with lifelike sensitivity. In January 2022, CMR Surgical's Versius Surgical Robot System was approved for thoracic surgery to support surgeons in providing MIS for patients undergoing lung, thymus, and esophageal surgeries. After gradually introducing specific cases and surgical selections, Versius is now used for both major and minor cases, including esophageal myotomy, lobectomy, and thymectomy.

The YuanHua Intelligent Orthopedic Surgical Robot System is one of the world's leading products in its field (Figure 7.7). It consists of arm carts, navigation carts, and main control console carts. This system achieves synergy

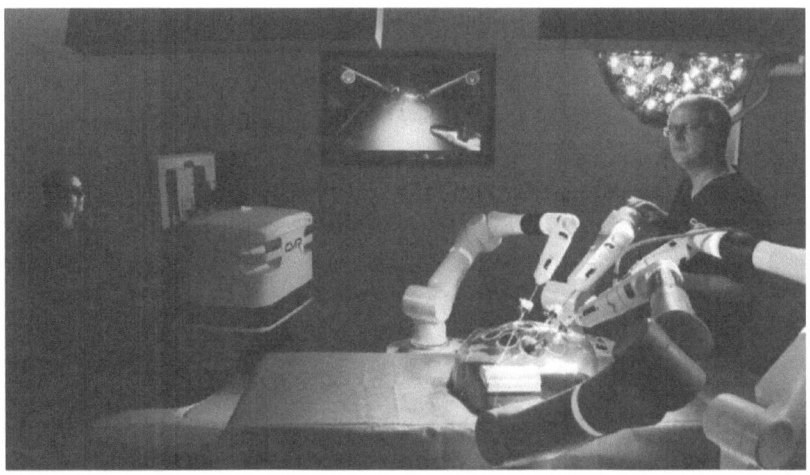

FIGURE 7.6   CMR Versius Surgical Robotic System.

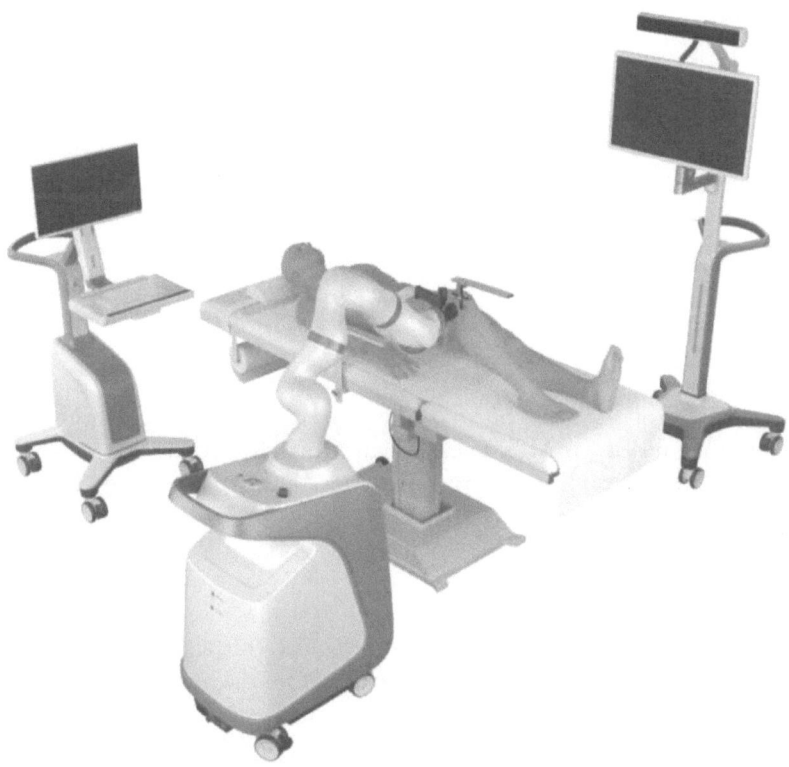

FIGURE 7.7   YH Orthopedic Surgical Robot System.

between "hands, eyes, and brain," allowing surgeons to perform intelligent, digital, and information-based surgeries through the robot's automatic CT modeling, precise measurement, and assisted implementation functions. The YH Orthopedic Surgical Robot System has independently developed navigation solutions and software systems. During the surgical process, there is no need for osteotomy plates (or similar tools) for assistance, and no need to use bone screws to fix the surgical site on the patient's legs. The robotic arms assist the surgeon throughout the precise osteotomy operation in an intelligent and interactive manner.

7.3 The working principle of minimally invasive surgical robots

As a revolutionary technology, the working principle of minimally invasive surgical robots determines their performance. These robots not only assist surgeons in performing complex operations but also minimize patient trauma and reduce recovery time to the maximum extent possible. In this chapter, we will delve into the working principle of minimally invasive surgical robots from four aspects: mechanical systems, motion mechanisms, control methods, and sensor systems.

7.3.1 Mechanical systems of robots

The mechanical system of minimally invasive surgical robots is one of its core components. These mechanical structures are designed to mimic the movements of a surgeon's hands and possess sufficient flexibility to adapt to different surgical environments. An excellent mechanical system enables surgical robots to achieve higher surgical precision, spatial controllability, and greater range of motion, allowing them to maneuver in more complex conditions and confined spaces. To achieve this purpose, researchers have proposed several different structures for robotic surgical systems, among which flexible robots based on snake-like, continuum, and soft mechanisms have been proposed for MIS. Each design provides reconfigurable capabilities, enhancing the ability of surgeons to access organs that are difficult to reach in traditional surgery.

7.3.1.1 Snake-like mechanisms

The application of flexible access robots requires mechanisms designed to reach deeper tissues and core hidden organs within the human body. The design mechanism of snake-like robots typically consists of three or more rigid segments connected by single or multiple joints for multi-degree-of-freedom (DoF) actuation. The bio-inspired snake-like robot developed by Owen et al. [12] remains one of the earliest qualitative design mechanisms. Additionally, early work by Chirikjian and Burdick [13] proposed flexible robots with snake-like mechanisms. While many research groups have developed flexible robots based on snake-like mechanisms, they have mainly been applied in monitoring and industrial inspection. However, recent research has paved the way for medical applications, particularly in MIS. Kim et al. [14] proposed a preliminary design of a direct-drive snake-like robot, while Li and Du [15] presented a design and analysis of a biomimetic multi-section flexible robot for MIS. Surgical robot systems with unique design mechanisms can be used for interventions such as diagnostic imaging, radiological surgery, or surgical repair of bodily target organs or tissues. Although achieving minimally invasive access to hidden locations imposes unique constraints on the design of such robots, many ingenious snake-like robot mechanisms have been developed to meet these constraints. Typically, snake-like surgical robots can be controlled using discrete micro-motor drives and/or tendon or cable drives at each joint.

7.3.1.2 Continuum mechanisms

The mechanisms provided by continuum robot designs offer some advantages over snake-like rigid link robots due to their compliant structures. Robots designed with continuum mechanisms can navigate and operate in hidden, confined, or complex spaces while conforming to curved paths in the operating area. Compared to snake-like mechanisms, continuum-based robots consist of tendons or cable/pulley devices controlled at one end by external actuators such as micro-motors or shape memory alloy (SMA). A common example is continuum robots constructed from a series of concentric tubes. This mechanism is driven by cumulative transmission of control signals from a fixed end. Continuum robots have demonstrated potential applications in cardiac arrhythmia ablation. Ota et al. [16] developed a robot probe for epicardial surgery. Flexible robots built on continuum mechanisms may suffer from redundancy and underactuation, as this structure typically offers more DoF with almost no direct drive. Additionally, completely passive structures exist, relying on the elasticity of the robot for actuation [17]. In the context of MIS, manufacturing quality, miniaturization, and the development of new actuators and functional materials are key driving factors. When creating robotic devices for MIS, connecting soft robots with appropriate user interfaces is another challenge that needs careful consideration, as surgeons need to maintain feedback loops.

7.3.1.3 Soft mechanisms

In the past two decades, interest in a new type of robot—soft robots—has surged. These novel robot structures have emerged from robot laboratories worldwide due to the demand for devices that can operate in unstructured and dynamic environments, as well as new developments associated with potential materials. Researchers have proposed a range of mechanisms to drive these structures, including fluids [18], dielectrics, SMAs, and tendons. Although soft robots have outstanding adaptability to the environment, their nearly infinite DoF enables them to bypass obstacles and can be relatively safely used within a patient's body, but it is well-known that soft robots are difficult to model, thus making navigation in a given environment challenging.

7.3.2 Motion mechanisms of robots

With the latest advancements in imaging and electromechanical integration, various simple yet efficient driving methods for minimally invasive surgical robots have been proposed. For example, motor-driven snake-like structures allow mechanical arms to achieve single-port access and navigation along complex and curved anatomical paths. The driving strategies of flexible surgical robots depend on the clinical applications they aim to achieve. Typically, driving strategies are characterized based on various factors such as the joint structure, kinematics, dynamics, and inverse driving performance of robot manipulators. A comprehensive review of existing systems has been observed from existing prototypes and considering these metrics and is discussed in this section.

7.3.2.1 Motor-driven driving

Micro-motor drive remains the most commonly used strategy in MIS robots; thus, it enhances the application of robots in single-port pathway surgery. Its feasibility for MIFS robots is related to the highly spatial deflection capability of the robot manipulator's unique part. This enhances flexible navigation along tortuous paths that can be modeled as internal pathways of the human body. Through this driving mechanism, the feasibility of safe and effective surgical procedures can be envisioned to achieve flexible pathway surgical interventions. The I2Snake is an early surgical robot utilizing a highly articulated snake-like design for flexible entry into robotic surgery [19, 20]. Additionally, Patel et al. [21] employed a flexible snake-like robot with a motion-driving strategy for intracavity gastrointestinal surgery. Most flexible robot devices feature manipulable modular designs with short rigid links connected to micro-motor or pulley-tendon strategies for driving. Salle and Morel [22] proposed an active flexible robotic tool for coronary artery bypass grafting surgery. The device has five DoFs driven by brushless motors. The modular design combines micro-motors with worm gear and gear transmission devices. The design enhances its agility with a $\pm 90°$ range of motion, but its intuitive internal motion is limited in terms of kinematics. Noonan et al. [23] also developed an extracorporeal 4-DoF robotic system for flexible probing. The mechanism has two universal joints and three yaw joints, with "twist-lock" interconnecting plates allowing it to maneuver flexibly in space. Later, it was integrated into a flexible surgical robot designed specifically for transvaginal peritoneal laparoscopy examinations [24].

7.3.2.2 Tendon-driven driving

Tendon-driven mechanisms, pioneered by Tanaka et al.'s biomechanical snake-like system [12], are another class of flexible surgical robots suitable for oral and anal surgery. One of the earliest flexible robots in this category was the highly articulated robotic probe (HARP) proposed in 2005 at Carnegie Mellon University for cardiac interventions [16]. The HARP's design mechanism consists of concentric tubes, cylindrical links connected by spherical joints, with each link capable of rotating $\pm15°$, thus providing the ability to twist in 3D with a curvature radius of 7.5 cm. It uses an external actuation source with six actuators and four cables to control the probe; thus, there is no electrical or heat generation inside the patient's body when inserted. While this is a major advantage of the robotic system, it limits the design's stiffness and curvature capability [25]. The HARP was later improved to Cardio-ARM [16] and MICS [26], which are highly articulated surgical robots for minimally invasive intrapericardial interventions. The CardioARM is more flexible, with over 100 DoF with continuous adjacent linkages, featuring $\pm10°$ relative rotational tricks. However, the design's curvature capability needs improvement for better maneuverability. In most cases, such flexible robot systems also use actuators located externally to the endoscope robot to manipulate its distal portion. Kato et al. [27] developed a tendon-driven continuum robot for neuroendoscopy examinations. The flexible robot has a miniaturized articulating channel with two skillful bending structures, each with one DoF. The tool channel has two sets of tendons, each set of three tendons extending away from the robot's center of mass and passing through holes in the wire guide. Li et al. [28] proposed a novel tendon- driven snake-like manipulator for spatially flexible and dexterous navigation during MIS. The snake-like design consists of short chain links and two adjacent vertebrae and a set of tendons. Agile manipulation of the tube is achieved through a minimum motion scheme based on stiffness control. Dupont et al. [29] demonstrated a combination of pre-bent elastic tubes as a design for a flexible robot system for MIS single-port access.

7.3.2.3 Cable and pulley-driven driving

In flexible surgical robots, a common alternative to motor-driven joints is the use of cable systems. These flexible robots are controlled by cables and/or wires; hence, they offer specific advantages such as remote driving, high flexibility, and lightweight design. The distal position and direction of steel wire robot systems are manipulated by manipulating cables or wires wound on pulleys and servo systems for flexible access surgery. The Phantom Omni (SensAble Technologies) is an electromechanical integrated device commonly used in medical robot research, which uses cable-driven transmission for various purposes such as remote and virtual operations during robot surgery and tactile interfaces [30]. To facilitate complex procedures with single-port access, Liang et al. [31] proposed an assumed compensation scheme for position control in surgical robots driven by cable pulleys. Similarly, Do et al. [32] proposed a new model of cable-driven and controlled snake manipulation during flexible robot surgery. In this driving strategy, the internal controller of the servo system can be adjusted to sense the power proportional to the control signal required for the robot's desired operation. Additionally, short-range navigation is achieved with minimal power, but lag remains a significant challenge [19, 33].

7.3.2.4   Other driving strategies

Many driving mechanisms have been proposed and applied to flexible surgical robots. The driving systems made using these strategies are unique and often differ from the systems mentioned above. Notable fluid and magnetic mechanisms explored in studies [34, 35], and [36] are worth mentioning. Similarly, hybrid driving mechanisms based on tendon-micro-motor strategies have been used for some MIFS robots [19, 24]. These strategies support flexible control of robot mechanisms with a large number of DoFs to reach all target points in high-dimensional space. The latest designs of snake-like and continuum-type flexible robots [37, 38] adopt hybrid driving strategies to improve spatial navigation and enhance tip force control.

7.3.3   Control systems of robots

7.3.3.1   Model-based control methods

As for model-based control methods, they mainly focus on snake-like robots and continuum robots. Researchers have provided physical models that characterize the characteristics of these robots, enabling the application of some traditional control methods. For snake-like robots, most research focuses on solving geometric approximations based on the DH method. For continuum robots, researchers have developed many different methods to describe the physical characteristics of the robot, each with its own characteristics. The most commonly used method is a physical model called the constant curvature model. This model assumes that the backbone of the continuum robot follows an approximately circular trajectory, allowing the control of the robot to be obtained by calculating its curvature [39–41]. In addition, finite element analysis has also been applied to the control of continuum robots. This model assumes that the robot is composed of several indivisible micro elements. By solving the interaction between each micro element, the final deformation shape of the robot is obtained. Additionally, researchers have proposed two special mechanical structures for describing continuum models, namely, the cosserat rod and cantilever beam model road. Currently, model-based control methods for continuum robots are still under development, and more and more related achievements are being proposed, making the operation and navigation of continuum robots in the body more precise.

7.3.3.2 Data-driven control methods

For traditional rigid-body robots, proposing a physical model, linearizing it, and calculating the Jacobian matrix are relatively straightforward tasks. Therefore, these methods have also been attempted for application to soft robots. However, due to the complexity of surgical robots, traditional methods are not still very effective.

Some researchers model robots using probability models. Probability models only consider the data of the robot as data in a probability distribution, without considering the physical properties of the robot. Regression methods are the most commonly used methods in soft robot modeling and control, such as linear regression, local weight regression (LWR), support vector regression (SVR), etc. In addition to regression methods, the Gaussian mixture model (GMM) is also a commonly used probability model. In addition, the Kalman filter integrates the results of modeling and measurement to better estimate the robot's state. Due to the nonlinearity of soft robots, the extended Kalman filter (EKF) is widely used in this field. Transition matrices, neural networks, and other models have been used as forward models of EKF, and the end position of the robot, force, and other state variables have been used as estimation quantities.

Neural networks are currently the most popular method in soft robot modeling and control. Due to the flexibility of soft robots, RNNs are very suitable for modeling and control tasks in this field. Bidirectional RNNs can handle spatial sequences of multiple robot segments. AE is used for feature extraction of robot images; CNN is used for image processing and for extracting temporal features of data matrices. In general, due to the nonlinearity of activation functions and complex network structures, neural networks are very suitable for use in soft robots. Due to the high demand of neural networks for data, they are often used as offline methods. There are various types of neural networks, and for most tasks, a suitable neural network solution can always be found.

7.3.3.2.1 Sensor systems of robots

The sensor system of a surgical robot is one of its core components, providing precise guidance for operations and real-time anatomical information to surgeons. First, cameras are one key sensor in this system. Placed at the end of the robot's tools, they offer high-definition images and zoom capabilities, allowing surgeons to clearly visualize details of the surgical area. These cameras can rotate 360 degrees and feature autofocus, ensuring surgeons have a clear view throughout the procedure.

Second, surgical guidance systems such as ultrasound are also vital components of the sensor system. Through technologies like ultrasound, surgical robots can acquire real-time structural information about internal tissues, aiding surgeons in precise localization and manipulation. This technology is particularly crucial in complex surgeries such as neurosurgery or minimally invasive procedures, helping surgeons avoid damage to surrounding tissues and improving surgical success rates.

In addition, magnetic control technology is widely used in the sensor systems of surgical robots. Magnetic sensors can perceive the position and movement of surgical instruments, allowing the robot to precisely follow the surgeon's maneuvers through magnetic field control, enabling highly flexible surgery. This technology is especially important in MIS requiring extreme precision, such as cardiac or ophthalmic surgeries, ensuring the accuracy and safety of surgical procedures.

Apart from these sensor systems, surgical robots are also equipped with various other sensors such as pressure sensors, temperature sensors, etc. These sensors provide comprehensive monitoring of the surgical environment and patient physiological parameters, helping surgeons promptly identify and address any potential risk factors. By leveraging these sensor systems, surgical robots can offer comprehensive surgical assistance to surgeons, enhancing the precision and safety of surgeries and improving treatment outcomes and patient experiences.

7.4 Clinical applications of minimally invasive surgical robots

In this section, we delve into the role of minimally invasive surgical robots in clinical applications. We will focus on two types of minimally invasive surgical robots: endoscopic surgical robots and intravascular surgical robots. Both types of robots have extensive applications in the medical field, not only enhancing the precision of surgeries but also significantly improving patients' recovery rates. Next, we will provide detailed insights into these two types of robots, including their working principles, key features, and specific applications in clinical settings.

7.4.1 Endoscopic surgical robots

The inception of MIS began with endoscopic surgical robots (Figure 7.8). MIS procedures involve precise surgeries on anatomical structures through small incisions or natural orifices. Continuum robots not only offer curved and flexible accessibility through these small incisions or orifices but are also capable of exerting considerable force at their distal end to support various operations [1, 4, 11, 42]. They are defined as manipulable structures whose constituent materials form curves with continuous tangent vectors [1], including concentric tube robots, actively cable/tendon-driven catheters, needles, single backbone, and multi-backbone continuum robots, as well as pneumatic and hydraulic-driven continuum robots. Their flexible structures exhibit high flexibility and precision, enabling them to reach target treatment sites. They can navigate complex morphologies and tortuous pathways within confined spaces to perform intricate surgeries through small incisions in the patient's body. These advantages facilitate reduced blood loss, minimal trauma, fewer postoperative complications, shorter recovery times for patients, and improvements in current clinical procedures, enabling new workflows [1, 4, 7].

In clinical practice, endoscopic minimally invasive surgical robots are increasingly and widely integrated into various MIS surgeries, including endoscopic mucosal biopsy via natural orifices, endoscopic procedures in the gastrointestinal tract, peroral endoscopic myotomy (POEM), endoscopic mucosal resection (EMR), endoscopic full-thickness resection (EFTR), endoscopic suturing, endoscopic submucosal dissection (ESD), renal transplantations, hepatic lobectomies, cholecystectomies/pancreatic/splenic resections, and other techniques. Overall, endoscopic surgical robots, as integral components of MIS, hold extensive prospects and value.

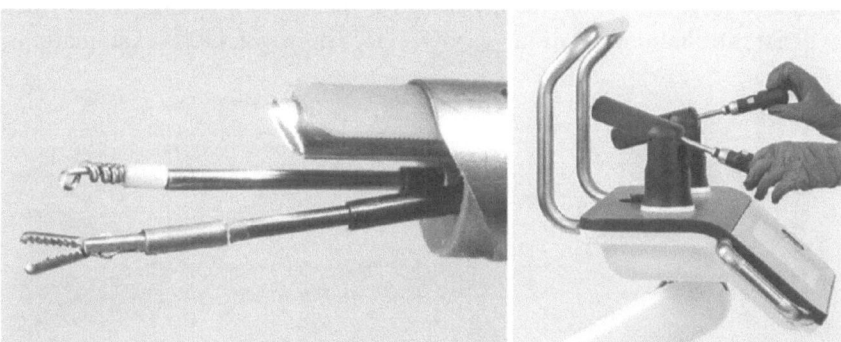

FIGURE 7.8 Endoscopic surgical robot.

7.4.2 Intravascular surgical robots

In recent years, cardiovascular diseases have been the leading causes of death and medical prescriptions. Robot-assisted endovascular surgery (RES) is an evolving therapeutic approach that, compared to open surgeries, alleviates patients' surgical pain and serves as a solution for MIS (Figure 7.9). Surgical robots have been incorporated into the field of intravascular surgery, providing a lower-risk alternative to open surgeries, assisting in disease localization, and expediting the planning of intravascular interventions. In robot-assisted procedures, serial link manipulators assist clinicians by manipulating cameras, lights, and medical instruments. Studies have shown that these surgeries, compared to traditional interventions, can reduce hospital stays, minimize incisions, and enhance accuracy. Take coronary stent placement as an example: first, physicians construct a three-dimensional model of the patient's vasculature based on preoperative and intraoperative imaging data and analyze features such as vascular bifurcations, bends, elasticity, and plaques. Then, the robot automatically constructs the intervention channel based on preoperative 3D information. During the surgery, contrast agents are injected to facilitate imaging for tracking catheters. Physicians distinguish the catheter from the arterial tree and precisely position it with reference to medical images, remotely operating interventional surgical instruments from the control room. While ensuring the continuous and stable execution of surgical actions, the robot can rapidly and accurately navigate complex trajectories to precisely reach the target vessels. Finally, vascular intervention surgery is completed under the physician's operation. The robot automatically and precisely delivers stents to occluded vessels, completing the treatment of two lesions. After the surgery, the robot conducts postoperative assessment and management. This process has been realized in clinical trials, where robotic manipulators can be remotely controlled with precision through operating devices such as handles and touch screens.

In clinical practice, intravascular surgical robots have been applied in various procedures, including coronary/carotid/renal/cerebral artery stenting, vascular interventional electrophysiological therapies or examinations (such as atrial fibrillation ablation, cardiac electrophysiological examinations,

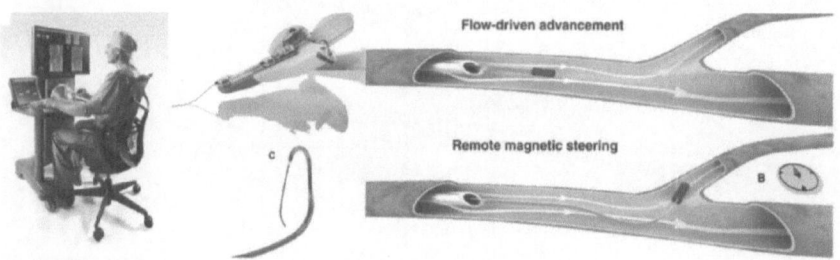

FIGURE 7.9   Endovascular surgical robot.

etc.), neurointerventional surgeries, and peripheral interventional surgeries, demonstrating extensive application value.

Apart from the aforementioned two types of surgical robots, there are other types of minimally invasive surgical robots in clinical practice, including orthopedic surgical robots, neurosurgical robots, and percutaneous puncture surgical robots, all of which share the common feature of minimizing patient harm while reducing the burden on physicians as much as possible. Meanwhile, an increasing number of minimally invasive surgical robots are being developed and utilized in diagnosis, treatment, care, and examination fields.

7.5 Challenges and future developments of minimally invasive surgical robots

Since the integration of RMIS into surgical procedures, it has continued to demonstrate progress. Sensors, computer vision, augmented reality, and other technologies have been utilized to compensate for the limitations of the RMIS experience, thereby creating safer and more efficient processes. The author believes that there are several trends in the future development of minimally invasive surgical robots.

7.5.1 Soft robotics

Over the past two decades, there has been a surge in interest in a new type of robot—soft robotics. Compared to traditional driving methods, soft robotics are attractive due to their high structural compliance and maneuverability. Due to the demand for devices that can operate in unstructured and dynamic environments, as well as new developments associated with potential materials, these novel robot structures have emerged from robotics labs around the world.

However, this field is still far from mature. Despite the exceptional adaptability of soft robots to the environment, their nearly infinite DoF enable them to maneuver around obstacles; they still face the following challenges: 1. Soft robots are difficult to model, making navigation in a given environment challenging. 2. Their performance is relatively poor when force needs to be applied to the environment, such as during tissue retraction in surgical procedures. Therefore, research on the insufficient precision and stiffness control of soft robots remains an important area that has not yet received sufficient attention.

7.5.2 Sensors

Robots operating in complex, unknown, and unstructured environments require sensors to understand their position in the environment and their physical interactions with it. Without sufficient perception capabilities, the navigational and positional accuracy of robots can be significantly compromised. Recent research has focused on developing sensor technologies that can be embedded within the structures of soft robots.

Currently, optical coherence tomography (OCT) has been widely used in minimally invasive robots. It offers real-time cross-sectional imaging of tissue microanatomy with micron-level resolution, providing further high-resolution three-dimensional and cross-sectional images. During actual procedures, OCT allows core biopsy needles to pass through the OCT imaging needle to reach the target area after identifying suspicious regions through structural imaging or quantifying the optical properties of tissues. However, the confined spaces constrain the practicality and robustness of OCT probes: 1. Miniature lenses are manually assembled within the needle, making it difficult to control the position of the lens relative to other miniature optical components. 2. Components such as fibers, lenses, and reflectors fail to provide sufficient mechanical strength, making it difficult to ensure robustness under high rigidity demands. To overcome these challenges, there is an urgent need for the design and development of new minimally invasive OCT imaging needles.

Photoacoustic sensors are considered one of the promising directions for the development of minimally invasive surgical robots. It is a hybrid technology combining the advantages of optical and ultrasound imaging. This imaging modality, with its optical contrast and excellent acoustic resolution, holds great potential for a wide range of clinical and preclinical applications. However, the intracavitary environment limits the further use of photoacoustic sensors: 1. The rotational imaging mode poses challenges in controlling bandwidth, making it difficult to achieve real-time control of endoscopes based on photoacoustic images. 2. Bending of optical components such as fibers limits the imaging capabilities of endoscopic photoacoustic probes. Nevertheless, photoacoustic imaging remains one of the research focuses in minimally invasive surgical robots.

Optical tactile sensors have become the preferred choice for RMIS due to their electrical passive nature and compatibility with MRI. Recent research has surpassed the limitations of optical tactile sensors, leading to the emergence of hybrid sensors. However, this new category of sensors aims to be more flexible for use in the operating room, such as working under static and dynamic forces, which is not possible with sensors based on electrical or optical principles. Machine learning and sensor fusion make hybrid sensor categories a more feasible area of research. However, the complex mechanical characteristics of minimally invasive surgical robots in confined environments make tactile sensors lack robustness. Overcoming the influence of external forces on optical tactile sensors is one of the current challenges in this field.

7.5.3 Computer vision and augmented reality

In today's medical technology domain, information technology has become a crucial innovative tool, reshaping our understanding and practice of surgery. Many breakthroughs and innovations in the field of information science have also been applied to surgical robots, driving not only the advancement of surgical robot technology but also opening up endless possibilities for future medical technology. Next, we will delve into the prospects of these areas in surgical robots in detail.

In the development of surgical robots, the application of computer vision technology has become an important trend. Computer vision can assist surgical robots in more accurately identifying and handling various situations during surgery, thereby enhancing the precision and efficiency of surgeries. Based on computer vision, surgical robots are allowed to carry out precise surgical planning. By scanning and analyzing the surgical area in detail, surgical robots can formulate precise surgical plans, thus avoiding unnecessary surgical risks. Furthermore, computer vision can also assist surgical robots in real-time surgical monitoring. By capturing and analyzing various information during the surgical process in real-time, surgical robots can adjust surgical strategies in a timely manner to address various issues that may arise during the surgery. Computer vision allows for surgical operations to be performed accurately. By precisely identifying and handling various situations during surgery, surgical robots can manipulate surgical instruments more accurately, thereby increasing the success rate of surgeries.

However, despite the vast prospects of computer vision in surgical robots, it also faces some challenges. For example, ensuring the accuracy and reliability of computer vision algorithms, handling large amounts of medical image data, and effectively integrating computer vision technology with other advanced technologies such as artificial intelligence and machine learning are all issues that require further research and resolution.

In modern medicine, surgeries are often performed through single-port natural or minimally invasive methods. The advantage of this surgical approach lies in its minimal trauma and quick recovery, but it also poses some challenges, with the most significant challenge being the limited information obtained from outside the surgical environment. To address this issue, researchers have begun to introduce augmented reality and virtual reality (AR/VR) technologies. This technology supplements information in the surgical environment by constructing artificial scenes and senses. This enables surgeons to perform surgeries in an artificial environment similar to what should be done in the patient's anatomical structures. This environment is an immersive but entirely artificial computer-simulated scene. In this scenario, surgeons and robots can interact in real-time, thus better controlling the surgical process.

In addition to surgical tasks, the introduction of virtual and augmented reality technologies significantly enhances the skills of surgeons, enabling them to better handle complex surgical procedures. For example, by simulating the surgical process in a virtual environment, doctors can anticipate problems that may arise during surgery in advance, thus being better prepared. Furthermore, virtual environments can also be used for teaching and learning. By transitioning the patient's anatomical structures into a virtual environment, doctors and students can better understand and appreciate structures in real space.

The application prospects of virtual reality (VR) and augmented reality (AR) technologies in the field of surgical robots are vast, but they also face some issues and obstacles in clinical applications. For surgeons who perform surgeries for several hours, current VR devices may have issues with comfort during prolonged use. Additionally, for remote surgeries, network latency is a significant concern. If surgeons are to perform remote surgeries, information needs to be displayed within approximately 70 milliseconds, requiring a reliable internet connection. Moreover, there is still a time gap between the movements and display of VR devices, and tracking is not accurate enough for surgical procedures. Furthermore, although VR and AR technologies have great potential, effectively integrating these technologies with other advanced technologies such as artificial intelligence and machine learning remains a challenge that requires further research and resolution.

7.5.4 Autonomy in surgical systems

Autonomy is one of the ultimate goals of minimally invasive surgical robots, and the industry categorizes the autonomy level of surgical robots from level 0 to level 5, representing increasing levels of autonomy (Figure 7.10). Level 0

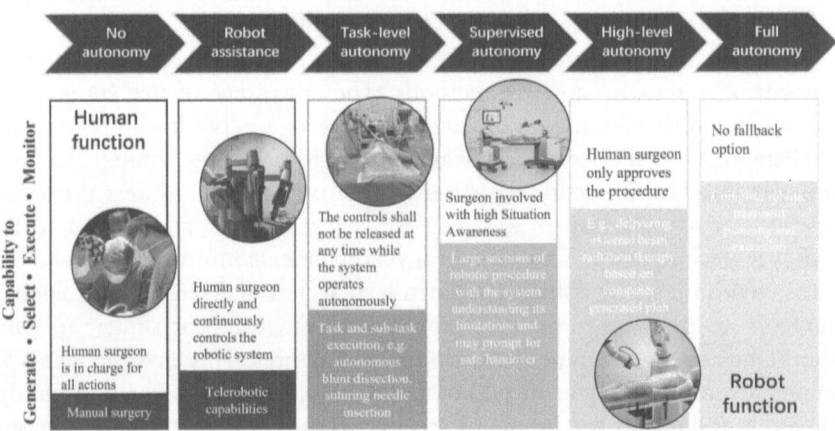

FIGURE 7.10 Autonomy in surgical systems.

signifies no autonomy, where the robot is fully controlled by a human operator, while level 5 represents full autonomy, where the robot can complete the entire surgery. These levels reflect possible directions for the future development of surgical robots.

In response to different autonomy requirements, flexible robot surgery typically adopts modular design and adds modules for specific functions based on the previous autonomy level to meet the requirements of the next level. Next, we will delve into the specific applications of these autonomy levels in surgical systems and their related technologies.

Level 0 autonomy refers to all system-level functions (generation, selection, execution, and monitoring of operations) being performed by human operators. Technically, this means that no active robot devices are used during the surgery, so it may be considered similar to non-robotic cases. Nevertheless, the robot still needs to have the capability to map from the surgeon's workspace to the task space within the body, thus possessing a certain level of control. Typical examples of Level 0 autonomy in minimally invasive surgical robots include controlled endoscopic examinations and coronary artery stent implantation procedures.

Level 1 autonomy, on the other hand, signifies that the robot operates without assistance, or with assistance only for specific low-level functions, such as remote operation systems, tremor filtering, or minor safety functions. Compared to the previous level, most Level 1 autonomy systems add positioning and recognition modules to monitor the current posture of the robot. A typical example is robot-assisted laparoscopic surgery, where systems like the handheld cooperative control system Micron provide active tremor compensation and image-guided aiming, e.g., in needle-based procedures, making it a Level 1 device.

Level 2 systems are trusted to autonomously complete certain tasks or subtasks, such as image-guided bone drilling or wound closure. This may only occur in a brief instance. These subtasks are directly provided by the operator, and compared to the previous level, most Level 2 autonomy systems add task planning modules to accomplish specific tasks. Various demonstrations of Level 2 types have been conducted using the open control platform created by Worcester Polytechnic Institute (WPI) and its partners. Through the Da Vinci Research Kit (DVRK), various Level 2 demonstrations have been performed: automatic suturing, anastomosis, injection, needle insertion, and many laparoscopic training tasks.

Level 3 systems can autonomously perform most of the surgical procedures while making low-level cognitive decisions. All operations are carried out under human supervision, assuming the operator has situational awareness. Compared to the previous level, this purpose requires Level 3 autonomy to add modules for autonomous decision-making to independently generate surgical processes, although this still requires experienced operators to implement supervision. The earliest typical system is ROBODOC, which already has autonomous image-to-robot registration, force-driven cutting feed, and virtual fixture-based safety functions. The robot can autonomously drill bones based on preoperative CT images.

Robotic systems at Levels 4 and 5 execute complete surgeries based on human-approved surgical plans. In Level 4, humans can only emergency stop (e-stop) surgeries. Even if humans fail to respond appropriately to intervention requests, the robot should be able to complete the task. In Level 5, the robot is deemed to succeed even in scenarios where even the most skilled human operators would fail, thus eliminating the need for human backup options. Compared to the previous level, Levels 4 and 5 autonomy adds modules for autonomous decision-making to independently generate surgical processes. Although there have been no Levels 4 and 5 robotic systems in the field of MIS, they have been applied in other simpler procedures. A typical application is Veebot, a recently developed autonomous blood collection robot that can find veins based on infrared camera images and then insert needles into veins using ultrasound. The robot has been proven to work well on a regular arm (finding the best vein for autonomous targeting 83% of the time). Since the entire workflow can be automated (given a simple program), Veebot can be considered at Level 4. Perhaps the most advanced autonomous functionality is integrated into the CyberKnife stereotactic radiosurgery system (Accuray Inc., Sunnyvale, CA, USA). It combines image guidance with robot positioning: a linear accelerator mounted on a KUKA KR 240 industrial robot arm. The primary deployment of CyberKnife is for the radiotherapy of brain and spinal tumors. X-ray cameras are used to track the patient's spatial displacement and compensate for any motion caused by breathing, etc. CyberKnife achieves highly autonomous operation, i.e., real-time image-guided radiation therapy, with only an emergency stop function available for human use once the treatment plan (designed by the system) is approved by humans (Level 4). If it is modified with additional computer supervision modules and an automated patient management environment, it could be classified as Level 5.

7.5.5 Training and techniques

Minimally invasive surgical robots have brought many benefits to the medical community and to those undergoing surgery, but challenges still exist in the implementation of minimally invasive procedures in certain cases. These challenges include technical difficulty, learning curves, lack of standardized training, and costs associated with different surgical procedures. Nonetheless, the advantages of robotic surgical platforms enable surgeons to perform more complex surgeries. However, many people lack access to robotic surgery assistance, especially in developing countries.

In developing countries like the Philippines, the number of hospitals offering robotic surgery is very limited, with St. Luke's Medical Center - BGC being one of the most renowned hospitals. Training for robotic surgery is key to addressing this challenge. Some surgical techniques using robotic surgery platforms, such as the TARUP technique, port placement, and autonomous camera navigation, have been introduced.

The TARUP technique is a surgery that assists in vertical incisional hernia repair using the da Vinci Xi platform, addressing issues that traditional surgery may struggle with. In MIS, proper port placement is crucial for the success of the surgery, which is also an important technique. Additionally, the introduction of autonomous camera navigation allows surgeons to have better visibility and tool control during the initial stages of training, optimizing the learning process.

7.6 Conclusion

Overall, training and application of minimally invasive surgical robots face multiple challenges. However, these challenges can be effectively overcome by introducing new surgical techniques and training methods, thereby improving the success rate and accessibility of MIS and providing safer and more effective medical services to a larger number of patients. In addition to the aforementioned points, researchers in this field also show interest in studying the ethical aspects of minimally invasive surgical robots. In general, minimally invasive surgical robots bring novel treatment modalities to the field of surgical robotics, advancing it toward autonomy, safety, and stability.

References

1 F. B. Chioson et al., "Recent advancements in robotic minimally invasive surgery: a review from the perspective of robotic surgery in the Philippines", 2020 IEEE 12th International Conference on Humanoid Nanotechnology Information Technology Communication and Control Environment and Management (HNICEM), pp. 1–7, 2020.
2 F. E. T. Munsayac et al., "Design and analysis of a robotic articulating laparoscopic instrument", 2020 IEEE 12th International Conference on Humanoid Nanotechnology Information Technology Communication and Control Environment and Management (HNICEM), pp. 1–5, 2020.
3 H. Takeishi, F. E. T. Munsayac, F. B. Chioson, R. G. Baldovino and N. T. Bugtai, "Design and force analysis of the robot end-effector of a semi-automated laparoscopic instrument using finite element analysis", 2018 IEEE 10th International Conference on Humanoid Nanotechnology Information Technology Communication and Control Environment and Management (HNICEM), pp. 1–4, 2018.
4 N. M. D. Espiritu, F. E. T. Munsayac, J. Reyes, L. J. A. F. Tan, R. G. Baldovino and N. T. Bugtai, "Design and testing of a robotic articulating laparoscopic instrument using the pig model simulation approach", 2020 IEEE 12th International Conference on Humanoid Nanotechnology Information Technology Communication and Control Environment and Management (HNICEM), pp. 1–5, 2020.

5 "St. Luke's unparalleled technology and expertise", October 2017, [online] Available: https://www.stlukes.com.ph.

6 H. Ashrafian, O. Clancy, V. Grover and A. Darzi, "The evolution of robotic surgery: Surgical and anaesthetic aspects", Brit. J. Anaesthesia, vol. 119, no. 1, pp. i72–i84, 2017.

7 B. Bardou, F. Nageotte, P. Zanne and M. Mathelin, "Design of a robotized flexible endoscope for natural orifice transluminal endoscopic surgery", in Computational Surgery and Dual Training, Berlin, Germany: Springer, pp. 155–170, 2009.

8 W. Tang and S. Hazen, "Atherosclerosis in 2016: Advances in new therapeutic targets for atherosclerosis", Nat. Rev. Cardiol., vol. 14, no. 2, pp. 71–72, 2017.

9 Z. Li, C. Yang and E. Burdet, "An overview of biomedical robotics and biomechatronics systems and applications", IEEE Trans. Syst. Man Cybern. Syst., vol. 46, no. 7, pp. 869–874, 2016.

10 R. Kneebone and A. Woods, "Recapturing the history of surgical practice through simulation-based re-enactment", Med. History, vol. 58, no. 1, pp. 106–121, 2014.

11 J. Dervaderics, "The beginnings of robotic surgery–from the roots up to the da Vinci telemanipulator system", Orvosi hetilap, vol. 148, no. 49, pp. 2307–2313, 2007.

12 T. Owen, "Biologically inspired robots: Snake-like locomotors and manipulators by Shigeo Hirose," Robotica, vol. 12, no. 3, p. 282, 1994.

13 G. S. Chirikjian and J. W. Burdick, "A modal approach to hyper-redundant manipulator kinematics", IEEE Trans. Robot. Autom., vol. 10, no. 3, pp. 343–354, 1994.

14 S. Kim, W. Xu and H. Ren, "Inverse kinematics with a geometrical approximation for multi-segment flexible curvilinear robots", Robotics, vol. 8, no. 48, pp. 1–14, 2019.

15 Z. Li and R. Du, "Design and implementation of a biomimetic wire-driven underactuated serpentine manipulator", Trans. Control Mech. Syst., vol. 1, no. 6, pp. 250–258, 2012.

16 T. Ota et al., "A highly articulated robotic surgical system for minimally invasive surgery", Ann. Thorac. Surg., vol. 87, no. 4, pp. 1253–1256, 2009.

17 M. Chikhaoui, S. Lilge, S. Kleinschmidt and J. Burgner-Kahrs, "Comparison of modeling approaches for a tendon actuated continuum robot with three extensible segments", IEEE Robot. Autom. Lett., vol. 4, no. 2, pp. 989–996, 2019.

18 M. Runciman, A. Darzi and G. P. Mylonas, "Soft robotics in minimally invasive surgery", Soft Robot, vol. 6, no. 4, pp. 423–443, 2019.

19 V. Vitiello, S. L. Lee, T. Cundy and G. Z. Yang, "Emerging robotic platforms for minimally invasive surgery", IEEE Rev. Biomed. Eng., vol. 6, pp. 111–126, 2013, [online] Available: https://ieeexplore.ieee.org/abstract/document/6392862.

20 P. Berthet-Rayne, K. Leibrandt, G. Gras, P. Fraisse, A. Crosnier and G.-Z. Yang, "Inverse kinematics control methods for redundant snakelike robot teleoperation during minimally invasive surgery", IEEE Robot. Autom. Lett., vol. 3, no. 3, pp. 2501–2508, 2018.

21 N. Patel, T. Cundy, A. W. Darzi, G. Z. Yang and J. Teare, "A novel flexible snake robot for endoluminal upper gastrointestinal surgery", Gastrointest. Endoscopy, vol. 79, no. 5, p. AB147, 2014.

22 D. Salle and G. Morel, "Optimal design of high dexterity modular MIS instrument for coronary artery bypass grafting", Proc. IEEE Int. Conf. Robot. Autom., pp. 1276–1281, 2004.

23 D. P. Noonan, V. Vitiello, J. Shang, C. J. Payne and G. Z. Yang, "A modular mechatronic joint design for a flexible access platform for MIS", Proc. Int. Conf. Intell. Robots Syst., pp. 949–954, 2011.

24 J. Shang et al., "An articulated universal joint based flexible access robot for minimally invasive surgery", Proc. IEEE Int. Conf. Robot. Autom., pp. 1147–1152, 2011.

25 A. Degani, H. Choset, A. Wolf, T. Ota and M. Zenati, "Percutaneous intrapericardial interventions using a highly articulated robotic probe", Proc. IEEE 1st Int. Conf. Biomed. Robot. Biomechatronics, pp. 7–12, 2006.

26 S. Thakkar et al., "A novel new robotic platform for natural orifice distal pancreatectomy", Surg. Innovat., vol. 22, no. 3, pp. 274–282, 2015.

27 T. Kato, I. Okumura, H. Kose, K. Takagi and N. Hata, "Tendon-driven continuum robot for neuroendoscopy: Validation of extended kinematic mapping for hysteresis operation", Int. J. Comput. Assist. Radiol. Surg., vol. 11, no. 4, pp. 589–602, 2016.

28 Z. Li, J. Feiling, H. Ren and H. Yu, "A novel tele-operated flexible robot targeted for minimally invasive robotic surgery", Engineering, vol. 1, no. 1, pp. 073–078, 2015.

29 E. Dupont, J. Lock, B. Itkowitz and E. Butler, "Design and control of concentric-tube robots", IEEE Trans. Robot., vol. 26, no. 2, pp. 209–225, 2010.

30 A. Mohammadi, M. Tavakoli and A. Jazayeri, "PHANSIM: A simulink toolkit for the sensable phantom haptic devices", Proc. 23rd Can. Congr. Appl. Mech. (CANCAM), pp. 787–790, 2011.

31 Y. Liang, Z. Du, W. Wang and L. Sun, "A novel position compensation scheme for cable-pulley mechanisms used in laparoscopic surgical robots", Sensors, vol. 17, no. 10, p. 2257, 2017.

32 T. Do, T. Tjahjowidodo, M. Lau and S. Phee, Performance control of tendon-driven endoscopic surgical robots with friction and hysteresis, 2017, [online] Available: http://arXiv:1702.02063.

33 J. M. Prendergast and M. E. Rentschler, "Towards autonomous motion control in minimally invasive robotic surgery", Expert Rev. Med. Devices, vol. 13, no. 8, pp. 741–748, 2016.

34 M. Cianchetti, C. Laschi, A. Menciassi and P. Dario, "Biomedical applications of soft robotics", Nat. Rev. Mater., vol. 3, pp. 143–153, 2018.

35 G. Gerboni, T. Ranzani, A. Diodato, G. Ciuti, M. Cianchetti and A. Menciassi, "Modular soft mechatronic manipulator for minimally invasive surgery (MIS): Overall architecture and development of a fully integrated soft module", Meccanica, vol. 50, no. 11, pp. 2865–2878, 2015.

36 C. Heunis, J. Sikorski and S. Misra, "Magnetic actuation of flexible surgical instruments for endovascular interventions", IEEE Robot. Autom. Mag., vol. 25, no. 3, pp. 71–82, 2018.

37 M. Loschak, Y. Tenzer, A. Degirmenci and R. D. Howe, "A 4-DoF robot for positioning ultrasound imaging catheters", Proc. ASME Int. Design Eng. Techn. Conf., p. 7, 2015.

38 O. M. Omisore, S. Han, L. Ren, N. Zhang and L. Wang, "A geometric solution for inverse kinematics of redundant teleoperated surgical snake robots", Proc. IEEE Int. Conf. Ind. Technol., pp. 710–714, 2017.

39 D. Camarillo, C. Carlson and J. Salisbury, Task-space control of continuum manipulators with coupled tendon drive. Experimental Robotics 2009: 271–280.

40 R. Penning, J. Jung, N. Ferrier and M. Zinn, "An evaluation of closed-loop control options for continuum manipulators", 2012 IEEE International Conference on Robotics and Automation, 2012., pp. 5392–5397.

41 A. Bajo and N. Simaan, "Hybrid motion/force control of multi-backbone continuum robots", Int. J. Robot. Res., vol. 35, pp. 422–434, 2015.

42 J. G. Fujimoto, "Optical coherence tomography for ultrahigh resolution in vivo imaging", Nat. Biotechnol., vol. 21, pp. 1361–1367, 2003.

8

AI-AIDED TOOLS FOR TEACHING AND RESEARCH IN MEDICAL RESEARCH

Charles Oretomiloye and Blessing Funmi Komolafe

8.1 Introduction

Teaching and research are focal points in the area of medical research. Both are crucial for driving innovation and advancing knowledge in the medical field. Effective teaching ensures that the next generation of scientists, clinicians, and medical practitioners are well-equipped with the theoretical, practical skills and artificial intelligence (AI)-aided tools necessary to tackle complex health challenges. This study builds a foundation for critical thinking, evidence-based practice, and ethical considerations in medicine.

Similarly, teaching within a research context has traditionally been defined as an intervention that leads to learning, with effective teaching methods resulting in improved, impactful learning outcomes and, ultimately, enhancing the quality of patient care (Arja et al., 2024). However, advancements in technology have given rise to various AI-aided teaching tools, such as hybrid teaching methods (Kokko et al., 2024) and fully online pedagogy during the COVID-19 pandemic (Komolafe et al., 2020).

Conversely, research plays a pivotal role in expanding the boundaries of medical science. It enables the discovery of new treatments, technologies, and methodologies that improve patient care and public health. By integrating teaching with research, medical education fosters a dynamic environment where students and professionals will not only acquire existing knowledge but also contribute to its growth and evolution.

Furthermore, medical research often involves interdisciplinary collaboration, drawing insights from fields such as biology, engineering, and data science. This collaboration reinforces the importance of educators staying at the forefront of their fields. The symbiotic relationship between teaching

DOI: 10.1201/9781003481959-8

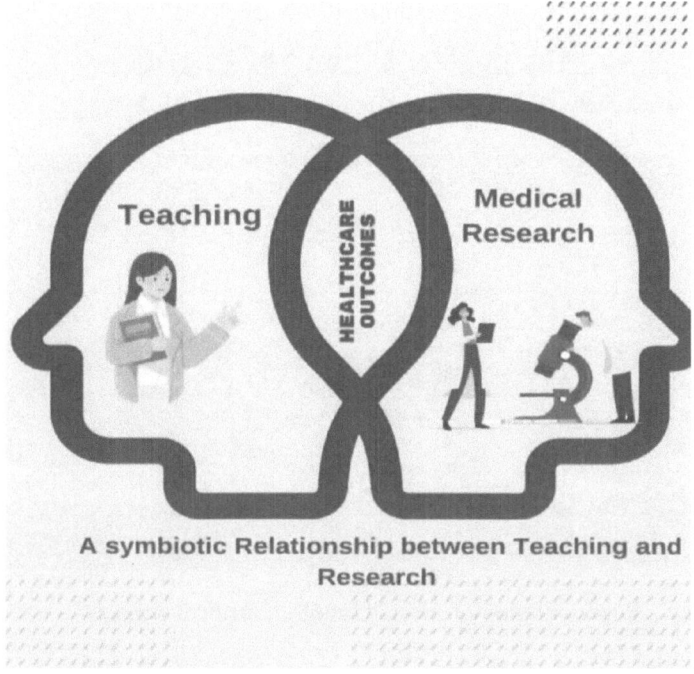

FIGURE 8.1 Schematic representation of the symbiotic relationship between teaching and research.

and research ensures continuous innovation and progress in medical science, ultimately leading to better healthcare outcomes, as illustrated in Figure 8.1.

Talaulikar et al. (2014) define medical research as focusing on understanding or treating diseases and health conditions, with the ultimate goal of improving human health and quality of life. To develop a more sustainable healthcare system, there has been a shift from traditional medical practices to more advanced healthcare management approaches, such as the use of AI-aided tools. Recent studies highlight various AI-aided tools in medical science, including "Machine Learning Algorithms for Real-Time Computing," "Edge AI Computing," and "AI Ecosystem Integration" (Li et al., 2024). Other examples include AI detection tools (Cooperman & Brandão, 2024), AI-based medical imaging technology, and cognitive perception models (Nirapai & Leelasantitham, 2024), as illustrated in Figure 8.2.

The advent of AI in research has ushered in a profound transformation across various sectors, with medicine experiencing one of the most significant shifts. This technological revolution has dramatically enhanced the accuracy and efficacy of diagnostic processes, therapeutic interventions, and medical education, marking a new era in medical practice and research.

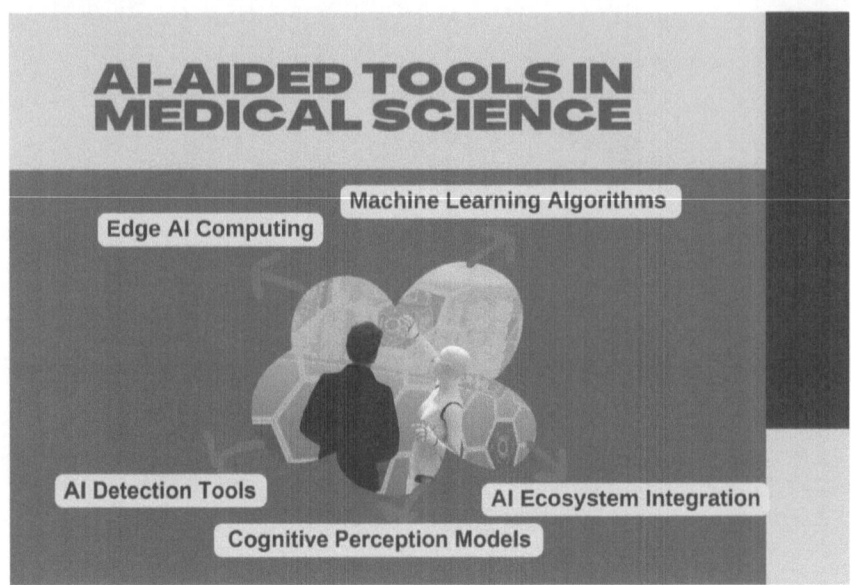

FIGURE 8.2 Representation of AI-aided tools in medical sciences.

AI has made substantial strides in improving the interpretation of diagnostic images and laboratory results. Esteva et al. (2019) report that AI models have achieved dermatologist-level accuracy in diagnosing skin cancer from images, showcasing AI's impressive capabilities in diagnostic imaging. This advancement significantly reduces the likelihood of human error, thereby enhancing diagnostic precision and improving patient survival rates. By minimizing the risk of misdiagnosis, AI ensures that patients receive the most appropriate treatment for their conditions, leading to better clinical outcomes.

In contrast to traditional treatment approaches, which often relied on generalized guidelines rather than individualized patient characteristics, AI has introduced a paradigm shift toward personalized medicine. Collins and Varmus (2015) highlight how AI enables the prediction of patient responses to various therapies through comprehensive data analysis. By evaluating a patient's genetic, environmental, and lifestyle factors, AI systems can recommend the most effective therapies tailored to individual needs. Chen et al. (2020) further elaborate on AI's role in predicting drug interactions and side effects, which helps ensure that medications are developed with minimized adverse effects, leading to faster and more effective recovery.

AI's predictive capabilities also extend to forecasting the likelihood of developing diseases such as cancer, heart disease, and diabetes. Dunn and Bailey (2022) discuss how AI models can anticipate these risks, enabling proactive treatment and preventive measures. This early identification of potential health issues allows for timely interventions, ultimately contributing to longer lifespans and improved health outcomes.

The traditional drug discovery process has long been labor-intensive, involving extensive trial and error and numerous laboratory and clinical trials that often span several years. AI has streamlined this process by analyzing large volumes of biological data to identify potential drug candidates more efficiently. AI models can also predict interactions between compounds and biological targets, significantly reducing the time and cost associated with drug development. This capability proved especially valuable during the COVID-19 pandemic, where AI facilitated rapid responses to the emerging health crisis (Chen et al., 2020).

In addition to clinical applications, AI is revolutionizing medical education and research. AI-driven simulations and virtual reality (VR) technologies are creating more immersive and interactive learning environments. Traditional educational methods, such as lectures and textbooks, have limitations in the scope and variability of training experiences. AI-powered platforms offer extensive practice scenarios and immediate feedback, enhancing the learning process. Sonntag, Roberts, and Anderson (2022) emphasize how VR and AI-driven simulations create realistic clinical scenarios, allowing students and professionals to gain practical experience in a controlled, risk-free setting.

AI has also made significant advancements in surgical training through virtual and augmented reality simulations. Tools like Touch Surgery provide detailed practice environments where medical students and professionals can refine their surgical skills without the risks associated with live surgeries. These AI-driven simulations help enhance procedural proficiency and prepare practitioners for real-world surgical challenges.

Moreover, AI's role in research is expanding through the use of natural language processing (NLP) to extract insights from vast amounts of medical literature. AI algorithms can analyze large volumes of text, identifying emerging research trends and generating hypotheses. This capability accelerates scientific discovery and contributes to the advancement of medical knowledge (Huang et al., 2021). Despite its numerous benefits, the integration of AI in medicine presents several challenges. These include concerns about data privacy, potential biases in AI algorithms, a lack of fundamental knowledge about AI principles, financial issues, resistance to change among practitioners who are not convinced of the benefits of AI, and a lack of standards for clinical evaluation and efficient decision-making in clinical diagnosis (Hah & Goldin, 2021; Stogiannos et al., 2024). Obermeyer et al. (2019) emphasize the importance of addressing these challenges to ensure the ethical use of AI.

8.2 AI-aided tools in teaching medical students

Effective factors for teaching processes in clinical medicine, as illustrated by Alweshahi and Cook (2009), include interaction/communication, appropriate pedagogy, specific objectives, coaching, and conclusion. For instance, a recent qualitative study conducted in Saudi Arabia on incorporating technology tools such as VR, AI, and telemedicine into medical education demonstrated significant potential in enriching learning experiences, advancing clinical skills, and broadening healthcare access (Alrashed et al., 2024). Additionally, AI-aided tools have shown improvements in students' performance and satisfaction, as well as in attitudes and perceptions (Sit et al., 2020; Wu et al., 2020). Studies have shown a shift from the traditional method of teaching, specifically cadaver-based instruction, which has remained the main instructional tool for hundreds of years. However, there is an ongoing debate about the most suitable methods for delivering anatomical knowledge, a debate that remains unresolved (Estai & Bunt, 2016). Figure 8.3 illustrates the transition from cadaver-based instruction to AI-assisted instruction for medical students. Studies supporting the use of AI-aided tools in medical education suggest several areas of application: teaching students to analyze large datasets, incorporating AI-driven simulators into anesthesia education curricula, using AI-generated insights, integrating adaptive learning platforms, adding machine learning algorithms and NLP to the curriculum, employing VR and augmented reality (AR) tools, utilizing intelligent

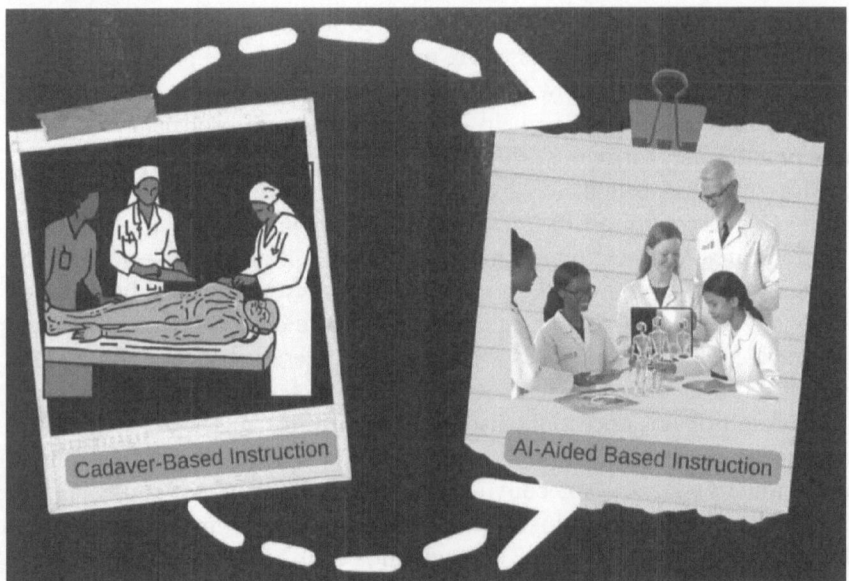

FIGURE 8.3 This is a schematic diagram showing the shift from cadaver-based instruction to AI-aided based instruction.

tutoring systems (ITS), applying deep learning models for medical imaging and diagnostics, and implementing AI-assisted clinical decision support systems (CDSS) (Chan & Zary, 2019; Davenport & Kalakota, 2019; Hinton & Sejnowski, 2019; Kurup & Herasevich, 2021; Topol, 2019; Wang, Casalino, & Khullar, 2020; Wartman & Combs, 2018; Zary & Alturkistani, 2020).

8.3 Discussion

The integration of AI-aided tools in medical sciences as shown in Figure 8.2 and research has undoubtedly transformed the landscape of medical practice and training. This study demonstrates how AI-driven tools not only enhance diagnostic accuracy and therapeutic interventions but also play a critical role in improving teaching methodologies. The adoption of AI tools such as machine learning algorithms, integrating adaptive learning platforms, VR, and NLP in medical training has expanded the capacity for students and practitioners to engage with more interactive and dynamic learning environments.

8.3.1 *Teaching and AI in medical education*

The role of AI in revolutionizing medical teaching is particularly significant. As highlighted in the literature, AI-powered simulations offer a risk-free environment for medical students to refine their skills and gain hands-on experience (see Figure 8.2). Platforms like Touch Surgery provide valuable opportunities for students to practice surgical procedures, improving their competency without compromising patient safety (Sonntag, Roberts, & Anderson, 2022). These AI-driven platforms are bridging the gap between theoretical knowledge and practical application, ensuring a more well-rounded medical education.

Additionally, the incorporation of AI tools like VR has been shown to enhance students' performance, satisfaction, and overall learning experience (Alrashed et al., 2024). The growing acceptance of these technologies indicates a shift in the perception of AI's role in education. However, resistance to change due to long time method of teaching "cadaver-based instruction" and the high cost of implementing such tools remain significant barriers to widespread adoption, particularly in regions with limited resources.

8.3.2 *Research and AI in medical innovation*

On the research front, AI is facilitating rapid advancements in drug discovery, disease prediction, and personalized medicine. By analyzing large datasets, AI can identify potential drug candidates more efficiently, reducing the time and cost associated with traditional drug development processes (Chen et al., 2020). This capability has been critical in addressing emergent health crises, such as the COVID-19 pandemic, where AI tools were used to accelerate vaccine and treatment development.

Despite these advancements, challenges related to data privacy, algorithmic bias, and the ethical use of AI in medical research persist (Obermeyer et al., 2019). Ensuring that AI systems are transparent, unbiased, and aligned with ethical standards is crucial for maintaining trust in these technologies. Moreover, the financial burden of integrating AI into research may limit access to these tools in underfunded institutions.

8.4 Challenges and future directions

Although AI has shown immense potential in both teaching and research, several challenges remain. These include concerns about data privacy, the lack of standardized clinical evaluation for AI tools, and general resistance to adopting new technologies. Additionally, AI's limitations in decision-making processes, particularly in clinical diagnosis, highlight the need for continuous improvement and regulation (Hah & Goldin, 2021; Stogiannos et al., 2024).

To address these challenges, future research should focus on developing more robust and transparent AI systems while ensuring that medical professionals are trained in the ethical and effective use of these tools. Regulatory frameworks must evolve to accommodate the growing influence of AI in healthcare, and educational institutions must invest in both the technology and training required to fully realize the benefits of AI-driven tools rather than compromise the quality of care.

8.5 Conclusion

The transformative power of AI in medical education and research cannot be overestimated. As this study has shown, AI-aided tools are reshaping the way medical students are trained and how research is conducted, leading to more efficient, personalized, and effective healthcare solutions. However, to fully harness the potential of AI, educators, researchers, and policymakers must work together to overcome the existing challenges, ensuring that AI's integration into the medical field is both equitable and ethical.

References

Alrashed, F. A., Ahmad, T., Almurdi, M. M., Alderaa, A. A., Alhammad, S. A., Serajuddin, M., & Alsubiheen, A. M. (2024). Incorporating technology adoption in medical education: A qualitative study of medical students' perspectives. Advances in Medical Education and Practice, 15, 615–625. doi: 10.2147/AMEP.S464555.

Alweshahi, Y., & Cook, D. (2009). Domains of effective teaching process: Students' perspectives in two medical schools. Medical Teacher, 31(4), e125–e130.

Arja, S. B., Arja, S. B., Ponnusamy, K., Kottath Veetil, P., Paramban, S., & Laungani, Y. C. (2024). Medical education electives can promote teaching and research interests among medical students. Advances in Medical Education and Practice, 15, 173–180. doi: 10.2147/AMEP.S453964.

Chan, K. S., & Zary, N. (2019). Applications and challenges of AI in medical education: Integrating artificial intelligence into medical training. Frontiers in Artificial Intelligence, 5(1), e13930.

Chen, J., et al. (2020). Artificial intelligence in drug discovery and development. Drug Discovery Today, 25(3), 682–691.

Collins, F. S., & Varmus, H. (2015). A new initiative on precision medicine. New England Journal of Medicine, 372(9), 793–795.

Cooperman, S. R., & Brandão, R. A. (2024). AI tools vs AI text: Detecting AI-generated writing in foot and ankle surgery. Foot & Ankle Surgery: Techniques, Reports & Cases, 4(1), 100367.

Davenport, T., & Kalakota, R. (2019). The potential for artificial intelligence in healthcare. Future Healthcare Journal, 6(2), 94–98.

Dunn, J., & Bailey, T. (2022). Predictive analytics in healthcare: A review. Healthcare Analytics Journal, 7(2), 45–58.

Estai, M., & Bunt, S. (2016). Best teaching practices in anatomy education: A critical review. Annals of Anatomy-Anatomischer Anzeiger, 208, 151–157.

Esteva, A., et al. (2019). Dermatologist-level classification of skin cancer with deep neural networks. Nature, 542(7639), 115–118.

Hah, H., & Goldin, D. S. (2021). How clinicians perceive artificial intelligence-assisted technologies in diagnostic decision making: Mixed methods approach. Journal of Medical Internet Research, 23(12), e33540.

Hinton, G., & Sejnowski, T. (2019). Artificial intelligence in healthcare education. Nature Medicine, 24(5), 581–586.

Huang, J., et al. (2021). Natural language processing for healthcare: A review. Journal of Biomedical Informatics, 117, 103788.

Kokko, M., Pramila-Savukoski, S., Ojala, J., Kuivila, H. M., Juntunen, J., Törmänen, T., & Mikkonen, K. (2024). The effect of educational intervention on hybrid teaching competence of health sciences and medical educators: A mixed methods study. Scandinavian Journal of Educational Research, 68(7), 1–16.

Komolafe, B. F., Fakayode, O. T., Osidipe, A., Zhang, F., & Qian, X. (2020). Evaluation of online pedagogy among higher education international students in China during the COVID-19 outbreak. Creative Education, 11(11), 2262.

Kurup, V., & Herasevich, V. (2021). Artificial intelligence and the future of anesthesia education. British Journal of Anaesthesia, 126(4), 569–572.

Li, Y., Nie, Y., Quan, Z., Zhang, H., Song, R., Feng, H., … & Wang, S. (2024). Brain-machine interactive neuromodulation research tool with edge AI computing. Heliyon, 10(12), e32609.

Nirapai, A., & Leelasantitham, A. (2024). A new adoption model for quality of experience assessed by radiologists using AI medical imaging technology. Journal of Open Innovation: Technology, Market, and Complexity, 10(3), 100369.

Obermeyer, Z., et al. (2019). Dissecting racial bias in an algorithm used to manage the health of populations. Science, 366(6464), 447–453.

Sit, C., Srinivasan, R., Amlani, A., Muthuswamy, K., Azam, A., Monzon, L., & Poon, D. S. (2020). Attitudes and perceptions of UK medical students towards artificial intelligence and radiology: A multicentre survey. Insights into Imaging, 11, 1–6.

Sonntag, G., Roberts, K., & Anderson, P. (2022). The role of virtual simulations in medical training. Journal of Medical Education and Curricular Development, 9, 238212052211054.

Stogiannos, N., Litosseliti, L., O'Regan, T., Scurr, E., Barnes, A., Kumar, A., ... & Malamateniou, C. (2024). Black box no more: A cross-sectional multi-disciplinary survey for exploring governance and guiding adoption of AI in medical imaging and radiotherapy in the UK. International Journal of Medical Informatics, 186, 105423.

Talaulikar, V. S., Hussain, S., Perera, A., & Manyonda, I. T. (2014). Low participation rates amongst Asian women: Implications for research in reproductive medicine. European Journal of Obstetrics & Gynecology and Reproductive Biology, 174, 1–4.

Topol, E. J. (2019). High-performance medicine: The convergence of human and artificial intelligence. Nature Medicine, 25(1), 44–56.

Wang, F., Casalino, L. P., & Khullar, D. (2020). Deep learning in medicine—Promise, progress, and challenges. JAMA, 324(22), 2352–2353.

Wartman, S. A., & Combs, C. D. (2018). Medical education must move from the information age to the age of artificial intelligence. Academic Medicine, 93(8), 1107–1109.

Wu, D., Xiang, Y., Wu, X., Yu, T., Huang, X., Zou, Y., ... & Lin, H. (2020). Artificial intelligence-tutoring problem-based learning in ophthalmology clerkship. Annals of Translational Medicine, 8(11).

Zary, N., & Alturkistani, A. (2020). The role of artificial intelligence in medical education: Current practices and future perspectives. International Journal of Medical Education, 11, 12–18.

9

DECODING NEURAL SIGNALS

Invasive BMI Review

Rezwan Firuzi, Ayub Bokani, Jahan Hassan,
Hamed Ahmadyani, Mohammad Foad Abdi,
Dana Naderi, and Diako Ebrahimi

9.1 Introduction

Over the centuries, our understanding of the human brain has increased significantly. Psychology and cognitive science are relatively new fields that have become involved in some of the most competitive research areas in contemporary times. Scientific approaches to treating, manipulating, and simulating human behavior have advanced by leaps and bounds in recent years. The complex and multiple functions of the brain such as perceptual interpretation, organ function regulation, and information processing capabilities have long been acknowledged by academia. Recent progress, especially in computer science and electrical engineering, allows the behavior of neurons to be easily captured, analyzed, and decoded. Such information can be used for creating real-world applications that can take our lives to a much higher level of comfort. From creating intelligent robot assistants for people with disabilities to efficiently curing brain damage or psychological disorders, invasive brain–machine interface (BMI) technology will play a vital role in human lives soon.

Since the introduction of electronic computers, the human brain has been increasingly seen as an organic carbon-based computer, rather than today's silicon-based electronic systems. This analogy has sparked a significant amount of study to create an analog computer of human consciousness [1]. Even the most elementary behavioral reactions are produced by the integrative activity of large networks in cortical and sub-cortical brain systems [2]. The central nervous system (CNS) has developed to provide efficient hormonal and muscle outputs and to keep pace with behavior adjustments continuously throughout life. BMIs provide the CNS with extra synthetic outputs generated from brain impulses [3].

DOI: 10.1201/9781003481959-9

In recent years, the development of a new stage of human evolution known as "AI Symbiosis" has emerged, indicating the establishment of mutually beneficial relationships between humans and artificial intelligence (AI). While true AI or uploading the contents of a human brain to an electronic equivalent may still be decades away, understanding electronic activities within brain cells has enabled us to design engineered systems like BMIs that can potentially replicate most of the capabilities of the human brain. To better understand the need for BMIs in research and development, it is important to review their relatively young history and initial development. While the terms BCI and BMI are often used interchangeably [3], BCI may be the more appropriate term as it recognizes the dynamic partnership between the system and the brain that is essential for successful BCI or BMI function, which goes beyond a fixed conversion of brain signals into outputs. Whether using externally recorded signals or signals recorded by implanted sensors, the ultimate goal of BMI technology is to enable communication between the brain and external devices, thus paving the way for the advancement of human-AI relationships in the future. Recent developments in machine learning make it possible to interpret neuron signals and perform a wide variety of tasks such as speech synthesis [4], motor imagery (MI) [5], emotion recognition [6], etc. Not only beneficial for patients with severe medical conditions, this technology can significantly impact different technologies and almost every aspect of human life. Such a deep understanding of neuron communications and the human mind can lead to a societal evolution and potentially initiate another civilization milestone. Despite its significant advantages, similar to all other emerging technologies, BMI comes with numerous challenges. The viability and reliability of this technology are highly dependent on the accuracy of collected brain signals. However, the sensitivity of the brain's neural network on the one hand and limitations on BMI devices on the other hand make data collection from neuron signals a challenging task for scientists. In addition to health-related risk factors, privacy concerns, and the accuracy of different decoding methods, the brain signals are also other barriers that slow down the progress in this domain. These are the key issues that are emerging or are becoming hot research topics in this area. Although the study of brain signals started in 1804, understanding and decoding its signals using BMI technology can open many opportunities for developing novel technologies in different domains. Decoding brain signals can be done via learning and classification methods. We dived into the cutting-edge machine learning models that are applied to different invasive neural signal interpretations. We studied supervised, unsupervised, semi-supervised, and other reinforcement learning methods, as well as federated learning (FL), to investigate opportunities in these areas that are not covered in other surveys. We have also dug through the literature to review all existing works that covered classification models. The main contributions of this chapter include:

- a comprehensive coverage of background knowledge, enabling technologies, and state-of-the-art scientific development on the applications of invasive BMI,
- an analysis of the brain structure and its signals from biological and engineering perspectives,
- a comprehensive review and analysis of possible applications of invasive BMI technology,
- an overview of different methods, including machine learning-based methods, devices for detecting and decoding brain signals, and possible options for stimulating signals into the human brain, and
- a discussion of challenges and opportunities of invasive BMI.

To have a clear understanding of the topics, we first discuss the brain structure and its signals from biological and engineering perspectives. Two major nervous systems, i.e., the CNS and peripheral nervous system (PNS), have been reviewed both functionally and anatomically, as well as action potentials (APs) in synapse formation. For neural signal detection, we focus on invasive methods due to the advancements in neurosurgery and minimized side effects of required operations. The related sections cover different aspects of brain signal processing, including signal generation, detection, acquisition, noise filtering, signal enrichment, feature extraction, decoding, encoding, and stimulation. Throughout this chapter, we consider different aspects of non-invasive BMI as a basis for developing invasive models and their applications.

Signal decoding models can be divided into two main categories: learning and classification. We systematically reviewed these models from invasive and non-invasive signal decoding perspectives. In the learning methods, we delved into some cutting-edge algorithms that are applied to different tasks and resulted in the state-of-the-art accuracy. To the best of our knowledge, such methods are not fully covered in existing surveys.

Different BMI applications might require different signal-detecting, decoding, or stimulating mechanisms. Therefore, we provide an overview and prediction of possible BMI applications in the future, most importantly in the field of medicine. As an example, we will look at the possibilities that BMI can offer patients with spinal cord injuries and other nervous system-related disabilities. We also discuss opportunities and threats of utilizing AI in areas such as learning, memory access, communications, virtualization, etc.

Table 9.1 highlights the main contributions of this survey and compares them with seven other surveys in this domain. We considered (A) noise filtering, (B) invasive and non-invasive models, (C) machine learning, and (D) applications and challenges in our comparison. As illustrated in the table,

TABLE 9.1 Summary of existing surveys on BMI

Ref.	Survey title	Year	Highlight	A	B	C	D
[7]	Recent Advances in Electrical Neural Interface Engineering: Minimal Invasiveness, Longevity, and Scalability	2020	• Large-scale, long-lasting neural recording • Wireless, miniaturized implants • Signal transmission, amplification, and processing	✓	×	×	✓
[8]	Neural Implants: A Review of Current Trends and Future Perspectives	2022	• Neurological disorders and the various types of BCIs used to address them • Possible future of DBS, Neuralink, motor and sensory neural prosthetics	✓	✓	✓	×
[9]	Signal Generation, Acquisition, and Processing in Brain Machine Interfaces: A Unified Review	2021	• Signal generation within the cortex, signal acquisition • Using invasive, non-invasive, or hybrid techniques, and the signal processing domain challenges and possible solutions	✓	✓	✓	×
[10]	Recent Approaches on Classification and Feature Extraction of EEG Signal: A Review	2021	• Robust techniques for feature extraction and classification • Comparative analysis of different classifiers	✓	×	✓	×
[11]	Review of Machine Learning Techniques for EEG Based Brain Computer Interface	2022	• Machine learning techniques applied in the brain computer interface • Classifying EEG signals for particular applications	✓	×	✓	✓
[12]	The Combination of Brain-Computer Interfaces and Artificial Intelligence: Applications and Challenges	2020	• Current state of AI as applied to BCIs • Advances in BCI applications, their challenges, and future	×	✓	✓	✓
[13]	Implantable Brain Machine Interfaces: First-In-Human Studies, Technology Challenges and Trends	2020	• Recent developments • Paradigm shift in BMI development	×	✓	✓	×
This chapter	Decoding Neural Signals: Invasive BMI Review	2024	• Anatomy and physiology of the brain • Noise filtering, signal enrichment and feature extraction methods • Signal decoding and signal encoding • Application and challenges • Learning strategies (self-supervised learning, semi-supervised learning, federated learning) • Adversarial attacks	✓	✓	✓	✓

A = Noise filtering, B = Invasive and non-invasive, C = Machine learning, D = Applications and challenges.

none of the existing survey papers provided such a comprehensive review of related concepts in BMI technology. In the noise filtering and signal enrichment parts, we discussed some methods, ranging from classical to deep learning-based models. It should be noted that due to the lack of significant work on invasive signals, we studied noise-filtering models in non-invasive BMI. Also, in the security and challenges section, adversarial attacks are primarily studied on non-invasive signals, whereas they are not studied very well on invasive signals. Summary of brain stimulation devices methods and effect and a list of abbreviated terms and their definitions are provided in tables in Sections 9.9 and 9.10.2.5. The rest of the chapter is organized as follows. The structure of the human brain is discussed in Section 9.2. A brief overview of artificial synapse technology is provided in Section 9.3. Section 9.4 discusses invasive and non-invasive methods. Reviews and analysis of possible applications of invasive BMI are provided in Section 9.5. Conducted techniques in the generation, detection, and acquisition of brain signals are discussed in Section 9.6. In Section 9.9, we discuss and compare various methods and devices for brain signal encoding, followed by ethical and implementation-related challenges of invasive BMI in Section 9.10. We finally conclude the book chapter in Section 9.11.

9.2   Human nervous system

The human nervous system consists of two main systems: CNS and PNS. Both systems work synchronously; for example, the PNS receives surrounding stimulation via many different types of sensors and transmits the sensation to the CNS. The CNS stores and interprets sensation stimulation. As well as sending interpretation messages, it transmits CNS messages to the target regions throughout the body by motor neurons. The anatomy of the CNS consists of the brain and the spinal cord. The brain is divided into three main regions: the forebrain, the brainstem, and the cerebellum. The forebrain is the largest part of the brain, including the cerebrum and diencephalon. The diencephalon is made up of the thalamus and hypothalamus. Furthermore, the large left and right cerebral hemispheres are formed by the cerebrum which includes the cerebral hemisphere and constitute four main lobes: frontal, temporal, parietal, and occipital lobes [14], which are shown in Figure 9.1.

9.2.1   The brain neural network

Neurons and glial cells, also known as supporting cells, are the two main biological components of the nervous system. The building block of the functionally human neuron system is a neuron which is an electrical and chemical signaling cell. A neuron has specialized membrane extensions called axons, dendrites, and tiny protrusions known as dendritic spines. Axons transmit

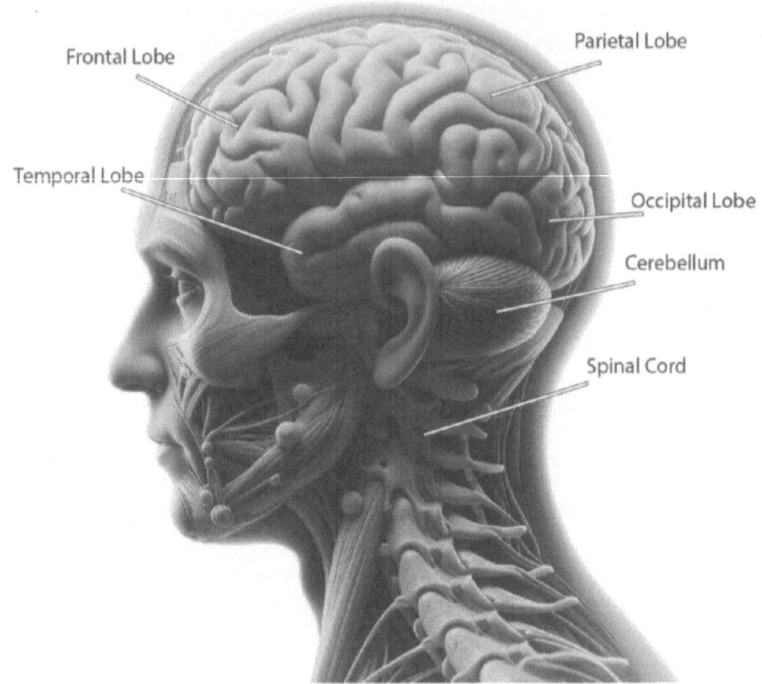

Frontal Lobe

Parietal Lobe

Temporal Lobe

Occipital Lobe

Cerebellum

Spinal Cord

FIGURE 9.1 Structure of the brain. Each human brain lobe performs a certain function.

information, while dendrites and tiny protrusions receive information. Between neurons, for example, axon to axon, axon to dendrites, and dendrites to dendrites is a cleft known as neuron synapses, which plays an important role during neural electrical activity. Several ion channels are involved in this process [14]. Ion transport across neuronal surface membranes is essential for neuronal signaling and computation. The multiple input stimulation is received by each neuron via activating and inhibiting ion transports. Multiple simulations are combined to decide whether the neuron will fire an AP, which sends the neuron message output to its target neurons. Thus, extracellular currents and voltage gradients are produced by all of these membrane currents and neural electrical activity, including action potentials. In the production of AP2, the Na^+ /K^+ channels are crucial. The Na^+ channel undergoes a conformational change followed by a dramatic increase in Na^+ permeability after a local depolarization of the membrane of approximately –20 mV to a threshold value of –70 mV. As a result, the membrane potential approaches the Na^+ resting-state potential (approximately +40 mV). Within 1 millisecond of the preceding events, the Na^+ channels are deactivated. Meanwhile, the K^+ channels begin to open and efflux K^+ from neurons as a result of resting membrane potential. The membrane is entirely refractory to a fresh

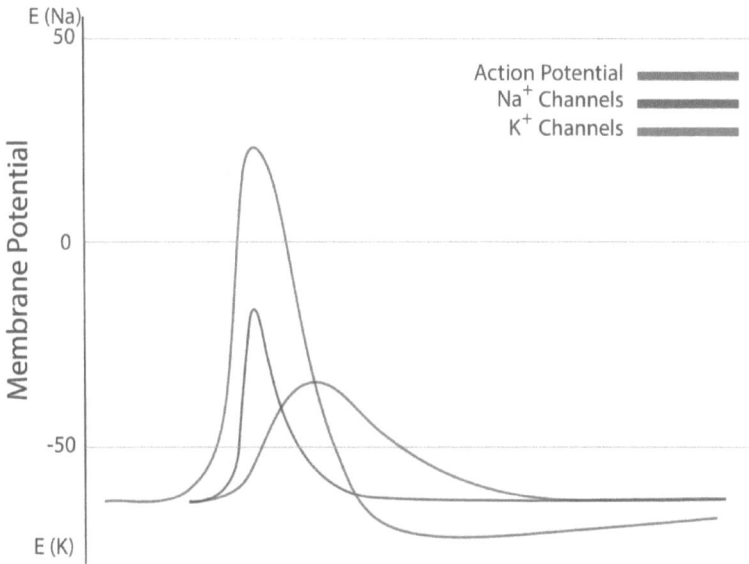

FIGURE 9.2 Permeability of potassium and sodium ions during an action potential (adapted from [16]).

depolarization during the interval of inactivation of the Na channels (absolute refractory phase) and afterward somewhat refractory. After a membrane potential is overshooted (hyperpolarization), the original equilibrium resurfaces (Figure 9.2). Finally, the firing of one neuron interacts with several neighboring neurons chemically and electrically [15]. Chemical and electrical synaptic transmission are the two main processes by which neurons interact.

9.2.1.1 Chemical connection

Chemical synapses are the most common type of synapses in the adult human nervous system. Chemical synapses are differentiated by the existence of a synaptic cleft, presynaptic vesicles near active zones, which serve as sites of neurotransmitter (NT) release, and postsynaptic membrane specializations. Extracellular matrix proteins are found in the cleft of many chemical synapses, and transmembrane proteins produced by the presynaptic neuron can bind to the partner on the postsynaptic cell across the synapse. The presynaptic electrical signal turns into a chemical signal, mainly NT, that binds to postsynaptic receptors and causes a response in the postsynaptic cell, which is typically an electrical signal, in chemical synapses (Figure 9.3). Because there are multiple metabolic stages involved, synaptic transmission at chemical synapses is slower than electrical signals with a range from 0.5 to 3.0 milliseconds. However, having biochemical stages has the advantage of making

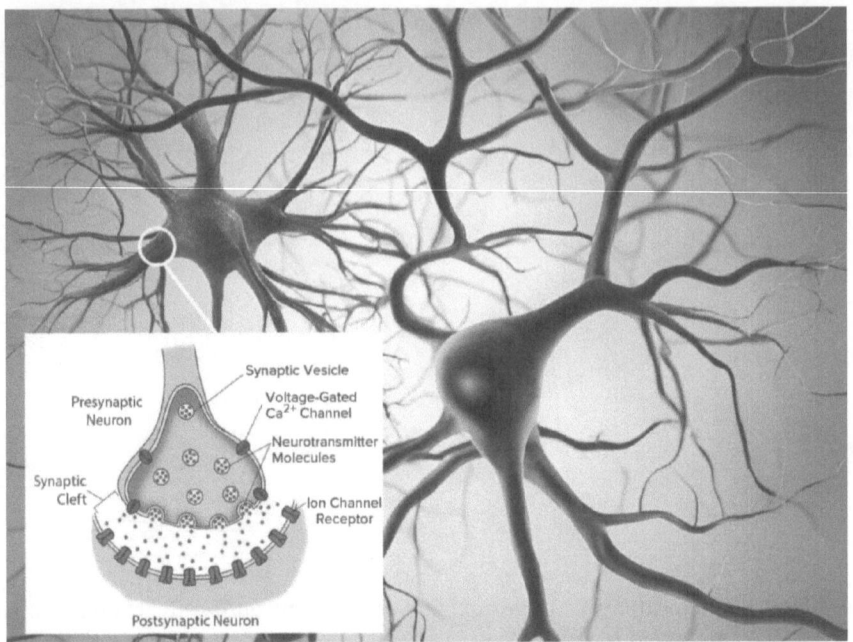

FIGURE 9.3 Structure of neuron and synapse.

chemical synapses more flexible. The reaction can be amplified, the electrical response's sign can be reversed, second messengers can be involved, and the response can be short-term or long-term. At chemical synapses, two forms of transmission can happen: fast/direct synaptic transmission and slow/indirect transmission. Fast/direct synaptic transmission is caused by binding of NT to ionotropic receptors, causing rapid changes in the postsynaptic membrane potential. Slow/indirect transmission (also known as neuromodulation) occurs when NT binds to metabotropic receptors, causing G proteins and second messengers to be activated, which can modify ion channels and/or cause long-term changes in excitability, metabolism, and gene expression. Because neurons contain both metabotropic and ionotropic receptors for NT, several NTs participate in both modes of transmission, whereas other NTs solely work through metabotropic receptors [14].

9.2.1.2 Electrical connection

Electrical synapses are the simplest and quickest type of synaptic transmission. Electrical synapses have been discovered in the retina, hypothalamus, and hippocampus and are thought to synchronize groups of neurons. The synaptic cleft in an electrical synapse has one or more domains where the postsynaptic and presynaptic plasma membranes are near enough to produce a gap junction (3–4 nm). Gap junctions, which include gap junction channels, link many different types of cells in the body. A transmembrane protein complex called a connexon in the presynaptic membrane links to a connexon in the postsynaptic membrane to produce the gap junction channel that joins the cytoplasm of the two neurons in electrical synapses. Current (ions) and second messengers can pass from the presynaptic to the postsynaptic neuron through these connexon channels. Because tiny ions diffuse rapidly, the delay between presynaptic and postsynaptic reactions is only 0.1 milliseconds. Electrical synaptic transmission has restrictions, despite being extremely fast. Because there is no conversion or gain, the postsynaptic reaction is always less than, and has the same sign as, the presynaptic response [14].

9.3   Artificial synapse technology

The term "memristor" or "memory resistance" refers to an artificial synapse unit that was first described in 1808 by Sir H. Davy and later formalized in 1971 by L. Chua. Following that, León Chua explored a new element of two-terminal circuits with a link between the electrical charge and the magnetic flux after a series of technical experiments. Modern memristors can mimic the synaptic mechanism and be tailored to the technical needs of neuromorphic computing systems. Today, some companies are investigating the development of experimental neurochips like Neuralink based on the characteristics of current memristors that can interpret brain activity via functional measurements of millions of neurons and their synapsis, allowing communication with the outside world. The technology is capable of translating the activity of the nervous system into real-world interaction, such as providing a sense of touch or proprioception to modify the movement of a human prosthetic limb [17].

9.4   Implantation of the devices

Today, research and applications of the brain–computer interface (BCI) and the BMI are among the most exciting interdisciplinary fields in science and technology. BMIs are divided into two categories: invasive and non-invasive. There are several types of invasive, non-invasive, and recording-stimulus technologies. Non-invasive methods do not require opening the skull of the implantation receiver. They act on the surface of the skin and can record an average of millions of neurons. However, non-invasive techniques are not able to detect the distinctive features of neurophysiological diseases in real time; therefore, one has to insert electrodes in certain areas of the brain to detect such features. In invasive procedures, electrodes are placed directly on the surface of the cortex. Useful signals can be recorded, which are the average activity of thousands of neurons. The authors in [18] discussed more information on all types of BMI.

The aggressive technologies are extremely interesting. Before we move on, let us discuss the neural network. The neural network (a phrase coined by novelist Ian M. Banks in 2000) is made up of arrays of microscopic electrodes that are attached to polymer wires or threads and injected into the brain. Neuralink has produced arrays of these strands, each of which is claimed to be considerably thinner than a hair and has 3072 electrodes dispersed among 96 strands. It has also built a neurosurgery robot that can connect six strands together, injecting 192 electrodes into the brain each minute while also preventing blood vessels from bleeding (this has yet to be tested on humans) [18].

9.5 Applications

Nowadays, BMI technology is used mainly in different areas of medicine to monitor neural communications. Most of the advances in BMI are done through academic research and are not yet available to the general public. In this section, we discuss applications of BMI in different areas which are expected to be among the most advanced technologies of the 21st century.

9.5.1 Medical

Currently, BMI devices are widely used to monitor brain signals, and among them, non-invasive ones are more common than the implanted type due to their simplicity and easier installation procedure. However, this technology is not yet the first choice of practitioners to treat patients with related medical conditions due to its numerous limitations [18]. In this section, we discuss a few examples to show how BMI technology can make a revolution by boosting human health to a much higher level.

9.5.1.1 Disease prediction

It is possible to imagine a world without the majority of current diseases if they can be predicted by BMI devices and prevented from occurring or affecting the human body. Brain signals that are produced via chemical and electrical communication of neurons can be recorded, decoded, and learned to prevent diseases prematurely.

9.5.1.2 Pain elimination

Perhaps, the pain phenomenon that is caused by injuries, burns, or illness is one of the most important reasons for human survival. Although its existence is highly crucial for our health, it can be minimized or completely eliminated during the treatment process as the cause of pain is already known. However, almost all pain relievers come with different side effects [19]. BMI technology makes it possible to communicate with the brain and send signals to eliminate pain.

9.5.1.3   Therapeutic

There is a wide range of medical conditions that can be treated using neural interfaces, also known as "Electroceuticals". This is a new category of therapeutic agents that target the neural circuits of organs. Such therapies involve mapping the neural circuitry and transmitting neural impulses to these specific organs [20]. Some remedies have been provided for many years in medical practice, such as cochlear implants, which many people with hearing impairment have benefited from, stimulants to help with stroke recovery, and deep brain stimulation (DBS) to improve crucial tremors in Parkinson's disease and dystonia [21]. Other remedies such as *transcranial direct current stimulation* (tDCS) for depression are still under investigation in the laboratory. Others are in the trial or initial phases of medical application. For example, DBS for *epilepsy* or the *Mollii Suit* is a body cloth that provides electrical stimulation to people who have muscle spasticity as a result of stroke or cerebral palsy [22].

In general, when conditions are resistant to drugs, interface treatments are frequently followed. For example, it is estimated that 20–30% of epilepsy patients are drug-resistant. These *electroceuticals* can be more efficient than drugs because they exactly target a specific part of the brain or body and also they do not have undesirable effects which are caused by ingesting chemical drugs [18]. Below, we discuss several practical examples.

9.5.1.4   Spinal cord injury (SCI)

It is a destructive occurrence, with symptoms ranging from loss of motor and sensory function to shortened life expectancy, with SCI survivors typically reliant on medical resources and social assistance [23]. The goal of many brain-computer (neural bypass) interfaces is to transform cerebral signals into peripheral motor responses, effectively bypassing SCI. Transcutaneous spinal cord stimulation is being investigated as a less invasive approach for activating local spinal circuitry. For neuromodulation, electrodes are inserted on the skin, and direct current stimulation is employed. As a result of this finding, researchers have worked to build algorithms that depend on non-invasive scalp electroencephalography (EEG) inputs [24]. However, due to the poor signal-to-noise ratio (SNR) of these signals, they are susceptible to artifact contamination. Electrocorticography (ECoG) signals obtained from the brain surface have been used in subsequent research. Because of the clinical justifications for ECoG (e.g., seizure mapping), these more recent attempts have been confined to brief implantation. Generally, research on the properties of brain signals (invasive and non-invasive) such as ERDs (event-related desynchronizations) and other frequency features is at the forefront of current efforts for various end-organ applications, including the manipulation of a computer cursor and the movement of paralyzed muscles [24].

9.5.1.4.1 Parkinson's disease (PD)

It is characterized by a gradual impairment of voluntary motor control caused by the buildup of α-synuclein-containing Lewy bodies in the brain's substantia nigra pars compacta and the death of dopaminergic neurons, resulting in a decrease in dopamine levels. [25, 26]. DBS can be used to treat it. A tiny electrode wire must be implanted in the area of the brain that causes aberrant movement via surgery. An implantable pulse generator (IPG) battery can be implanted in the belly or under the collarbone, requiring a second surgical surgery. The IPG sends electrical impulses to the brain, which can aid in the control of various motor symptoms [27].

- **Autism:** It is a neurodevelopmental disease that has a significant impact on verbal and nonverbal communication, as well as social interaction [28]. TMS has also shown promise in aiding autistic people in improving their social skills [18]. tDCS has been presented as a novel ASD therapeutic approach with the potential to improve cognitive, motor, and social communication abilities by addressing particular underlying neural abnormalities [29].
- **Body parts replacements:** After losing a limb, a person's life can be transformed by bionic limbs. These devices communicate directly with the remaining neurological or neuromuscular system. There has been a long history of making bionic limbs for disabled people due to the need to improve their lives [30]. When the user flexes, a bionic limb, such as an arm, recognizes minuscule impulses generated by the body. Recently, the Neuralink company showed how their app converts residual limb muscles into movements using the bionic limb. On the other hand, advanced BMIs can use this technique a step further by allowing us to use "the brain to transmit our intentions, without having to go through an extra, physical step of converting those intentions into text, speech, or gestures". It is possible to make interactions easier, faster, and more natural [27].

9.5.1.4.2 Epilepsy

In 2005, the International League Against Epilepsy (ILAE) suggested a conceptual definition of epilepsy as a brain illness marked by an enduring susceptibility to create epileptic seizures and its psychosocial repercussions [31]. BMIs can be used to diagnose and cure neurological problems as well as expose brain functioning. Karageorgos et al. [32] have presented HALO (Hardware Architecture for LOW-power BCIs), an architecture for implanted BCIs that can be used to treat illnesses like epilepsy. HALO also collects and analyses the information that can be utilized to better understand the brain. Epilepsy is characterized by uncontrolled and excessive electrical activity in neurons, which results in epileptic seizures. Seizures are predicted by analyzing neuronal signals [33]. The brain requires inhibitory synapses to tone down and regulate the activity of other cells when brain stimulation increases. BMIs then use electrical stimulation to reduce the intensity of seizures. The period between seizure initiation and stimulation, on the other hand, must be very short, in the tens of milliseconds range. Low-power hardware is also required for long-term implantation. The Neuralink BMI chip is based on prior methods; however, it provides better bandwidth brain connection in real-time while using less power [27].

9.5.1.4.3 Depression

It is one of the most common mental health conditions and almost one-third of depression cases are treatment resistant. Due to their severe side effects such as weight gain and decreased libido, mental health medications are not the best option. While BMIs also come with challenges, they are much safer than drugs [27]. High frequency repetitive transcranial magnetic stimulation (rTMS) to the left dorsolateral prefrontal cortex (DLPFC) is an authorized therapy for depression based on its safety and effectiveness factors [34]. On the other hand, it has side effects, such as discomfort at the head site, magnet effects on the muscles, etc. Advanced BMI technologies can stimulate neurons of the frontal cortex to release dopamine hormones which can directly target neurons related to depression with fewer side effects rather than rTMS.

9.5.2 *Hybrid human*

With the advancements of machine learning and AI, robotics moved to a much higher level in the last few decades. In 1997, Gary Kasparov, the world Chess champion, was defeated by an IBM supercomputer in a highly publicized match. Since then, we have witnessed how fast robots replaced humans in different sectors. They become faster and more intelligent while getting cheaper year by year, as their CPU power gets doubled every two years based on Moore's law. Although such advanced computers make our lives much easier, they can become threats. The well-known theoretical physicist, Stephen Hawking warned once about the rise of AI that if we are not careful, they can be the worst thing that has ever happened to us. There is no doubt that robots are much faster and more intelligent than humans today. With the current exponential development pace, theoretically, they can reach a point where they will not need our programs and will be able to reproduce themselves.

In any competitions against them, the relatively super slow humans will be defeated readily. In many ways, AI could outperform and replace us, but there is no possible global governance model for the shift from artificial narrow intelligence (ANI) to artificial general intelligence (AGI). If they do not establish the first situation correctly, an artificial super intelligence (ASI) might come out of AGI and our future may be endangered. So as an alarm we have to investigate international rules for transitions [35]. This also urges the need for a more advanced BMI that enables humans using machines to empower their decision-making system, and paying more attention to establish a consensus internationally about shifting [36].

Not only in theory, combined biological brain and AI systems are already developed and passed their initial trials. Neuralink's BMI chip, for example, can connect our brain to a synthetic neocortex, so we can be merged with an AI-based machine. Such models may result in the birth of hybrid species. Transhumanists anticipate that new technologies will improve the human condition by providing them more intellectual ability and longer life, endless memory, and faster communication. Mankind may evolve into post-human, and the human era may come to an end by 2045 [36].

9.5.3 Virtualization

Researchers believe that the investment and speed of development in the gaming world enable these technologies to thrive with benefits for a variety of applications among people with severe disabilities. Invincibility on the next generation, such as the decline of social skills and drowning in online and cyberspace, is advancing very fast. In the past few years, we have witnessed great advancements in the context of entertainment. From virtual reality (VR) and augmented reality (AR) to 3D holography, each has taken this experience one step beyond. Playing a video game with virtual/AR or holding a conference with a holographic projection of remote people has been a thrilling experience. As another example, we have experienced looking into our desired house to buy or going on a virtual tour of the Louvre museum with VR.

However, the sky is the limit for our future possibilities. In the near future, there will be no need for the above technologies because advanced BMI technologies such as Link (i.e., the Neuralink chip) promise a different experience, a whole new experience to be specific.

Consider there are cloud-based games designed specifically for Link. In this case, just a 5G or fiber internet connection would be enough for players around the world to not only play together but also share their feelings, emotions, intentions, and decisions. Additionally, we will be able to have the exact five senses of sight, smell, hearing, taste, and touch in the context of a virtual tour of, for example, a zoo, museum, or even the International Space

Station (ISS); just having someone in charge of doing our desired actions would be enough as it seems. Apparently, we are much closer than expected to experience everything we have seen in Sci-Fi movies.

9.5.4   Communications

Advanced BMIs such as Link allow communicating with a messenger app without typing or even touching a button. This possibility is already available for disabled people to help them communicate easily. While typing is not straightforward for them, they can think about the message they are about to send, and their Link system will handle the rest in milliseconds. They could even be enabled to be active on social media platforms, web surfing, and email responding. This capability becomes even more interesting when we understand that the high rate of data transfer can accelerate their routine jobs dramatically.

This amazing possibility can even encourage us to think about developing custom-designed apps only for the human brain. Instead of making use of a messenger app control feature of Link, we can develop special apps only for this goal. Consider there are many cloud-based servers hosting these apps around the world, and humans can connect to them in order to connect to a mesh of millions or billions of Links. In this case, not only we will be enabled to face a whole new social life, but also we can share what we see, feel, or experience with our peers simultaneously.

9.5.5   Advanced education

BMIs can provide opportunities to improve the entire brain's functionality. Our memories and decision-making abilities could be enhanced significantly when our brain is empowered by AI. This will enable us to access different memory layers and solve much more complex problems in a very short time. Information could be encoded into neuron signals and uploaded to our brain and become our new memories. We could easily upload new skills to our brain, similar to the Neo Matrix movie, instead of practicing hard for a long time. Students can benefit from neural interfaces in order to achieve educational goals by learning better and focusing more. All our knowledge which in fact is memorized information could be safely encoded to digital signals and stored on digital devices or uploaded to the cloud safely [27].

Education sector will be one of those areas that benefit the most from advanced BMI as it enables us to transfer not only data and information to our brains, but experience, knowledge, and wisdom as well. Consider a very special situation, when several aircraft pilots are needed and due to the time and geography constraints summoning registered pilots is not an option. Theoretically, it is viable to train pilots using advanced BMIs in a very short period of time as all necessary tools for knowledge transmission to the brain are available. However, there is always a downside for every innovation. While currently it requires years of hardworking, patience, and persistence to learn a particular skill, any changes in this traditional learning process can change the definition of morality and social values. We will discuss such challenges in more detail in Section 9.10.

9.5.6   Civilization shift

The extraction of information and knowledge associated with the help of AI is often biased. Technology influences individual decision-making, and this will have implications for the future of community democracy. We must be able to use technology to democratize processes through the digital platforms that build communities. The ability of machines and AI to solve problems quickly is one of their greatest advantages, which has already surpassed human capabilities. It is predicted that humans and super-intelligent creatures will live together in the future [37]. The relationship between humans and robots can be balanced by a cyber minister, and the future society may consist of a combination of human–machine systems, a community of forces brought together by the machine-human environment [36]. However, human civilization has evolved gradually over thousands of years and such changes will have a huge impact on many components of our civilization including our cultures, languages, and the entire industry.

9.6   Signals and devices

The five BMI steps—signal collection, signal processing, feature extraction, data categorization, and control interfaces—are covered in this section (Figure 9.4 shows an observation of these steps). We also cover the methods for generating, detecting, and acquiring signals, as well as their underlying concepts. Additionally, we explore the comparison of spatial and temporal resolution for BMI methods, both invasive and non-invasive.

9.6.1   Signal generation

Electrical signaling is a cardinal feature of the nervous system and endows it with the capability of quickly reacting to changes in the environment. Although synaptic communication between nerve cells is perceived to be mainly chemically mediated, electrical synaptic interactions also occur. Two different strategies are responsible for electrical communication between neurons. One is the consequence of low resistance intercellular pathways, called "gap junctions", for the spread of electrical currents between the interior of two cells. The second occurs in the absence of cell-to-cell contacts

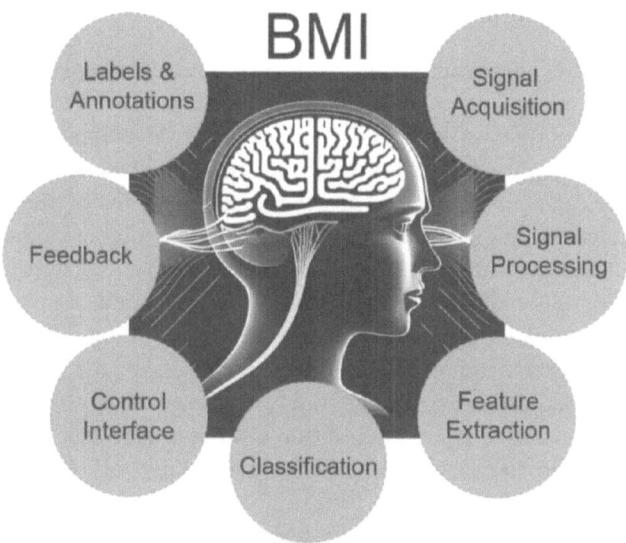

FIGURE 9.4   Schematic illustration of a BMI using five stages including signal acquisition, signal processing, feature extraction, data classification, and the control interface.

and is a consequence of the extracellular electrical fields generated by the electrical activity of neurons [38].

The first attempts to translate neuronal activity into commands to control external devices were made in monkeys in the 1960s. After that, during 1960–1970, the biological feedback was realized in monkeys, to provide voluntary control of the firing rate of cortical neurons [39].

We also distinguish between recording and stimulating activities. Recording, also mentioned as brain-to-computer interface (BCI), attempts to read brain signals and interpret them. Stimulating, also mentioned as computer-to-brain interface (CBI), goes in the opposite direction and tries to stimulate or control the brain [27]. These intelligent systems can decipher brain signals using five consecutive stages: signal acquisition, preprocessing, feature extraction, classification, and control interface as shown in Figure 9.4.

9.6.2 Signal detection

Synchronization of neuronal activity in the brain underlies the emergence of neuronal oscillations termed "brain waves", which serve various physiological functions and correlate with different behavioral states. It has been postulated that at least ten distinct mechanisms are involved in the formulation of these brain waves, including variations in the concentration of extracellular NTs and ions, as well as changes in cellular excitability [40].

9.6.3 *Signal acquisition*

Since the first EEG recording in 1938, numerous neural implants to stimulate and record electrical activity in the brain have been developed [41]. Over the past years, a number of technologies have been developed to measure the activity of the human brain. Some of the techniques measure the variation of the electrical activities related to the different states of the brain while some other techniques measure other parameters. Available modalities can be classified under two categories based on their invasiveness: non-invasive and invasive. The major difference between these two techniques is that invasive techniques require surgery to implant electrodes within the brain's cortex while non-invasive techniques rely on recordings over the skull. Generally, non-invasive methods have poor spatial resolution but show reasonable temporal resolution. Also, signal attenuation is a big problem in such techniques due to the limited electrical conductivity of the skull [42]. Recently, another class of BMIs has also emerged, utilizing the benefits of both invasive and non-invasive techniques, appropriately termed hybrid BMIs [43]. Figure 9.5 provides a hierarchical classification of BMIs.

9.6.3.1 *Invasive techniques*

To precisely record neuronal data with a higher degree of freedom for neuroprostheses, the development of BMIs will require invasive recording techniques [44] such as ECoG and intracortical electrodes.

The ECoG technique requires surgery to place electrodes in extracortical areas either inside or outside the dura mater, called subdural ECoG and epidural ECoG, respectively [45]. This technique is like EEG but with a higher

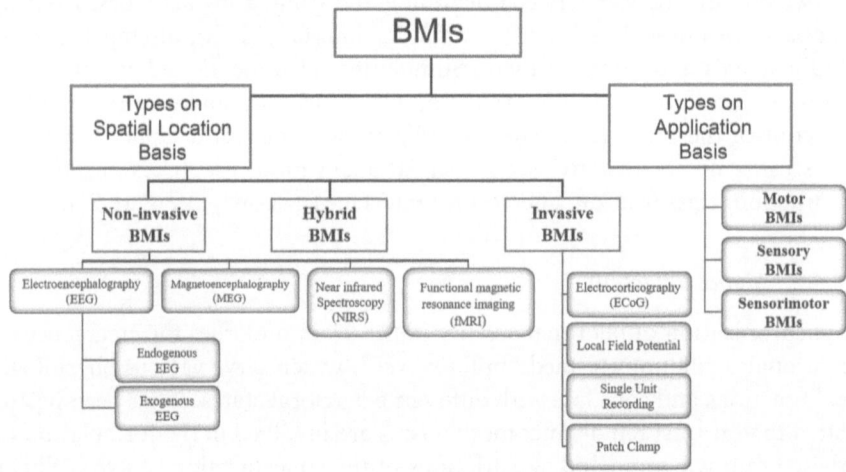

FIGURE 9.5 Hierarchical classification of BMIs based on their spatial position and application.

SNR as the electrode grid is placed directly above the cortex surface avoiding the skull. The brain's electrical activity can be recorded intracellularly and extracellularly depending on the position of the electrode. Extracellular activities of neurons can be called APs. Also, in nervous and other tissues, local field potentials (LFPs) arise from the summation and synchronization of the electrical activity of individual neurons. ECoG records an average of thousands of neurons and can also be referred to as LFPs; however, it is not suitable for obtaining deep brain signals [46]. However, AP readings from a group of functionally linked single neurons are required for high precision and increased data fidelity [47]. To achieve this, microelectrodes are used to record single unit activity (SUA) as well as multi-unit activity (MUA). However, even with SUA, a specific number of neurons must be recorded to derive some consistent and trustworthy meaning from the readings. Although opinions vary, a good estimate for a minimum number of readings can be anywhere between 15 and 30 neurons [48]. Hence, intracortical SUA and MUA recordings using microelectrodes are very important.

9.6.3.2 Non-invasive techniques

One of the most used neural recording techniques is EEG, in which electrodes are simply placed on the surface of the scalp at specific points to record averaged neuronal signals from different intracortical regions [49]. EEG-based systems are portable and are usually cheap. They have a good temporal resolution as they directly measure the neural activity while it lacks in spatial resolution as the signal has to pass through a number of physical barriers including the skull, scalp, and cerebrospinal fluid (CSF) [49, 50]. Also, EEG recordings are susceptible to artifacts that can be mechanical, electromyographic, or electrooculographic in nature [51]. Magnetoencephalography (MEG) is another technique that records postsynaptic activity of neurons using magnetic fields. Its spatial resolution is reasonably better than EEG and has a high temporal resolution [52]. Functional magnetic resonance imaging (fMRI) is a method used widely in medical science to create 3D maps of brains. As a result of neuronal activity, it detects changes in the magnetic field caused by changes in hemoglobin oxygenation levels. The signal generated by fMRI is also called "blood oxygen level dependence" (BOLD) [53]. It can be used to obtain full brain scans covering all brain areas unlike EEG or MEG [54].

Other than using electrical signals, neural data can be obtained using photons in the wavelength range of 650–900 nm that can penetrate cortical areas and show contrasts based on oxygenation/deoxygenation of hemoglobin. The method is called near infrared spectroscopy (NIRS) [55]. Functional near infrared topography (fNIRT) is another modification of NIRS that renders 3D images of the brain [56]. Some other known methods include positron emission tomography (PET), single positron emission computed tomography (SPECT), and computer axial tomography [57, 58].

Non-invasive techniques are widely used and well established; however, the major shortcomings of almost all the non-invasive techniques are low signal specificity, low SNR, and signal distortion. The hindrance due to the skull and intermediate brain layers between the cortex and the electrodes reduces the SNR of the recordings, leading to an average signal of millions of neurons. Moreover, any of the above-mentioned techniques cannot record a single or even a few hundred neurons, which is highly critical for practical BMI applications. Hence, a logical step forward for obtaining a specific high-resolution signal is to put electrodes directly outside or inside the cortex.

9.6.4   *Invasive vs. non-invasive*

Electrical activity in brain cells is regulated by ionic currents, the superposition of which is called the LFP which is recorded by an electrode and is dominated by populations with substantial synaptic processes. The main sources are APs and synaptic transmission. There is a widespread belief that high-frequency components (more than 500 Hz) originate from APs and low-frequency components from synaptic transmissions. Brain tissue exhibits different types of impedance. Although brain tissue is usually thought to have high-pass properties, there are signs that it may also have low-pass properties.

BMI technologies allow us to record APs up to LFPs. Neurons can form connections through electrical synapses, and action potentials (spikes) can modulate LFPs through synaptic input. These electric fields can influence the LFPs. Information in the LFPs and APs can be different [59]. But there is a misunderstanding that information between invasive and non-invasive is the same and obstacles cannot affect non-invasive BMI. This may have been influenced by studies that showed similar performance for intracortical BMIs based on APs versus LFPs [60]. Although invasive and non-invasive signals may originate from the same source, there are differences. Several factors are involved, such as the fact that some neuronal clusters are difficult to detect or record with EEG. Additionally, tissue acts as a low-pass filter that reduces high-frequency signals to bury them in the background noise [61]. Additionally, the electrophysiological properties of extracellular media influence how LFPs propagate in extracellular spaces [62, 63]. Through EEG, these limitations cannot be overcome. EEG, however, can monitor neural activity in areas adjacent to the neurocranium with a low cost and without risk. Invasive recordings, however, can be deeper, but do not cover the entire neocortex, as they require surgical intervention.

9.7   Signal decoding

The most important component of BMI technology is signal translation and decoding. After collecting a massive amount of brain signals, it is time to understand them using different decoding and signal processing methods that are reviewed in this section.

9.7.1 Noise filtering and signal enrichment

For achieving better results during processing data, identifying noises generated by different sources during the data collection process is crucial. These are usually caused by natural factors, such as muscle movements located near the brain, the effect of environmental signals or internal movements, interrupting sensations, hardware, and data collection. However, sometimes noises can be created intentionally by someone to attack the device, which is related to the security and privacy of BMI devices. We will discuss the robustness of models against the attacks in Section 8.4. The goal of noise filtering applications is to leverage brain signals to enhance them through noise filtering and signal enhancement so that devices and applications utilizing brain signals are more accurate and robust.

A variety of methods have been proposed to remove artifacts. For general noise filtering and signal enhancement, lots of work have been done in signal processing using classical methods (like wavelet, PCA, etc.) and neural network-based models. Obviating noisy segments manually results in missing information on these segments. Two main methods of automatic signal removal are [64]:

  i estimating using the reference channel and
  ii decomposition of the brain signal into other domains.

The lack of research into invasive signal filtering led us to discuss invasive and non-invasive denoising and enrichment techniques in this section. Methods applied to non-invasive signals can be applied to invasive signals. In the following, we discuss invasive and non-invasive noise filtering methods with available methods ranging from classical to deep learning-based algorithms.

* *Non-invasive signals*

For denoising non-invasive signals, both classical and deep learning methods are used. In the following, we will review them.

9.7.1.1 Classical methods

Classical methods include regression [65], blind source separation (BSS) [66], empirical-mode decomposition (EMD) [67], wavelet transform algorithm [68], as well as hybrid methods such as canonical correlation analysis (CCA) [69], blind source separation (BSS), and EMD-BSS, EEMD-CCA [64]. One of the most common methods researchers use is the common average reference (CAR) spatial method, which filters common noises out [70]. However, this method may share noises between channels that can cause significant signal interference.

9.7.1.2 Deep learning methods

Nowadays, deep learning methods provide state-of-the-art (SOTA) results in various tasks. SOTA algorithms for signal denoising, use deep learning algorithms to accomplish one of these tasks. Most of the recent works used autoencoder-decoder and generative adversarial networks (GANs), which we will describe in the following.

A well-known denoising architecture is deep convolutional autoencoders. This method is used in refs. [71, 72] which were previously used for music and voice enrichment. Also, from another perspective, signal denoising can be designed for a specific task in order to prevent reducing accuracy. For instance, ref. [73] tries to improve the quality of EEG signals to avoid reducing the performance of steady-state visually evoked potential (SSVEP)-based BMI against noises using autoencoders. As a recommendation for improving the results of these algorithms, data augmentation could be helpful to compensate for training data shortages.

Another algorithm used for signal decoding is GAN. The study in [74] uses a GAN-based denoising method to denoise the multichannel EEG signals and also defines a new loss function to ensure that the filtered signal can retain as much effective original information and energy as possible.

- *Invasive signals*

The number of studies conducted on noise filtering and signal enrichment is limited due to problems like lack of data and no available public dataset. In the following, some recent works will be discussed, as well as suggestions for solving problems in this field.

For detecting LFP artifacts, ref. [75] attempted to solve this issue by an adaption of Alexnet [76]. Also, ref. [77] solved the problem using LSTM neural network architectures. SANTIA [78] is a tool that tries to simplify machine learning training steps for offline artifact identification in invasive signals.

There has been little work in this area because of the lack of datasets for signal noise enrichment and filtering. Adding different types of noises to signals can be considered a solution to this problem which is a data augmentation technique. In addition, works like ref. [71] show that by applying speech noise filtering methods to brain signals, accurate results could be achieved.

9.7.2 Feature extraction

BMI systems perform much better when an appropriate feature extraction technique is employed. The main goal of feature extraction is to make it easier to identify patterns and improve the accuracy of the BMI using supervised or unsupervised methods. Another related goal is data dimensionality reduction. The majority of these feature extraction techniques have different domains such as time, frequency, time-frequency, and spatial as discussed below.

9.7.2.1 Time domain features

Using time domain features will allow employing signal values at distinct intervals of time. Following the preprocessing of lowpass filtering, bandpass filtering, and down sampling, the time domain features are extracted. These features are used to quantify the temporal variations in time-locked brain signal amplitudes.

Hjorth Parameters: Hjorth parameters allow computing the activity, mobility, and complexity of time-varying signals [79].

Statistical Features: The signals' time series are characterized by a variety of statistical metrics. Energy, entropy, mean, standard deviation, skewness, and kurtosis are six statistical parameters commonly employed in BMI investigations [80].

Fractal Dimension: The fractal dimension (FD) is a statistical metric that measures a signal's self-similarity across a given spatial or time interval. The nature of brain signals is fractal; hence, fractal pieces can be used to determine the features [81, 82].

- **Kalman Filter:** It is important for BMI to represent the uncertainty associated with an estimation before committing to a decision in order to prevent potentially disastrous actions based on poor estimations. Signal properties and their uncertainty can be estimated statistically using Bayesian filtering techniques. One of the most well-known Bayesian filtering algorithms is the Kalman filter [83].
- **Particle Filter:** In nonlinear non-Gaussian processes, particle filters are used in order to derive a posterior distribution over the hidden state. Human signals are nonlinear, so linear regression models will not reflect the nonlinearity of those signals. Particle filter, as an alternative nonlinear decoding model, can be used to overcome this problem [84].

9.7.2.2 Frequency domain features

Frequency domain features describe the signal power at a particular frequency band. Some of the most important features are listed below:

Discrete Fourier Transform: Decomposing a signal into a weighted sum of sinusoidal and cosine waves of different frequencies is known as Fourier analysis. Fourier decomposition, rather than expressing a signal in terms of time, does it in terms of frequency content. The original signal can be reconstructed using the inverse Fourier transform (IFT). For BMI applications, brain signals are frequently recorded at discrete periods. In the discrete Fourier transform (DFT), the Fourier series is changed and applied to discretely sampled data [85].

Fast Fourier Transform: The fast Fourier transform (FFT) effectively computes the DFT with fewer calculations, making processing more efficient. Many BMI systems use characteristics collected from the power spectrum of a brain signal across time, such as EEG or ECoG. Welch's approach (based on FFT) is a frequently used method for power spectrum estimate, and the power of a certain frequency band is utilized as a spectral characteristic in subsequent analysis such as classification [86].

9.7.2.3 Time-frequency domain features

Time-frequency methods can be useful in understanding brain signals that are non-stationary because they consider dynamic changes to provide useful information.

- **Matched Filtering (MF):** It is a feature extraction approach that detects a specific pattern from unknown signals by comparing it to known signal templates [87].
- **Autoregression Model (AR):** It is a type of statistical modeling that uses a natural tendency of the signals to correlate over time or across various dimensions such as space. Thus, it is possible to predict future measurements based on a few historical values [88].
- **Short Time Fourier Transform:** The Fourier transform represents an original signal with as a sum of basis functions, namely, sines and cosines of different frequencies. The Fourier transform, however, does a poor job of capturing signals that are finite and non-periodic or have sharp peaks and discontinuities since sines and cosines have an indefinite temporal breadth. However, the assumption of a stationary signal in Fourier analysis is broken by brain signals which are often non-stationary (i.e., statistical features change with time). One solution is to perform Fourier analysis over short-time windows, a procedure known as short-term Fourier transform (STFT). The STFT addresses the issue of window size, where tiny windows offer high temporal resolution and poor frequency resolution, and wide windows offer superior frequency resolution but worse temporal resolution. This insight produces the wavelet transform, which successfully balances temporal and frequency resolution [89, 90].
- **Wavelet:** Wavelet transform modifies the shape of the simple sine and cosine functions of the Fourier transform. In a wavelet, the mother wavelet function is finite in time in contrast to Fourier where sine and cosine run from $(-\infty, +\infty)$. Unlike a Fourier decomposition which always uses complex exponential basis functions, a wavelet decomposition uses a time-localized oscillatory function as the analyzing or mother wavelet [91].

9.7.2.4 The common spatial pattern

The common spatial pattern (CSP) is a prominent feature extraction approach that emphasizes differences while minimizing similarities between classes. CSP finds spatial filters which can transform the input data into resulting feature vectors that enhance the discriminability between classes. Although CSP was primarily designed to handle multichannel data related to two-class problems, a few extensions have also been proposed for multi-class BMI data. Additionally, the spatial resolution influences CSP performance since the few electrode positions offer more discriminating data for specific brain activity compared to others. Considering these issues, the following strategies for improving CSP performance have been proposed: common sparse spectral-spatial pattern (CSSP), common spatio-spectral pattern (CSSP), and wavelet common spatial pattern (WCSP) [92, 93].

9.8 Machine learning

The purpose of this section is to provide an overview of machine learning techniques that are relevant for signal decoding (classification and learning methods) as well as adversarial attacks. As part of signal decoding, various learning strategies are also discussed for learning representations in the various conditions from data, such as learning from unlabeled data, lack of labeled data, learning representations of data without supervision, privacy, etc. In the adversarial attack part, we challenge the robustness of machine learning-based models against different attacks on BMI signals.

9.8.1 Signal decoding: Classifications methods

The next stage of the functional model is to decode a BMI signal into meaningful representations in order to learn a model for a specific task. Signal decoding is important to understanding relationships between neural signals and the world. It can be used to determine how much information neural activity contains about an external variable (e.g., sensation or movement) [94], and how this information differs across brain areas [95], experimental conditions [96], disease states [97], speech recognition and speech synthesis [98, 99], sleep spindle identification [100, 101], emotion recognition [102], etc. When the goal is to determine how much information a neural population has about an external variable, regardless of the form of that information, then using ML will generally be beneficial. It is extremely important to be careful with the scientific interpretation of decoding results, both for ML and other models [103]. Decoding can tell us how much information a neural population has about a variable X. However, high decoding accuracy does not mean that a brain area is directly involved in processing X or that X is the purpose of the brain area [104].

Different classifiers are used to translate the features extracted from brain signals to control commands. These classifiers range from the simplistic linear classifiers to complex nonlinear classifiers. Some of the commonly used classifiers are (i) K-nearest neighbor (KNN), (ii) linear discriminant analysis (LDA), (iii) support vector machine (SVM), (iv) artificial neural network (ANN), (v) extreme learning machine (ELM), and (vi) naive Bayes (NB). These classifiers are discussed in detail below, highlighting their suitability for specific situations and example usage from the literature.

- **K-Nearest Neighbor:** In KNN, training samples are identified and classified into the dominant class based on their proximity to an unobserved point. Nearest neighbors for BMI are often found using a distance measure. The Euclidean distance metric was used in [105] to calculate the distance between the target sample and other samples using the equation given below:

$$d(x,y) = \sqrt{\sum_{i=1}^{n} (x_i - y_i)^2} \tag{9.1}$$

where n is the number of features, x_i, y_i is the sample's ith feature, and $d(x, y)$ indicates the distance between x and y samples.

KNN was used to classify EEG signals in [106–108] and employed in [109, 110] for categorizing ECOG signals. In order to classify the signals, Euclidean distance was calculated between them, and a further majority class was assigned to the test signal among its K neighbors. In [111–113], the KNN approach provided better accuracy for classification tasks with improved specificity and sensitivity percentages by non-invasive techniques for detecting epileptic seizures. Moreover, in [109, 113, 114], the invasive technique KNN was found to be more efficient than other classifiers for motor imagery (MI) tasks and decoding finger movements. A subspace KNN technique was used for MI classification in [115]. Each time an arbitrary subspace was chosen, the subspace KNN scheme calculated a new set of KNN. Aggregating K near neighbors in each chosen subspace was used to conduct the majority voting on the test sample's class membership. Recent research [116] used a combined method of recurrent neural network (RNN) and KNN algorithm in human emotion recognition.

- **Linear Discriminative Analysis:** LDA is a type of linear classifier. The major benefits of using LDA are as follows. First, the computational complexity of LDA is less, and hence the time taken for the classification is reduced. This is useful when using the algorithm in an online session. Second, LDA is a simple classifier to use and visualize. Linearity can be a limitation while handling nonlinear data. On the other hand, simpler techniques like

LDA are suitable when small training dataset is available. LDA is used in a number of BMI-controlled humanoid applications for classification. For LDA, decision boundaries are singly connected and convex.

LDA was used by the authors in [117, 118] to categorize EEG signals and in [119, 120] to categorize acquitted ECOG signals by invasive technique.

LDA as an efficient classifier was used in [121] to decode hand flexion and extension and also in [119] to epileptic seizure detection based on ECOG signals. In [122], an aggregated sparse LDA method was used to classify ERP data. By exploiting the conformity between least-squares regression and LDA, the aggregated sparse LDA acquired several discriminant vectors for classification. This method outperformed the traditional LDA and produced superior results for single-test ERP categorization.

- **Support Vector Machine:** SVM is a nonlinear classifier. It is useful in cases when the training data is less. Most of the time, it generalizes better and this makes its use advantageous for BMI systems as the classifiers, once trained, classify brain signals for multiple sessions. The features generated during multiple sessions may vary even for a single user. Hence, the models that are less sensitive to over-fitting may perform better. SVM also performs well with high dimensionality data. However, SVM is sometimes slower than other classifiers, which becomes an issue while dealing with large data. SVM was employed in [107, 108, 123] for classifying EEG signals. The authors in [124–126] used the SVM approach for the identification of children with autism spectrum disorder, seizure detection, and for decoding pilot behavior consciousness based on EEG. EEG signals linked with random words and right and left body movements were classified robustly in [127] using the multi-class SVM approach. The authors in [128] employed a fuzzy kernel-SVM approach for classifying EEG signals. EEG signals were classified by radial basis function (RBF) kernel with the SVM approach in [129].

To categorize ECOG-based signals, [130–132] used the SVM algorithm. SVM for hand and motor can be applied in a wide variety of use-cases. Unfortunately, ANNs are prone to over-fitting, and thus the selection of the parameters/architecture and regularization needs to be done carefully [133].

The authors in [108] employed ANNs for EEG signal categorization and in [134–136] for ECoG signal categorization. It was noticed that the ANNs provided superior classification outputs than other compared techniques. Authors in [137] compared ANN with other classifiers (KNN, LDA, NB, SVM) which is ANN consequences much better accuracy. In [138], ANNs trained using a classical back-propagation scheme were exploited for categorizing EEG signals connected with diverse mental tasks such as math, baseline, figure rotation, visual counting, and letter composing. In [136, 139], ANN was used for decoding of finger movement and activation from ECoG data and it outperformed linear models such as the linear regression model (LRM). In [140], ANNs were used for categorizing six distinct emotions, namely, satisfied, pleasant, happy, frustrated, sad, and fear along with different ML schemes such as KNN, NB, and SVM. The ANN structure employed six outputs and ten hidden layers for classifying distinct emotional states. Results signified that among the exploited ML schemes, ANN displayed good classification performance by providing greater accuracy.

Naive Bayes: In NB, features are assumed to be independent in every class. It forecasts the class C of an arriving instance Z consisting of features $[z_1, ..., z_n]$ through estimating the highest probability using Equation (9.2):

$$p(C_i|Z) = \frac{p(C_i)\prod_j p(z_j \mid C_j)}{p(Z)} \tag{9.2}$$

Imagery recognition shows a significant increment in accuracy in [141–143] compared with other tasks.

The NB method was mainly used in [140, 144] for classifying non-invasive signals like EEG data and in [145] for classifying EGOG data of invasive techniques. It was applied for classifying MI in [146, 147]. The probabilistic NB method was employed in [148] for limb movement classification. In [149], a multinomial NB classifier was used as one of the classification methods for Seizure detection and Prediction of motor and somatosensory functions. The authors in [150] used a weighted NB algorithm to classify EEG-MI signals by assigning a weight for every extracted feature where this approach performed better than various competing techniques in existing works. In [151], the Gaussian naive Bayes (GNB) method was used to categorize EEG-MI signals. By using the NB and the Gaussian distribution, the EEG-MI signals were classified. The experimental assessment reported that GNB showed better performance than two other classical classifiers, namely, SVM and LDA.

9.8.2 Signal decoding: Learning methods

Machine learning, a subset of computational intelligence, relies on patterns in the data extracted by algorithms to explore a specific task without using explicit instructions. Machine learning tasks are generally categorized into several models, such as supervised learning, semi-supervised learning, unsupervised learning, self-supervised learning (SSL), reinforcement learning (RL), FL, etc. The training data for unsupervised machine learning does not have any classifications or labels. An input function or learned representation of data to describe hidden structures, such as clustering or grouping, consists only of input data. The following sections discuss different strategies for learning data from different perspectives, starting with learning from labeled data to unlabeled data. This section will explore learning strategies that can be applied with little labeled data, such as semi-supervised learning, SSL, and unsupervised learning. The reinforcement learning section focuses on the interaction between an agent and brain signals, as well as recent advancements in RL. Due to sensitivity to the privacy of users, we will also discuss some work done on privacy preserving FL opportunities in the FL area. Throughout this section, we will discuss various learning strategies and their applications.

- **Supervised Learning:** With supervised learning, classification and regression tasks can be performed based on the results of the training stage with labeled examples, now that the new data (testing data) has been processed to identify types of events or predict future events. In general, supervised machine learning approaches can be divided into classical algorithms (like linear regression, SVM, etc.) and deep learning-based approaches that use neural networks.

  Some tasks such as emotion recognition [4, 102] and detecting neurodegenerative diseases [152, 153] are examples of classification tasks, while others like speech synthesis [98, 99] and signal enrichment [71, 72, 75, 77] are examples of regression tasks.

  Deep Learning: In the traditional neural network, the weights of the model have to be chosen very carefully. This is a major obstacle in the effective use of the neural network in many applications of BMI. In recent studies, researchers have been using a deep learning approach as deep neural network has high descriptive power and thus improves the accuracy of the system. Deep learning has successful performance in the field of computer vision and in recent years has also been applied in the classification of MI tasks [154, 155]. Deep learning algorithms play an important role in decoding brain signals into tasks such as classification, regression, etc. These algorithms can be used for recognition and speech synthesis [98, 99], sleep spindle identification [100, 101, 156], emotion recognition [4, 102], and for categorizing neurodegenerative diseases [152, 153].

  Nowadays, researchers use many deep learning-based architectures such as DNN, CNN [157], LSTM [158], RNN [159, 160], transformers [161], etc. Classical algorithms require few data and low computation resources compared to deep learning-based models, but they are not as accurate as deep learning-based models. On the other hand, deep learning-based models are more accurate and have more parameters to consider more data features. But training these parameters requires more computation resources and data.

The use of deep learning faces several challenges. To develop a reliable model, the parameters need to be more precise, high-quality features need to be included, and a real dataset is needed. Deep learning models especially require large labeled datasets for training. Creating a dataset with high-quality labels is difficult, expensive, or time-consuming to obtain. However, these issues can be addressed by alternative solutions, which are discussed in the following paragraphs.

- **Semi-Supervised Learning:** The supervised model cannot be efficiently trained without expert labeling, which is one of the major limitations. It is a time-consuming analysis of multiple human experts that is necessary to produce labels, especially for medical tasks that need expensive machinery. By using a few labeled samples, it is difficult to build a successful learning system. Building a successful learning system with a few labeled samples is a challenging task. Comparatively, unlabeled data are publicly available and can be obtained easily or inexpensively. Learning performance can be enhanced by using a large amount of unlabeled data and a few labeled samples. Using semi-supervised learning training strategies can be helpful in such cases; these algorithms have been at the forefront of research in recent years [162–164].

  The difference in existing approaches is on what information to gain from the structure of the unlabeled data. There are many standards for evaluating semi-supervised learning algorithms. In one common approach, we start with a labeled dataset; keep only a few percentages of the labels and treat the rest as unlabeled. Even though this method does not guarantee realistic settings for semi-supervised learning [165], it continues to be the standard evaluation methodology for semi-supervised learning. Recent studies show that adding discrepancies between predictions made on perturbed unlabeled data points to loss function can improve results on standard baselines [166].

  Hence, collecting labeled invasive data is very expensive and labeling them requires neurologists; it is a time-consuming process, but there are lots of unlabeled invasive signals, as such using this method can improve the accuracy of models. For example, [167] uses this method to train an electrographic seizure classifier. On the other hand, this method is widely used for BMI applications using non-invasive signals for tasks such as abnormal signal classification [168], spelling [169], emotion recognition [6], MI recognition [5], effective computing [170], etc.
- **Unsupervised Learning:** Extracting meaningful information from data without supervision or target labels is a challenging area in machine learning. Basic algorithms can be mainly divided into two categories: clustering algorithms (like K-means, DBSCAN, etc.) and dimension reduction

methods (PCA, ICA, t-SNE, etc.). The objective of clustering algorithms is to cluster data that are similar to each other, and the objective of dimension reduction methods is to reduce the dimension of data with keeping important information under many constraints.

A number of breakthroughs have been achieved in machine learning benchmarks as a result of the rise of deep neural networks. Typically, successful models are trained through supervised learning, which requires large datasets annotated for the specific task at hand. The cost of obtaining annotated data can often be prohibitive or even impossible in some cases. As such, there has been increasing attention being paid to unsupervised learning in recent years [171, 172]. These methods mainly try to maximize the mutual information between the input and output of the model. There are various techniques to learn neural networks, and latent representation of data in an unsupervised manner, such as Autoencoder and Contrastive Learning, to name but a few.

Although this type of learning can be helpful for applications of BMI, few projects are done using this strategy. There are lots of invasive and non-invasive unlabeled data, and these methods can be applied to them, especially for invasive data for which collecting labeled records is hard. Here, we mention some works that were done for non-invasive datasets. In EEGGFuseNet [173], authors presented an unsupervised hybrid convolutional recurrent GAN-based characterization and fusion of EEG features. The EEGFuseNet is trained unsupervised, and its spatial and temporal capabilities are automatically characterized. The performance of this model was evaluated in an unsupervised emotion recognition application. As a method for determining latent factors from multichannel EEGs, [174] proposed utilizing an unsupervised deep generative model based on variational autoencoders. By using a sequence modeling approach, we examine how well we can recognize emotions based on latent factors we have learned.

- **Self-Supervised Learning:** Nowadays self-supervised learning is a common technique because data labeling is expensive, and thus high-quality labeled datasets are limited and expensive. Hence, learning a good representation of data structure makes it easier to transfer useful information to a variety of downstream tasks as downstream task has only a few examples and it can be used for zero-shot transfer to new tasks. There have been impressive advancements in SSL methods on a wide range of tasks, including vision [171, 175–179], speech [180], graphs [181, 182], natural language processing [183, 184], and RL [185, 186].

SSL makes use of the underlying data structure to obtain supervisory signals from the data itself. Predicting any unseen or hidden component (or property) of the input from any visible element of the input is the general approach of SSL. For instance, from the current frames in a video (observed data), we can also predict previous or future frames. SSL may employ a range of supervisory signals for a variety of co-occurring modalities and for big datasets without depending on labels by utilizing the structure of the data itself. It is important to note that SSL requires a much greater number of feedback signals than standard supervised learning does, despite its unsupervised nature [187].

Various methods are available for SSL, and here we discuss some of them. The BERT method [184] randomly masks words of the document and tries to predict masked words given the context of the document and tries to predict the next sentence in the training procedure. In GPT [188], training mechanism tries to predict the next word in the document in an auto-regressive way. In MYOW [189], an adaptive selection technique is presented to obtain additional similar views by fitting examples from the entire dataset for augmentation of neural population activity. An augmentation can take two forms: temporal jitter (coupling samples with close timing) and dropout (masking a subset of input channels randomly). The Swap-VAE [190] disentangles the latent representations of multi-unit neural recordings from nonhuman primates according to the latent representations of their augmentation-based self-supervised information maximization latent representations.

Data collection (and labeling) is one of the most challenging tasks in neuroscience. While plentiful labeled data exist, it is rarely clear that these variables—such as behavior or environment—truly reflect an individual's underlying brain state. This is why SSL appeals to neuroscientists in two ways: it has the capacity to represent brain activity robustly without labels, and it can unbiasedly predict an unknown (rather arbitrary) set of variables [191].

Brain signals, in contrast to multicellular recordings, which record the activity of individual neurons, measure general activity in a variety of brain locations. To create representations of these macro-scale brain data, authors in [192] examined various physiological datasets using augmentation and adversarial training techniques, including EEG [193]. Another work examined a variety of temporal pretext tasks used with EEG for patient pathology screening and sleep decoding [194]. Authors in that work proposed a cross-modal deep clustering approach that constructs representations of EEG, ECoG, and behavior in a self-supervised way. Transformer-based models such as BENDR [195] compute latent representations of EEG signals using self-supervised sequence modeling approaches like wave2vec 2.0 [196].

- **Reinforcement Learning:** RL is a learning procedure characterized by trial-and-error search and delayed reward. The goal of RL is to optimize a reward signal by learning what to do in situations and how to take action. By trying various activities, the learner, instead of being told which actions to take, learns which ones yield the maximum reward. Actions may affect not only the immediate reward but also the next situation and, through that, all following rewards [197].

In [198], a framework is presented for integrating a deep reinforcement learning (DRL) model with an implicit human feedback mechanism (with EEG signals) in a practical and sample-efficient way. For the purpose of human-assisted RL algorithms, [198] takes a game as a proxy for a real-life environment. Authors in [199] use EEG signals as features of a Q-learning-based system in order to recommend music as music therapy to improve clinical depression and anxiety. For controlling games, error-related potentials (ErrPs) are used in [198] as feedback of the RL algorithm. Authors in [198] propose and validate an experimentally zero-shot method of learning ErrPs, where ErrPs can be learned for one game and then transferred to other unseen games. The intersection of RL and BMI has various applications that can help humans in various applications such as controlling robots, controlling emotions, VR, etc. Existing works mainly use non-invasive signals as input; however, since invasive signals have better quality and can capture specific zones of brain and neuron connections, the use of invasive signals can therefore lead RL based agents to reach better results.

- **Federated Learning:** FL is a machine learning setting where multiple entities work together under the supervision of a central provider or server to solve a machine learning problem. In order to accomplish the learning objective, focused updates destined for immediate aggregation are used instead of exchanging or transferring raw data between clients. To reduce data consumption, focused updates have a high degree of focus on the minimum necessary information for the particular learning task at hand. Aggregation is performed as early as possible to minimize data usage. According to this definition, FL from fully decentralized (peer-to-peer) learning techniques is different. FL can mitigate many systemic privacy risks and costs associated with traditional, centralized machine learning through focused collection and data minimization. Due to this feature of FL, there has been a significant increase in research and applications in this area in recent years [200].

The success of deep learning-based BCI models is restricted by the lack of large datasets. Because of the high cost of collecting brain signal data and privacy concerns, it is difficult to create a large enough dataset by combining multiple small datasets. Considering that brain signals can reflect brain activity from multiple angles, abuse of brain data can result in serious privacy violations. Thus, organization data exchanges without explicit user approval are prohibited by regulations like the General Data Protection Regulation (GDPR) [201]. In order to protect privacy while analyzing brain signals, it is important to conduct a joint analysis. Thus, FL frameworks may be used to solve this problem [202, 203].

Machine learning can be trained using data from multiple sources without any actual sharing of data due to FL, which is a powerful and emerging technique [204].

According to [204], a deep learning architecture is proposed based on the spatial correlation matrix of EEGs. To protect data privacy, it was adapted to multi-device learning settings based on FL frameworks. An analysis of PhysioNet EEG Motor Movements/Imagery Dataset [205] is also done subject-specifically and subject-adaptively. The results show that FL can achieve the same classification accuracy as state-of-the-art methods without sharing EEG data with others.

FL can be also applied to invasive signals. Furthermore, existing deep learning models can be trained by the FL strategy. As we know, invasive brain data is very sensitive; therefore, due to serious concerns about these data such as data privacy, it is an important learning strategy to learn from multiple devices and protect the privacy of users' data.

9.8.3 Large language models (LLMs) for invasive BMI

Since the introduction of LLMs like GPT-3 and its variants, including Chat-GPT, there has been remarkable growth in their development and application across various domains, such as natural language processing, machine translation, content generation, and more [188]. Naturally, a focus on the use of LLMs in the medical domain has emerged, and the idea of using them in the BMI or BCI tasks has been shared [206]. One of the early works is by Cui et al. [206] which presented Neuro-GPT. Neuro-GPT combines an EEG encoder with a GPT model to process brain signal data. It utilizes both pre-training on large datasets and fine-tuning on specific BCI tasks to achieve robust performance in real-world applications.

In [207], the authors introduced an end-to-end framework for brain signal decoding using LLMs, demonstrating its potential to revolutionize assistive communication technologies. This framework significantly enhances speech neuroprosthetics by integrating LLMs with invasive brain signal decoding. This framework enables the direct conversion of neural signals into speech outputs, removing the need for intermediate processing steps. This innovation holds the potential to enhance communication restoration for individuals with speech impairments.

9.8.4 Adversarial attacks

A BCI provides direct access to external devices via brain signals, typically recorded using brain activity. Those with severe paralysis can use it to communicate or to assist in rehabilitation [208]. In addition to medical applications, recent advancements in devices have made BCIs adaptable for consumer equipment, may provide stress relief [209], or Emotive headsets that may control ground vehicles and drones [210]. A failure of a BCI system could result in misdiagnoses, user frustration, or even physical harm while driving a wheelchair or operating a drone [211, 212]. Even though deep learning models have state-of-the-art performance, recent studies have demonstrated their vulnerability against adversarial examples, which can degrade the performance of a well-trained model by adding small imperceptible perturbations. For example, in a classification task, an adversarial perturbation can be attached to the other labels sometimes that are irrelevant to data, and the attacker does this in order to cause disorder or crash the system [213]. Using adversarial examples to classify images can deceive a deep learning model into giving incorrect labels for images [214, 215]. In addition to speech recognition and malware classification, semantic segmentation and many other techniques have also been subjected to adversarial attacks [216–218]. Adversarial attacks can be divided into two classes, white-box and black-box attacks. In the white-box attack, the attacker has full control of the model architecture and parameters. A gradient-based strategy or an optimization-based strategy can, therefore, be used to attack by adding perturbations to the calculated direction. Various algorithms have been proposed to generate adversarial examples, including the fast gradient sign method (FGSM) [214], the C&W method [219], L-BFGS [215], the basic iterative method [220], Deep Fool [221], etc. In the black-box attack scenario, the attacker only observes how a target model responds to inputs but does not know anything about the model's architecture, parameters, and training data. In order to generate adversarial examples, the attacker must limit the magnitude of perturbations and limit the number of queries. They were however inefficient when it came to querying: to build a substitute model sufficiently similar to the target model, they typically required a large number of queries. Based on the transferability, authors in [222] presented an adversarial attack method for creating black-box substitute models and attacking black-box target models. Some works have been done in order to attack non-invasive based models. Due to a lack of invasive data and hard-to-access invasive data sets, there is not such work in models that take invasive signals as input, but attacks on invasive devices can cause dangerous effects, especially when the device stimulates brain neurons. Next, we review some related work on models that exploit non-invasive signals.

According to [223], adversarial examples for black-box attacks on EEG-based BCIs can be done using unsupervised fast gradient sign methods (UFGSM). Authors in [224] introduce a query synthesis-based active learning strategy to transferability-based black-box attacks of EEG-based BCIs. Authors in [225] provide a practical adversarial example. An EEG trial can be preprocessed with this signal before the square-shaped signal is added. An interesting aspect of the attack is that it is described as a backdoor key, which implies that the attacker could have access directly to the training dataset and pollute it with adversarial examples.

9.9 Signal encoding and stimulation

Electrical brain stimulation and other neuromodulation techniques can be used as a treatment for a variety of neurological disorders including movement disorders, pain, and epilepsy. These therapies are carried out by activating or inhibiting the brain with electricity. The electricity can be induced by either implanting electrodes directly in the brain or placing them on the scalp. Also, applying magnetic fields to the head can induce brain neurons. Although these types of therapies are less frequently used than medication and psychotherapies, they hold promise for treating certain mental disorders that do not respond to other treatments.

There are some methods for brain stimulation, including electroconvulsive therapy (ECT) [226], vagus nerve stimulation (VNS) [227], rTMS [228, 229], magnetic seizure therapy (MST) [230], and DBS [231]. A summary of methods and side effects of these devices can be found in Table 9.2.

TABLE 9.2 Summary of brain stimulation devices, methods, and their side effects

Device	Side effects	Method
Electroconvulsive Therapy	Headache, upset stomach, muscle aches, memory loss	Non-invasive
Repetitive Transcranial Magnetic Stimulation	Some patients actually get worse, with voice changes, hoarseness, cough or sore throat, neck pain, difficulty swallowing discomfort, or tingling in the area	Non-invasive
Repetitive Transcranial Magnetic Stimulation	Discomfort at the head site, mild headaches, brief lightheadedness, or seizure; during the treatment, the scalp, jaw, or face muscles may contract with the magnet and have some effects on them	Non-invasive
Magnetic Seizure Therapy	Same as ECT, MST has risks that can be caused by anesthesia exposure and the induction of a seizure	Non-invasive
Deep Brain Stimulation	Side effects form of brain surgery, bleeding in the brain or stroke, infection; disorientation or confusion, unwelcome mood changes, movement difficulties, lightheadedness, and difficulty sleeping are all possible	Invasive
Neuralink	Side effects form of brain surgery	Invasive

9.9.1   Electroconvulsive therapy

ECT is an electric current used to treat mental disorders. Typically, this type of treatment is used when all other treatments (such as antidepressant medications or psychotherapy) have failed to improve the patient's condition. On the other hand, this therapy has some side effects such as headache, upset stomach, muscle aches, and memory loss.

ECT is a non-invasive procedure that uses electrodes placed at specific sites on the head. A current of electricity passes through the electrodes into the brain causing a seizure that lasts less than a minute [226].

9.9.2   Vagus nerve stimulation

VNS works through a device implanted under the skin that sends electrical pulses through the left vagus nerve, half of a prominent pair of nerves that run from the brainstem through the neck and down to each side of the chest and abdomen. The vagus nerves carry messages from the brain to the body's major organs (e.g., heart, lungs, and intestines) and to areas of the brain that control mood, sleep, and other functions.

Electrical pulses are sent to the left vagus nerve through a device which is inserted under the skin to deliver the therapy. A major function of the nervous system is sending signals to the body's organs and to various parts of the brain related to moods, sleep, and other functions. For this therapy, a small device is surgically implanted in the upper left side of the chest called a pulse generator. There is an electrical lead wire connected to the left vagus nerve to drive the pulse generator [227]. VNS treatment is used to reduce symptoms of depression; some patients will not respond to this method, and some actually get worse. Also, VNS has some side effects such as voice changes or hoarseness, cough or sore throat, neck pain, discomfort or tingling in the area where the device is implanted, breathing problems, especially during exercise, and difficulty swallowing [226].

9.9.3   Repetitive transcranial magnetic stimulation

This method is a non-invasive method that tries to stimulate the brain by using a magnate. rTMS has been studied as a treatment for depression, psychosis, anxiety, and other disorders.

This treatment includes holding a coil against the forehead near the area of the brain associated with mood control. The magnetic pulses that are transmitted from the coil easily pass through the skull and cause small electrical flows that stimulate nerve cells in the targeted brain region [228]. During the treatment, scientists can select which parts of the brain will be affected and which will not. The magnetic field in this treatment has the same strength as that of a magnetic resonance imaging (MRI) scan. An rTMS session usually lasts between 30 and 60 minutes without requiring anesthesia.

In some cases, the patient may have discomfort at the head site, especially at the place of the magnet, and during the treatment, the scalp, jaw, or face muscles may contract with the magnet and have some effects on them. Also, it may result in the mild headaches, brief lightheadedness, or seizure; however, long-term side effects are unknown.

The main advantage of this method over ECT is that rTMS can be targeted to a specific region in the brain because focusing on a specific part of the brain decreases the chances of side effects associated with ECT [226].

9.9.4 Magnetic seizure therapy

MST is an alternative to ECT that may not adversely affect memory. MST tries to keep the effectiveness of ECT and reduce its cognitive side effects. This method is like both ECT and rTMS, for stimulating a specific target in the brain, uses magnetic pulses instead of electricity, and aims to induce a seizure-like ECT. Hence, the pulses have a higher frequency than that used in rTMS. Therefore, like ECT, in order to prevent movement and muscle relaxation, the patient should be anesthetized.

Same as ECT, MST has risks that can be caused by anesthesia exposure and the induction of a seizure. MST produces fewer memory side effects, shorter seizures, and allows for a shorter recovery time than ECT [226, 230].

9.9.5 Deep brain stimulation

DBS was developed for treating Parkinson's disease symptoms such as tremors, stiffness, walking difficulties, and uncontrollable movements. In this method, a generator that is inserted in the chest controls a pair of electrodes implanted in the brain, sending out continuous signals customized to fit the individual.

During DBS, the brain is surgically shaved and then attached to a sturdy frame to prevent the head from moving. During the procedure, the head is fixed to this frame and the patient is awake to give feedback to the surgeon. Two holes are drilled into the head, then a thin tube is threaded into the brain by the surgeon to place electrodes on either side of a specific brain area. This is followed by general anesthesia. In the chest, electrode wires are attached to battery-operated generators and transmit electrical pulses to brain electrodes [232].

DBS comes with similar risk factors as any other form of brain surgery. Bleeding in the brain or stroke, infection, disorientation or confusion, unwelcome mood changes, movement difficulties, lightheadedness, and difficulty sleeping are all possible side effects of the operation. Other adverse effects that have not been documented yet are possible because the method is currently being researched. Long-term benefits and adverse effects have yet to be determined [226].

9.9.6 Neuralink chips

Elon Musk unveiled Neuralink's implantable brain chip, the Link version 0.9, in 2019 [233]. It is undoubtedly the most advanced BCI designed to be implanted directly into the brain by a surgical robot (Figure 9.6e). The chip plugs into many areas of the brain directly by tiny microscopic threads (Figure 9.6c). They are about 1/20th of the width of a human hair. Link can process, stimulate, and transmit brain signals wirelessly (Figure 9.6d). The entire operation is done by the robot with tiny arms (Figure 9.6a, 9.6b) precisely instead of human hands to completely eliminate associated risks. It is the same-day surgery, performed without a large incision or general anesthesia. They remove about a coin sized piece of skull and the person can walk around right after the surgery. [234] Neuralink enables its users to control their phone, keyboard, and mouse directly with the brain by recording and analyzing brain signals with the smartphone applications. For doing this process, they built an application exercise for users to control the device [233]. Many strategies meant to control the activity of whole-brain regions, rather than to transport information to and from the brain, have been considered. As a result, they have fewer electrodes (fewer than ten) and are substantially thicker than Neuralink threads. For example, DBS leads have just four to eight electrodes and are 800 times thicker. With over 1024 channels of input from the brain, Neuralink can deliver unparalleled scalable data. The Link will also detect spikes in real-time on each channel, and this information will be relayed wirelessly.

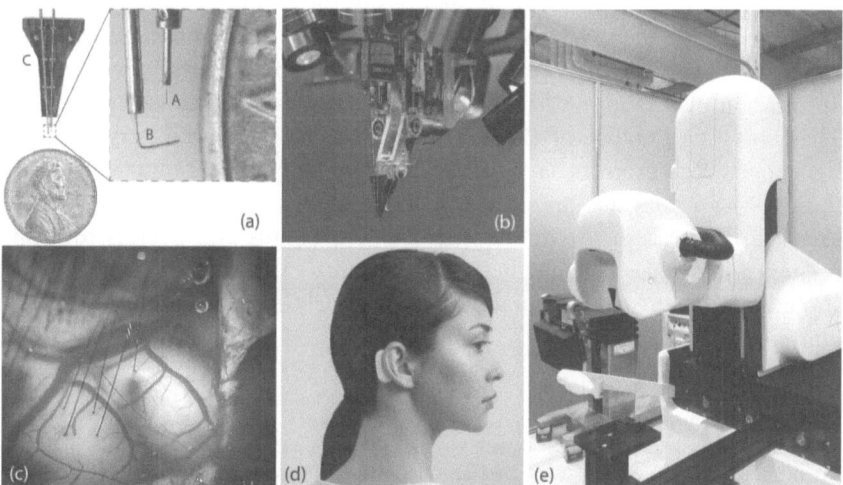

FIGURE 9.6   The Neuralink robotic system for brain implant insertion: (a) Close-up of ultra-thin robotic needles, (b) Robotic implantation device, (c) Implanted microscopic electrode threads in brain tissue, (d) External wearable Neuralink device, (e) Full Neuralink robotic system (reproduced from Neuralink [234]).

9.10   Challenges

The development and deployment of BMI applications face non-technical and technical challenges. Ethical concerns are major non-technical hindrances of the development and deployment of technology that directly interact with the human body, and BMI is no exception. Implementation challenges include cost, data privacy, machine capability, etc. We elaborate on these challenges next.

9.10.1   Ethical challenges

AI is gradually merging with neurotech and has the potential to have an impact not only on quality of life, particularly for someone suffering from diseases such as SCI, Parkinson's disease, paralysis, etc., but also on the development of new technologies. Ethical concerns are rising about whether the technology will serve medical and industrial sector or like other technology being involved in the privacy, security, and stability concerns. Combining current advances in technology with neuroscience may lead to progress in different areas of human existence and may lead to global uniform regulation.

9.10.1.1   Bias

The development of these technologies has seen some limitations. The challenges stem from the initial target markets of these applications or the nature of their training data, which may result in biases, including those related to gender or race, particularly evident in AI-based applications. For example, an application may work well on men but does not perform as well on women. These may be because of their training data or their brain structure, etc. Recent research projects have focused on finding ways to remove or prevent these biases in various applications. In addition, we suggest that potential users be involved in the development of algorithms and devices to ensure prejudice is discussed from the very beginning of their development which should lead to greater acceptability, particularly for those who are already marginalized.

9.10.1.2   Privacy and security

Today, due to the sensitivity of brain-related datasets, concerns about information misuse can arise, and protecting the privacy of users is a challenging task. When the neuro data of a person is protected from seeing, intrusion, analysis, accumulation, or interference by third parties or unlicensed neurotech gadgets, it is called "brain shielding" [235]. Applications should be designed to give access to information only to persons to whom they give permission, such as doctors. However, storing these datasets is another problem due to their volume, transferability, and other factors. The information is useful for training models or someone who wants their neuron's activities. It is better for applications to adapt these activities to the users on the device without any connection from other servers or sources. Additionally, companies can use FL methods instead of directly collecting data, and applications can be designed to encrypt the information on the device for security.

Another challenge of the applications is the model robustness, especially applications that are based on machine learning and are noise sensitive. They can be fooled by noises as discussed in adversarial attacks. Neuroimplants with impaired or disabled functionality may have disastrous effects, so data security is essential. "Brainjacking" or malicious changes in the algorithms may be caused by exploiting several vulnerabilities in the system. Models can be robust by various techniques that are discussed in the machine learning literature. These attacks can be done in a targeted way to force or encourage users distributing their actions.

Neuro data protection is a set of technologies, standards, and guidelines that protect neuro data and data inferred from neurotech from unapproved users' entry, disclosure, alteration, or damage [235]. Creating justice in protecting the privacy of individuals leads to gaining popularity and legal acceptance in all countries of the world.

9.10.1.2.1 Human Identity

Personal, complicated, and dynamic manifestation of different fields of human reality is not restricted to biology, culture, ecology, experiences, and historic sociopolitical situations. All these things build each person's distinct concept about meaning, in relation to people and the world as well as self-concepts and possession, a phenomenon which is both special and literally imprinted within the nervous system while also being affected by outer pressure and societal constructs [235].

9.10.1.2.2 Fairness

This technology could be available to every person in the world and be treated fairly and justly. Products designed for neurotech can't be designed to meet the needs of a specific social class. There can be limitations that make it difficult for neurotech capabilities and participation in neurotech design to be accessed. Neurotech gives solutions to those limitations and neuro data explanation is another factor that causes discrimination [235].

9.10.1.2.3 Accuracy and Efficiency

Even though applications can be helpful, they can also be harmful, especially in the applications that stimulate the brain or can lead the user to dangerous situations. Applications can misclassify signals or encode them incorrectly. This can stimulate neuron signals completely wrong, resulting in chromatic nerves or even irreparable damage and the user's death.

When assessing neuro data, neurotech [235] provides explanations, as well as code designed by them to modify the nervous system. They are forthright and honest about neurotechnology's capabilities and their application of neuro data, as well as any conclusions that are drawn.

9.10.1.2.4 Well-Being

When designing or implementing neurotech (or using related neural data) products, the application should satisfy the user to a physical and mental state (including health, safety, happiness, and comfort) as a priority. It is very important to be able to create this feeling of satisfaction in people who use this technology.

9.10.1.2.5 Social Issues

Interaction with machines increases as a result of BMI, which leads to a diminishing interaction among people. Moreover, as technology tends to widen inequalities in society, BMIs will do the same, by providing benefits to those who can afford them [27].

9.10.2 Implementation Challenges

Clearly, all of the above-mentioned ideas come with their design and implantation issues. We are at the early stages of development currently; however, this fascinating project drives us to come up with mind-blowing ideas that require managing the implementation challenges to use the technology for human benefits.

9.10.2.1 Cost

Gradually, with the advancement of this technology and the emergence of newer and more expensive versions, it may cause class distance and at the same time lead to the domination of the richer group to other classes due to affordability of the newer versions. The manufacturers of this technology should support their software from older models that may reduce this domination.

9.10.2.2 Implant monitoring

Data security, data ownership, and handling large amounts of data are some of the challenges in this field. When 250 channels are recorded at 30 kHz, micro-electrode recordings generate 115 GB of data per hour which is a significant volume [236]. This amount of data is beyond the capacity of many hospital systems currently in place. High-performance computing (HPC) systems and cloud-based computing may provide solutions that scale with increasing data storage and processing demands [236]. The use of distributed algorithms or FL algorithms (as discussed in Section 8.2) in device computing cores is another solution.

9.10.2.3 Chips

The little electrical impulses that each electrode records must be transformed by the Link into current neuronal information. High-performance signal amplifiers and digitizers are required for the Link since the neural signals in the brain are tiny (micro-volts). Additionally, when the number of electrodes rises, the amount of information included in these raw signals is too large to upload using low power devices. These technologies must be able to identify and characterize brain spikes on a real-time basis in the chip. While significantly decreasing per-channel chip size and power consumption in comparison to the existing technologies, Link's customized chips can achieve such real-time analysis [234].

9.10.2.4 Hermetic packaging

It is important to keep the fluid and salts in the brain away from the Link. An enclosure made from biocompatible materials, replacing the skull physically, and having over 1,000 electrical channels can be challenging to make water-proof, but the challenge is multiplied when it is made from biocompatible materials, replaces the skull, and has over 1,000 electrical channels. Neuralink is developing cutting-edge techniques to construct and seal each significant component of the package. By creating components as a single component, it can reduce device size and remove failure points by replacing the connection between several components [234].

9.10.2.5 Neural decoding

In order to use brain spikes for computer control, the spikes must first be decoded. Scientists in academic labs have created computer programs that decode hundreds of neurons' activity to control a virtual computer mouse. This technology will enable electrical gadgets to be controlled more accurately and realistically by capturing more neurons. Through this method, they seek to increase the effectiveness and robustness of neural decoding by leveraging current developments in statistics and algorithm design. The implanted device is controlled using these algorithms in real-time. A challenging aspect of designing adaptive algorithms is ensuring that they remain reliable and stable while improving over time [234]. List of abbreviations presented in Table 9.3.

TABLE 9.3 List of abbreviations used in this chapter

Number	Abbreviations	Definition	Number	Abbreviations	Definition
1	AI	Artificial Intelligence	42	EMD	Empirical-Mode Decomposition
2	BMI	Brain–Machine Interface	43	CCA	Canonical Correlation Analysis
3	CNS	Central Nervous System	44	CAR	Common Average Reference
4	PNS	Peripheral Nervous System	45	GAN	Generative Adversarial Network
5	BCI	Brain–Computer Interface	46	SSVEP	Steady State Visually Evoked Potential
6	DBS	Deep Brain Stimulation	47	LFP	Local Field Potential
7	tDCS	transcranial Direct Current Stimulation	48	LSTM	Long Short Term Memory
8	SCI	Spinal Cord Injury	49	FD	Fractal Dimension
9	EEG	Electroencephalography	50	IFT	Inverse Fourier Transform
10	ECoG	Electrocorticography	51	DFT	Discretely Sampled Data
11	ERD	Event-Related Desynchronization	52	FFT	Fast Fourier Transform
12	PD	Parkinson's Disease	53	MF	Matched Filtering
13	IPG	Implantable Pulse Generator	54	STFT	Short-Time Fourier Transform
14	TMS	Transcranial Magnetic Stimulation	55	CSP	Common Spatial Pattern
15	ASD	Autism Spectrum Disorder	56	CSSP	Common Sparse Spectral-Spatial Pattern
16	ILAE	International League Against Epilepsy	57	WCSP	Wavelet Common Spatial Pattern
17	DLPFC	Dorsolateral Prefrontal Cortex	58	LDA	Linear Discriminant Analysis
18	rTMS	repetitive Transcranial Magnetic Stimulation	59	SVM	Support Vector Machines
19	ANI	Artificial Narrow Intelligence	60	ANN	Artificial Neural Network
20	AGI	Artificial General Intelligence	61	LDA	Linear Discriminant Analysis
21	ASI	Artificial Super Intelligence	62	NN	Neural Network
22	HMM	Hidden Markov Model	63	DNN	Deep Neural Network
23	MS	Multiple Sclerosis	64	KNN	K-Nearest Neighbor
24	CBI	Computer-to-Brain Interface	65	MI	Motor Imagery

(Continued)

TABLE 9.3 (Continued)

Number	Abbreviations	Definition	Number	Abbreviations	Definition
25	NIRS	Near Infrared Spectroscopy	66	RNN	Recurrent Neural Network
26	fMRI	functional Magnetic Resonance Imaging	67	ERP	Event-Related Potential
27	PET	Positron Emission Tomography	68	RBF	Radial Basis Function
28	SNR	Signal-to-Noise Ratio	69	LRM	Linear Regression Model
29	LFP	Local Field Potential	70	GNB	Gaussian Naive Bayes
30	AR	Augmented Reality	71	ICA	Independent Component Analysis
31	SUA	Single Unit Activity	72	t-SNE	t-Distributed Stochastic Neighbor Embedding
32	MUA	Multi-Unit Activity	73	SSL	Self-Supervised Learning
33	CSF	Cerebrospinal Fluid	74	DRL	Deep Reinforcement Learning
34	MEG	Magnetoencephalography	75	RL	Reinforcement Learning
35	BOLD	Blood Oxygen Level Dependence	76	ErrP	Error-related Potential
36	fNIRT	functional Near Infrared Topography	77	GDPR	General Data Protection Regulation
37	SPECT	Single Positron Emission Computed Tomography	78	FGSM	Fast Gradient Sign Method
38	AP	Action Potential	79	UFGSM	Unsupervised Fast Gradient Sign Methods
39	VR	Virtual Reality	80	VNS	Vagus Nerve Stimulation
40	PCA	Principal Component Analysis	81	MST	Magnetic Seizure Therapy
41	BSS	Blind Source Separation	82	ECT	Electroconvulsive Therapy

9.10.2.6 Mechanical damage

Although current devices have considered many aspects, mechanical damages to electrodes, stems, ligaments, and other implant components still need to be considered. Recent reports show evidence of mechanical damage to parts of the recording system during or after planting. Crisp materials are more prone to failure, so it is recommended to use harder and more flexible materials. The first barrier to new achievements is their so-called "adaptive decoding algorithm"; the algorithm is implemented on the device itself with the task of processing APs in real-time. Algorithm time and battery usage optimization can increase its efficiency dramatically. Another challenge they face is security issues because all of the device's connections are based on Bluetooth wireless communication technology, from charging the link to its outside connections [234].

9.11 Conclusions

Invasive BMI is an emerging technology that has an enormous potential beyond the obvious applications, such as improving the lives of patients with SCI or Parkinson's disease. Beyond the medical applications, this technology can provide immense benefits in other applications, such as advanced AI-based education, communication among human–machine systems, etc. To develop innovative applications of invasive BMI, an understanding of biological and engineering key concepts that underpin this technology is necessary. In this chapter, we highlighted the recent developments in the field of BMI by analyzing recent literature. Specifically, we have provided the developing signal sensing technologies and discussed applying computational approaches to interpret and decode brain signal data. In this chapter, we systematically surveyed the recent advancements in dry sensors, wearable devices, signal enhancement, signal decoding, deep learning, etc., for BMIs. We focused on explaining the brain structure and studied computational methods and strategies, especially machine learning-based methods, for decoding brain signals with a focus on invasive signals. Furthermore, we addressed brain signal stimulation and discussed challenges of implementing these technologies including ethical issues. The various computational intelligence approaches enable us to learn reliable brain cortex features and understand human knowledge from signals. We summarized the recent brain signal encoding and decoding methods, followed by discussing dominant machine learning-based models for BMI applications. We also provided an overview of healthcare applications and pointed out the open challenges and future directions.

References

1 T Liam Herman, Michael-Brian C Ogawa and Martha E Crosby. Utilizing current technologies to foster augmented on-line learning. In *International Conference on Human-Computer Interaction*, pages 400–406. Springer, 2021.

2 Eduardo López-Larraz, A Sarasola-Sanz, N Irastorza-Landa, N Birbaumer and A Ramos-Murguialday. Brain-machine interfaces for rehabilitation in stroke: A review. *NeuroRehabilitation*, 43(1):77–97, 2018.

3 Jonathan R Wolpaw, José del R Millán and Nick F Ramsey. Brain-computer interfaces: Definitions and principles. *Handbook of clinical neurology*, 168:15–23, 2020.

4 Salma Alhagry, Aly Aly Fahmy and Reda A El-Khoribi. Emotion recognition based on EEG using LSTM recurrent neural network. *Emotion*, 8(10):355–358, 2017.

5 Minjie Liu, Mingming Zhou, Tao Zhang and Naixue Xiong. Semi-supervised learning quantization algorithm with deep features for motor imagery EEG recognition in smart healthcare application. *Applied soft computing*, 89:106071, 2020.

6 Guangyi Zhang and Ali Etemad. Deep recurrent semi-supervised EEG representation learning for emotion recognition. In *2021 9th International Conference on Affective Computing and Intelligent Interaction (ACII)*, pages 1–8. IEEE, 2021.

7 Lan Luan, Jacob T Robinson, Behnaam Aazhang, Taiyun Chi, Kaiyuan Yang, Xue Li, Haad Rathore, Amanda Singer, Sudha Yellapantula, Yingying Fan, et al. Recent advances in electrical neural interface engineering: Minimal invasiveness, longevity, and scalability. *Neuron*, 108(2):302–321, 2020.

8 Munima Haque, Salman Khan Promon, et al. Neural implants: A review of current trends and future perspectives. Europe PMC 2022. Preprint, doi: 10.20944/ preprints202202.0050.v1.

9 Usman Salahuddin and Pu-Xian Gao. Signal generation, acquisition, and processing in brain machine interfaces: A unified review. *Frontiers in neuroscience*, 15: 1174, 2021.

10 SK Pahuja and Karan Veer, et al. Recent approaches on classification and feature extraction of EEG signal: A review. *Robotica*, 40(1): 1–25, 2022.

11 Swati Aggarwal and Nupur Chugh. Review of machine learning techniques for EEG based brain computer interface. *Archives of computational methods in engineering*, 29(5): 1–20, 2022.

12 Xiayin Zhang, Ziyue Ma, Huaijin Zheng, Tongkeng Li, Kexin Chen, Xun Wang, Chenting Liu, Linxi Xu, Xiaohang Wu, Duoru Lin, et al. The combination of brain-computer interfaces and artificial intelligence: Applications and challenges. *Annals of translational medicine*, 8(11), 2020.

13 Adrien B Rapeaux and Timothy G Constandinou. Implantable brain machine interfaces: First-in-human studies, technology challenges and trends. *Current opinion in biotechnology*, 72:102–111, 2021.

14 Franklin R. Amthor, Anne B. Theibert, David G. Standaert and Erik D. Roberson. *Essentials of Modern Neuroscience*. McGraw Hill, New York, NY, 2020.

15 Kerry R Mills. *Oxford Textbook of Clinical Neurophysiology*. Oxford University Press, 2017.

16 Charles Frye. What is the ionic basis of the basic features of an action potential? Foundational Neuroscience, 2016. Retrieved from https://charlesfrye.github.io/ FoundationalNeuroscience//23/.

17 Alejandra T Rabadán. Neurochips: Considerations from a neurosurgeon's standpoint. *Surgical neurology international*, 12, 2021.

18 Royal Society. *iHuman: Blurring Lines between Mind and Machine*. Royal Society, 2019.

19 Yurt Kıymet Kubra and Suleyman Kaplan. As a painkiller: A review of pre-and postnatal non-steroidal anti-inflammatory drug exposure effects on the nervous systems. *Inflammopharmacology*, 26(1):15–28, 2018.

20 Arshad Majid. *Electroceuticals*. Springer, 2017.

21 Matthew D Johnson, Hubert H Lim, Theoden I Netoff, Allison T Connolly, Nessa Johnson, Abhrajeet Roy, Abbey Holt, Kelvin O Lim, James R Carey, Jerrold L Vitek, et al. Neuromodulation for brain disorders: Challenges and opportunities. *IEEE transactions on biomedical engineering*, 60(3):610–624, 2013.

22 Iona Novak, Catherine Morgan, Michael Fahey, Megan Finch-Edmondson, Claire Galea, Ashleigh Hines, Katherine Langdon, Maria Mc Namara, Madison CB Paton, Himanshu Popat, et al. State of the evidence traffic lights 2019: Systematic review of interventions for preventing and treating children with cerebral palsy. *Current neurology and neuroscience reports*, 20(2):1–21, 2020.

23 Louis DV Johnson, Mark R Pickard and William EB Johnson. The comparative effects of mesenchymal stem cell transplantation therapy for spinal cord injury in humans and animal models: A systematic review and meta-analysis. *Biology*, 10(3):230, 2021.

24 Iahn Cajigas and Aditya Vedantam. Brain-computer interface, neuromodulation, and neurorehabilitation strategies for spinal cord injury. *Neurosurgery clinics*, 32(3):407–417, 2021.

25 Pedro Cruz-Vicente, Luís A Passarinha, Samuel Silvestre and Eugenia Gallardo. Recent developments in new therapeutic agents against Alzheimer and Parkinson diseases: In-silico approaches. *Molecules*, 26(8):2193, 2021.

26 Sharvari Lotankar, Kedar S Prabhavalkar and Lokesh K Bhatt. Biomarkers for Parkinson's disease: Recent advancement. *Neuroscience bulletin*, 33(5):585–597, 2017.

27 Dimitri Gurtner. Neuralink and beyond: Challenges of creating an enhanced human. 2021. Retrieved from https://folia.unifr.ch/unifr/documents/309154.

28 Malinda L Pennington, Douglas Cullinan and Louise B Southern. Defining autism: Variability in state education agency definitions of and evaluations for autism spectrum disorders. *Autism research and treatment*, 2014 (1), 2014.

29 Christina Luckhardt, Sara Boxhoorn, Magdalena Schütz, Nikola Fann and Christine M Freitag. Brain stimulation by tDCS as treatment option in autism spectrum disorder—A systematic literature review. *Progress in brain research*, 264:233–257, 2021.

30 Khan Academy. overview of neuron structure and function. https://www.khanacademy.org/science/biology/human-biology/neuron-nervous-system/a/overview-of-neuron-structure-and-function

31 Robert S Fisher. Redefining epilepsy. *Current opinion in neurology*, 28(2):130–135, 2015.

32 Ioannis Karageorgos, Karthik Sriram, Ján Veselý, Michael Wu, Marc Powell, David Borton, Rajit Manohar and Abhishek Bhattacharjee. Hardware-software co-design for brain-computer interfaces. In *2020 ACM/IEEE 47th Annual International Symposium on Computer Architecture (ISCA)*, pages 391–404. IEEE, 2020.

33 Mladen Veletić and Ilangko Balasingham. Synaptic communication engineering for future cognitive brain–machine interfaces. *Proceedings of the IEEE*, 107(7):1425–1441, 2019.

34 Stephanie H Ameis, Daniel M Blumberger, Paul E Croarkin, Donald J Mabbott, Meng-Chuan Lai, Pushpal Desarkar, Peter Szatmari and Zafiris J Daskalakis. Treatment of executive function deficits in autism spectrum disorder with repetitive transcranial magnetic stimulation: A double-blind, sham-controlled, pilot trial. *Brain stimulation*, 13(3):539–547, 2020.

35 Jerome C Glenn. *Work/technology: 2050 Scenarios and Actions*. Millennium Project, 2019.

36 Mara Di Berardo. A global discussion about our possible futures during the 2021 world future day. *Futures*, 136: 102905, 2022.

37 Jennifer Preece. Citizen science: New research challenges for human–computer interaction. *International journal of human-computer interaction*, 32(8):585–612, 2016.

38 Donald S Faber and Alberto E Pereda. Two forms of electrical transmission between neurons. *Frontiers in molecular neuroscience*, 11: 427, 2018.

39 Alexander N Pisarchik, Vladimir A Maksimenko and Alexander E Hramov. From novel technology to novel applications: Comment on "an integrated brain-machine interface platform with thousands of channels" by Elon Musk and Neuralink. *Journal of medical internet research*, 21(10):e16356, 2019.

40 Yossi Buskila, Alba Bellot-Saez and John W Morley. Generating brain waves, the power of astrocytes. *Frontiers in neuroscience*, 13:1125, 2019.

41 James A Frank, Marc-Joseph Antonini and Polina Anikeeva. Next-generation interfaces for studying neural function. *Nature biotechnology*, 37(9):1013–1023, 2019.

42 Marcel Van Gerven, Jason Farquhar, Rebecca Schaefer, Rutger Vlek, Jeroen Geuze, Anton Nijholt, Nick Ramsey, Pim Haselager, Louis Vuurpijl, Stan Gielen, et al. The brain–computer interface cycle. *Journal of neural engineering*, 6(4):041001, 2009.

43 Gert Pfurtscheller, Brendan Z Allison, Günther Bauernfeind, Clemens Brunner, Teodoro Solis Escalante, Reinhold Scherer, Thorsten O Zander, Gernot Mueller-Putz, Christa Neuper and Niels Birbaumer. The hybrid BCI. *Frontiers in neuroscience*, 4:3, 2010.

44 Mikhail A Lebedev and Miguel AL Nicolelis. Brain–machine interfaces: Past, present and future. *Trends in neurosciences*, 29(9):536–546, 2006.

45 Gerwin Schalk, Jan Kubanek, Kai J Miller, NR Anderson, Eric C Leuthardt, Jeffrey G Ojemann, Dave Limbrick, Daniel Moran, Lester A Gerhardt and Jonathan R Wolpaw. Decoding two-dimensional movement trajectories using electrocorticographic signals in humans. *Journal of neural engineering*, 4(3):264, 2007.

46 Taro Kaiju, Keiichi Doi, Masashi Yokota, Kei Watanabe, Masato Inoue, Hiroshi Ando, Kazutaka Takahashi, Fumiaki Yoshida, Masayuki Hirata and Takafumi Suzuki. High spatiotemporal resolution ECoG recording of somatosensory evoked potentials with flexible micro-electrode arrays. *Frontiers in neural circuits*, 11:20, 2017.

47 Rafael Yuste. From the neuron doctrine to neural networks. *Nature reviews neuroscience*, 16(8):487–497, 2015.

48 Miguel AL Nicolelis and Mikhail A Lebedev. Principles of neural ensemble physiology underlying the operation of brain–machine interfaces. *Nature reviews neuroscience*, 10(7):530–540, 2009.

49 Donald L Schomer and Fernando Lopes Da Silva. *Niedermeyer's Electroencephalography: Basic Principles, Clinical Applications, and Related Fields*. Lippincott Williams & Wilkins, 2012.

50 Claudio Babiloni, Claudio Del Percio, Paolo M Rossini, Nicola Marzano, Marco Iacoboni, Francesco Infarinato, Roberta Lizio, Marina Piazza, Mirella Pirritano, Giovanna Berlutti, et al. Judgment of actions in experts: A high-resolution EEG study in elite athletes. *Neuroimage*, 45(2):512–521, 2009.

51 Mehrdad Fatourechi, Ali Bashashati, Rabab K Ward and Gary E Birch. EMG and EOG artifacts in brain computer interface systems: A survey. *Clinical neurophysiology*, 118(3):480–494, 2007.

52 Malcolm Proudfoot, Mark W. Woolrich, Anna C. Nobre, and Martin R. Turner. *Magnetoencephalography*. Practical Neurology, 14(5):336–343, 2014.

53 Seiji Ogawa, Tso-Ming Lee, Asha S Nayak and Paul Glynn. Oxygenation-sensitive contrast in magnetic resonance image of rodent brain at high magnetic fields. *Magnetic resonance in medicine*, 14(1):68–78, 1990.

54 Nikos K Logothetis, Jon Pauls, Mark Augath, Torsten Trinath and Axel Oeltermann. Neurophysiological investigation of the basis of the fMRI signal. *Nature*, 412(6843):150–157, 2001.

55 H Owen-Reece, M Smith, CE Elwell and JC Goldstone. Near infrared spectroscopy. *British journal of anaesthesia*, 82(3):418–426, 1999.

56 Leonardo Rodrigues Limongi, Radu Bojoi, Giovanni Griva and Alberto Tenconi. Digital current-control schemes. *IEEE industrial electronics magazine*, 3(1):20–31, 2009.

57 GT Herman. Image reconstruction from projections. The fundamentals of computerized tomography, 316, 1980.

58 Jeffrey A Fessler and John M Ollinger. Signal processing pitfalls in positron emission tomography. *IEEE signal processing magazine*, 14(1):43–55, 1997.

59 Andrei Belitski, Arthur Gretton, Cesare Magri, Yusuke Murayama, Marcelo A Montemurro, Nikos K Logothetis and Stefano Panzeri. Low-frequency local field potentials and spikes in primary visual cortex convey independent visual information. *Journal of neuroscience*, 28(22):5696–5709, 2008.

60 Carsten Mehring, Jörn Rickert, Eilon Vaadia, Simone Cardoso de Oliveira, Ad Aertsen and Stefan Rotter. Inference of hand movements from local field potentials in monkey motor cortex. *Nature neuroscience*, 6(12):1253–1254, 2003.

61 Gunnar Waterstraat, Martin Burghoff, Tommaso Fedele, Vadim Nikulin, Hans Jürgen Scheer and Gabriel Curio. Non-invasive single-trial EEG detection of evoked human neocortical population spikes. *Neuroimage*, 105:13–20, 2015.

62 Christoph M Michel and Micah M Murray. Towards the utilization of EEG as a brain imaging tool. *Neuroimage*, 61(2):371–385, 2012.

63 Stephan Waldert. Invasive vs. non-invasive neuronal signals for brain-machine interfaces: Will one prevail? *Frontiers in neuroscience*, 10:295, 2016.

64 Xiao Jiang, Gui-Bin Bian and Zean Tian. Removal of artifacts from EEG signals: A review. *Sensors*, 19(5):987, 2019.

65 Ali H Husseen Al-Nuaimi, Emmanuel Jammeh, Lingfen Sun and Emmanuel Ifeachor. Complexity measures for quantifying changes in electroencephalogram in Alzheimer's disease. *Complexity*, 2018(1), 2018.

66 Ana R Teixeira, Ana Maria Tomé, Elmar Wolfgang Lang, Peter Gruber and A Martins Da Silva. Automatic removal of high-amplitude artefacts from single-channel electroencephalograms. *Computer methods and programs in biomedicine*, 83(2):125–138, 2006.

67 Kevin T Sweeney, Tomás E Ward and Seán F McLoone. Artifact removal in physiological signals—Practices and possibilities. *IEEE transactions on information technology in biomedicine*, 16(3):488–500, 2012.

68 Ben Somers and Alexander Bertrand. Removal of eye blink artifacts in wireless EEG sensor networks using reduced-bandwidth canonical correlation analysis. *Journal of neural engineering*, 13(6):066008, 2016.

69 Christopher J James and Christian W Hesse. Independent component analysis for biomedical signals. *Physiological measurement*, 26(1):R15, 2004.

70 Y Liu, WG Coon, A De Pesters, P Brunner and G Schalk. The effects of spatial filtering and artifacts on electrocorticographic signals. *Journal of neural engineering*, 12(5):056008, 2015.

71 Niago Moreira Nobre Leite, Eanes Torres Pereira, Edmar Candeia Gurjao and Luciana Ribeiro Veloso. Deep convolutional autoencoder for EEG noise filtering. In *2018 IEEE International Conference on Bioinformatics and Biomedicine (BIBM)*, pages 2605–2612. IEEE, 2018.

72 Arthur Sena Lins Caldas, Eanes Torres Pereira, Niago Moreira Nobre Leite, Arthur Dimitri Brito Oliveira and Ellen Ribeiro Lucena. Towards automatic

EEG signal denoising by quality metric optimization. In *2020 International Joint Conference on Neural Networks (IJCNN)*, pages 1–7. IEEE, 2020.

73 Yeou-Jiunn Chen, Pei-Chung Chen, Shih-Chung Chen and Chung-Min Wu. Denoising autoencoder-based feature extraction to robust SSVEP-based BCIs. *Sensors*, 21(15):5019, 2021.

74 Yang An, Hak Keung Lam and Sai Ho Ling. Auto-denoising for EEG signals using generative adversarial network. *Sensors*, 22(5):1750, 2022.

75 Marcos Fabietti, Mufti Mahmud, Ahmad Lotfi, Alberto Averna, David Guggenmos, Randolph Nudo and Michela Chiappalone. Signal power affects artefact detection accuracy in chronically recorded local field potentials: preliminary results. In *2021 10th International IEEE/EMBS Conference on Neural Engineering (NER)*, pages 166–169. IEEE, 2021.

76 Alex Krizhevsky, Ilya Sutskever and Geoffrey E Hinton. Imagenet classification with deep convolutional neural networks. *Advances in neural information processing systems*, 25, 2012.

77 Marcos Fabietti, Mufti Mahmud, Ahmad Lotfi, Alberto Averna, David Guggenmos, Randolph Nudo and Michela Chiappalone. Artifact detection in chronically recorded local field potentials using long-short term memory neural network. In *2020 IEEE 14th International Conference on Application of Information and Communication Technologies (AICT)*, pages 1–6. IEEE, 2020.

78 Marcos Fabietti, Mufti Mahmud, Ahmad Lotfi, M Shamim Kaiser, Alberto Averna, David J Guggenmos, Randolph J Nudo, Michela Chiappalone and Jianhui Chen. Santia: A MATLAB-based open-source toolbox for artifact detection and removal from extracellular neuronal signals. *Brain informatics*, 8(1):1–19, 2021.

79 Seung-Hyeon Oh, Yu-Ri Lee and Hyoung-Nam Kim. A novel EEG feature extraction method using Hjorth parameter. *International journal of electronics and electrical engineering*, 2(2):106–110, 2014.

80 L Vega-Escobar, AE Castro-Ospina and L Duque-Muñoz. Feature extraction schemes for BCI systems. In *2015 20th Symposium on Signal Processing, Images and Computer Vision (STSIVA)*, pages 1–6. IEEE, 2015.

81 Niferiti Aminuddin, Anusha Achuthan, Nur Intan Raihana Ruhaiyem, Che Mohd Nasril Che Mohd Nassir, Nur Suhaila Idris and Muzaimi Mustapha. Reduced cerebral vascular fractal dimension among asymptomatic individuals as a potential biomarker for cerebral small vessel disease. *Scientific reports*, 12(1):1–11, 2022.

82 J Montalvo Aguilar, J Castillo and D Elias. EEG signals processing based on fractal dimension features and classified by neural network and support vector machine in motor imagery for a BCI. In *VI Latin American Congress on Biomedical Engineering CLAIB 2014, Paraná, Argentina 29, 30 & 31 October 2014*, pages 615–618. Springer, 2015.

83 Zheng Li, Joseph E O'Doherty, Timothy L Hanson, Mikhail A Lebedev, Craig S Henriquez and Miguel AL Nicolelis. Unscented Kalman filter for brain-machine interfaces. *PloS one*, 4(7):e6243, 2009.

84 Sile Hu, Qiaosheng Zhang, Jing Wang and Zhe Chen. Real-time particle filtering and smoothing algorithms for detecting abrupt changes in neural ensemble spike activity. *Journal of neurophysiology*, 119(4):1394–1410, 2018.

85 Stefan Haufe, Paul DeGuzman, Simon Henin, Michael Arcaro, Christopher J Honey, Uri Hasson and Lucas C Parra. Elucidating relations between fMRI, ECoG, and EEG through a common natural stimulus. *NeuroImage*, 179:79–91, 2018.

86 Hindarto Hindarto and Sumarno Sumarno. Feature extraction of electroencephalography signals using fast Fourier transform. *CommIT (communication and information technology) journal*, 10(2):49–52, 2016.

87 José C Principe and Dennis J McFarland. BMI/BCI modeling and signal processing. In *Brain-Computer Interfaces*, pages 47–64. Springer, 2008.

88 Imali T Hettiarachchi, Thanh Thi Nguyen and Saeid Nahavandi. Multivariate adaptive autoregressive modeling and Kalman filtering for motor imagery BCI. In *2015 IEEE International Conference on Systems, Man, and Cybernetics*, pages 3164–3168. IEEE, 2015.

89 Dechun Zhao, Xiaoxiang Li, Xiaorong Hou, Mingyang Feng and Renping Jiang. Synchrosqueezing with short-time Fourier transform method for trinary frequency shift keying encoded SSVEP. *Technology and health care*, 29(3):505–519, 2021.

90 Zijian Wang, Lei Cao, Zuo Zhang, Xiaoliang Gong, Yaoru Sun and Haoran Wang. Short time Fourier transformation and deep neural networks for motor imagery brain computer interface recognition. *Concurrency and computation: Practice and experience*, 30(23):e4413, 2018.

91 Shixian Wen, Allen Yin, Po-He Tseng, Laurent Itti, Mikhail A Lebedev and Miguel Nicolelis. Capturing spike train temporal pattern with wavelet average coefficient for brain machine interface. *Scientific reports*, 11(1):1–10, 2021.

92 Ebrahim A Mousavi, Jerome J Maller, Paul B Fitzgerald and Brian J Lithgow. Wavelet common spatial pattern in asynchronous offline brain computer interfaces. *Biomedical signal processing and control*, 6(2):121–128, 2011.

93 Guido Dornhege, Benjamin Blankertz, Matthias Krauledat, Florian Losch, Gabriel Curio and K-R Muller. Combined optimization of spatial and temporal filters for improving brain-computer interfacing. *IEEE transactions on biomedical engineering*, 53(11):2274–2281, 2006.

94 Erin L Rich and Jonathan D Wallis. Decoding subjective decisions from orbitofrontal cortex. *Nature neuroscience*, 19(7):973–980, 2016.

95 Adrián Hernández, Verónica Nácher, Rogelio Luna, Antonio Zainos, Luis Lemus, Manuel Alvarez, Yuriria Vázquez, Liliana Camarillo and Ranulfo Romo. Decoding a perceptual decision process across cortex. *Neuron*, 66(2):300–314, 2010.

96 Joshua I Glaser, Matthew G Perich, Pavan Ramkumar, Lee E Miller and Konrad P Kording. Population coding of conditional probability distributions in dorsal premotor cortex. *Nature communications*, 9(1):1–14, 2018.

97 Martin Weygandt, Carlo R Blecker, Axel Schäfer, Kerstin Hackmack, John-Dylan Haynes, Dieter Vaitl, Rudolf Stark and Anne Schienle. fMRI pattern recognition in obsessive–compulsive disorder. *Neuroimage*, 60(2):1186–1193, 2012.

98 Gautam Krishna, Co Tran, Jianguo Yu and Ahmed H Tewfik. Speech recognition with no speech or with noisy speech. In *ICASSP 2019-2019 IEEE International Conference on Acoustics, Speech and Signal Processing (ICASSP)*, pages 1090–1094. IEEE, 2019.

99 Gopala K Anumanchipalli, Josh Chartier and Edward F Chang. Speech synthesis from neural decoding of spoken sentences. *Nature*, 568(7753):493–498, 2019.

100 Lars Kaulen, Justus TC Schwabedal, Jules Schneider, Philipp Ritter and Stephan Bialonski. Sumo: Advanced sleep spindle identification with neural networks. *arXiv preprint arXiv:2202.05158*, 2022.

101 Jiaxin You, Dihong Jiang, Yu Ma and Yuanyuan Wang. SpindleU-Net: An adaptive U-Net framework for sleep spindle detection in single-channel EEG. *IEE transactions on neural systems and rehabilitation engineering*, 29:1614–1623, 2021.

102 Jiyao Liu, Li Zhang, Hao Wu and Huan Zhao. Transformers for EEG emotion recognition. *arXiv preprint arXiv:2110.06553*, 2021.

103 Sebastian Weichwald, Timm Meyer, Ozan Özdenizci, Bernhard Schölkopf, Tonio Ball and Moritz Grosse-Wentrup. Causal interpretation rules for encoding and decoding models in neuroimaging. *Neuroimage*, 110:48–59, 2015.

104 Zheng Wu, Ashok Litwin-Kumar, Philip Shamash, Alexei Taylor, Richard Axel and Michael N Shadlen. Context-dependent decision making in a premotor circuit. *Neuron*, 106(2):316–328, 2020.

105 Amir Ahangi, Mehdi Karamnejad, Nima Mohammadi, Reza Ebrahimpour and Nasoor Bagheri. Multiple classifier system for EEG signal classification with application to brain–computer interfaces. *Neural computing and applications*, 23(5):1319–1327, 2013.

106 MNAH Sha'Abani, N Fuad, Norezmi Jamal and MF Ismail. KNN and SVM classification for EEG: A review. *InECCE2019*, 555–565, 2020.

107 Rabel Guharoy, Nanda Dulal Jana and Suparna Biswas. An efficient epileptic seizure detection technique using discrete wavelet transform and machine learning classifiers. *arXiv preprint arXiv:2109.13811*, 2021.

108 Abdulkadir Saday and Ilker Ali Ozkan. Classification of epileptic EEG signals using DWT-based feature extraction and machine learning methods. *International journal of applied mathematics electronics and computers*, 9(4):122–129, 2021.

109 Sudip Paul, Ishmam Zabir, Tanmoy Sarker, Shaikh Anowarul Fattah and Celia Shahnaz. Higher order statistics of bispectrum and MRP of ECoG signals for motor imagery tasks classification. In *2017 IEEE Region 10 Symposium (TENSYMP)*, pages 1–4, 2017.

110 Erdem Erkan and Ismail Kurnaz. A study on the effect of psychophysiological signal features on classification methods. *Measurement*, 101:45–52, 2017.

111 Lal Hussain. Detecting epileptic seizure with different feature extracting strategies using robust machine learning classification techniques by applying advance parameter optimization approach. *Cognitive neurodynamics*, 12(3):271–294, 2018.

112 Muhammad Bilal Qureshi, Muhammad Afzaal, Muhammad Shuaib Qureshi, Muhammad Fayaz, et al. Machine learning-based EEG signals classification model for epileptic seizure detection. *Multimedia tools and applications*, 80(12):17849–17877, 2021.

113 Seyede Mahya Safavi, Alireza S. Behbahani, Ahmed M. Eltawil, Zoran Nenadic and An H. Do. A cortical activity localization approach for decoding finger movements from human electrocorticogram signal. In *2015 49th Asilomar Conference on Signals, Systems and Computers*, pages 930–934, 2015.

114 Liu Chong, Zhao Hai-bin, Li Chun-sheng and Wang Hong. Classification of ECoG signals for motor imagery tasks. In *2010 2nd International Conference on Signal Processing Systems*, volume 3, pages V3–185. IEEE, 2010.

115 Shalu Chaudhary, Sachin Taran, Varun Bajaj and Siuly Siuly. A flexible analytic wavelet transform based approach for motor-imagery tasks classification in BCI applications. *Computer methods and programs in biomedicine*, 187:105325, 2020.

116 Shashank Joshi and Falak Joshi. Human emotion classification based on EEG signals using recurrent neural network and KNN. *arXiv preprint arXiv:2205.08419*, 2022.

117 Mamunur Rashid, Norizam Sulaiman, Mahfuzah Mustafa, Bifta Sama Bari, Md Golam Sadeque and Md Jahid Hasan. Wink based facial expression classification using machine learning approach. *SN applied sciences*, 2(2):1–9, 2020.

118 Susan Aliakbaryhosseinabadi, Ernest Nlandu Kamavuako, Ning Jiang, Dario Farina and Natalie Mrachacz-Kersting. Classification of EEG signals to identify

variations in attention during motor task execution. *Journal of neuroscience methods*, 284:27–34, 2017.

119 Marcin Kołodziej, Andrzej Majkowski, Remigiusz Jan Rak, Paweł Tarnowski and Andrzej Rysz. Epileptic seizure detection based on ECoG signal. In *International Conference on Artificial Intelligence and Soft Computing*, pages 193–202. Springer, 2019.

120 Debadatta Dash, Paul Ferrari and Jun Wang. Role of brainwaves in neural speech decoding. In *2020 28th European Signal Processing Conference (EUSIPCO)*, pages 1357–1361, 2021.

121 Tianxiao Jiang, Tao Jiang, Taylor Wang, Shanshan Mei, Qingzhu Liu, Yunlin Li, Xiaofei Wang, Sujit Prabhu, Zhiyi Sha and Nuri F. Ince. Investigation of the influence of ECoG grid spatial density on decoding hand flexion and extension. In *2018 40th Annual International Conference of the IEEE Engineering in Medicine and Biology Society (EMBC)*, pages 3052–3055, 2018.

122 Yu Zhang, Guoxu Zhou, Jing Jin, Qibin Zhao, Xingyu Wang and Andrzej Cichocki. Aggregation of sparse linear discriminant analyses for event-related potential classification in brain-computer interface. *International journal of neural systems*, 24(01):1450003, 2014.

123 I. Ignacio A. Zapata, Yan Li and Peng Wen. Rules-based and SVM-Q methods with multi-tapers and convolution for sleep EEG stages classification. *IEEE access*, 10, 71310, 2022.

124 Jiannan Kang, Xiaoya Han, Jiajia Song, Zikang Niu and Xiaoli Li. The identification of children with autism spectrum disorder by SVM approach on EEG and eye-tracking data. *Computers in biology and medicine*, 120:103722, 2020.

125 Inung Wijayanto, Achmad Rizal and Annisa Humairani. Seizure detection based on EEG signals using Katz fractal and SVM classifiers. In *2019 5th International Conference on Science in Information Technology (ICSITech)*, pages 78–82, 2019.

126 Xiashuang Wang, Guanghong Gong, Ni Li, Li Ding and Yaofei Ma. Decoding pilot behavior consciousness of EEG, ECG, eye movements via an SVM machine learning model. *International journal of modeling, simulation, and scientific computing*, 11(04):2050028, 2020.

127 Catur Atmaji, Agfianto Eko Putra and Irvan Albab Tontowi. Three-class classification of EEG signals using support vector machine methods. In *2018 4th International Conference on Science and Technology (ICST)*, pages 1–4. IEEE, 2018.

128 K Yasoda, RS Ponmagal, KS Bhuvaneshwari and K Venkatachalam. Automatic detection and classification of EEG artifacts using fuzzy kernel SVM and wavelet ICA (WICA). *Soft computing*, 24(21):16011–16019, 2020.

129 Weijie Ren and Min Han. Classification of EEG signals using hybrid feature extraction and ensemble extreme learning machine. *Neural processing letters*, 50(2):1281–1301, 2019.

130 Haitham S Mohammed, Hagar M Hassan, Michael H Zakhari, Hassan Mostafa and Ebtesam A Mohamad. Linear and non-linear feature extraction from rat electrocorticograms for seizure detection by support vector machine. *Biomedical engineering/Biomedizinische Technik*, 66(6):563–572, 2021.

131 Yueqiu Sun, Daniel Friedman, Patricia Dugan, Manisha Holmes, Xiaojing Wu and Anli Liu. Machine learning to classify relative seizure frequency from chronic electrocorticography. *Journal of clinical neurophysiology*, 40(2): 2021.

132 Ming-Ai Li, Lin Nan and Yu-Xin Dong. A novel multi-period multivariate multi-scale phase locking value and its application. In *Proceedings of the 2020 12th International Conference on Computer and Automation Engineering*, pages 145–149, 2020.

133 Shivam Sharma and Rishi Raj Sharma. Variational mode decomposition-based finger flexion detection using ECoG signals. In *Artificial Intelligence-Based Brain-Computer Interface*, pages 261–282. Elsevier, 2022.

134 Lin Yao and Mahsa Shoaran. Enhanced classification of individual finger movements with ECoG. In *2019 53rd Asilomar Conference on Signals, Systems, and Computers*, pages 2063–2066, 2019.

135 Jessica Centracchio, Antonio Sarno, Daniele Esposito, Emilio Andreozzi, Luigi Pavone, Giancarlo Di Gennaro, Marcello Bartolo, Vincenzo Esposito, Roberta Morace, Sara Casciato, et al. Efficient automated localization of ECoG electrodes in CT images via shape analysis. *International journal of computer assisted radiology and surgery*, 16(4):543–554, 2021.

136 Guillaume Jubien, Marie-Caroline Schaeffer, Stéphane Bonnet and Tetiana Aksenova. Decoding of finger activation from ECoG data: A comparative study. In *2019 International Joint Conference on Neural Networks (IJCNN)*, pages 1–8, 2019.

137 Nguyen The Hoang Anh, Tran Huy Hoang, Vu Tat Thang, TT Quyen Bui, et al. An artificial neural network approach for electroencephalographic signal classification towards brain-computer interface implementation. In *2016 IEEE RIVF International Conference on Computing & Communication Technologies, Research, Innovation, and Vision for the Future (RIVF)*, pages 205–210. IEEE, 2016.

138 MM El Bahy, M Hosny, Wael A Mohamed and Shawky Ibrahim. EEG signal classification using neural network and support vector machine in brain computer interface. In *International Conference on Advanced Intelligent Systems and Informatics*, pages 246–256. Springer, 2016.

139 Ali Marjaninejad, Babak Taherian and Francisco J. Valero-Cuevas. Finger movements are mainly represented by a linear transformation of energy in band-specific ECoG signals. In *2017 39th Annual International Conference of the IEEE Engineering in Medicine and Biology Society (EMBC)*, pages 986–989, 2017.

140 Mostafa Mohammadpour, Seyyed Mohammad Reza Hashemi and Negin Houshmand. Classification of EEG-based emotion for BCI applications. In *2017 Artificial Intelligence and Robotics (IRANOPEN)*, pages 127–131. IEEE, 2017.

141 Fangzhou Xu, Wenfeng Zheng, Dongri Shan, Qi Yuan and Weidong Zhou. Decoding spectro-temporal representation for motor imagery recognition using ECoG-based brain-computer interfaces. *Journal of integrative neuroscience*, 19(2):259–272, 2020.

142 Md Nahidul Islam, Norizam Sulaiman, Mamunur Rashid, Bifta Sama Bari, Md Jahid Hasan, Mahfuzah Mustafa and Mohd Shawal Jadin. Empirical mode decomposition coupled with fast Fourier transform based feature extraction method for motor imagery tasks classification. In *2020 IEEE 10th International Conference on System Engineering and Technology (ICSET)*, pages 256–261, 2020.

143 Wenfeng Zheng, Fangzhou Xu, Minglei Shu, Yingchun Zhang, Qi Yuan, Jian Lian and Yuanjie Zheng. Classification of motor imagery electrocorticogram signals for brain-computer interface. In *2019 9th International IEEE/EMBS Conference on Neural Engineering (NER)*, pages 530–533, 2019.

144 Jordan J Bird, Luis J Manso, Eduardo P Ribeiro, Anikó Ekárt and Diego R Faria. A study on mental state classification using EEG-based brain-machine interface. In *2018 International Conference on Intelligent Systems (IS)*, pages 795–800. IEEE, 2018.

145 Carlos H. Mendoza-Cardenas and Austin J. Brockmeier. Shift-invariant waveform learning on epileptic ECoG. In *2021 43rd Annual International Conference*

of the IEEE Engineering in Medicine & Biology Society (EMBC), pages 1136–1139, 2021.

146 Fatemeh Shahlaei, Niraj Bagh, Madhukar Sarvottam Zambare, RamasubbaReddy Machireddy and Arvind Digamber Shaligram. Detection of event related patterns using Hilbert transform in brain computer interface. In *2019 IEEE Canadian Conference of Electrical and Computer Engineering (CCECE)*, pages 1–4. IEEE, 2019.

147 Mohammad Khubeb Siddiqui, Md Zahidul Islam and Muhammad Ashad Kabir. A novel quick seizure detection and localization through brain data mining on ECoG dataset. *Neural computing and applications*, 31(9):5595–5608, 2019.

148 Arnab Rakshit, Anwesha Khasnobish and DN Tibarewala. A naïve Bayesian approach to lower limb classification from EEG signals. In *2016 2nd International Conference on Control, Instrumentation, Energy & Communication (CIEC)*, pages 140–144. IEEE, 2016.

149 Seokyun Ryun, June Sic Kim, Donghyuk Lee and Chun Kee Chung. Prediction of motor and somatosensory function from human ECoG. In *2018 6th International Conference on Brain-Computer Interface (BCI)*, pages 1–4, 2018.

150 Minmin Miao, Hong Zeng, Aimin Wang, Changsen Zhao and Feixiang Liu. Discriminative spatial-frequency-temporal feature extraction and classification of motor imagery EEG: An sparse regression and weighted naïve Bayesian classifier-based approach. *Journal of neuroscience methods*, 278:13–24, 2017.

151 SR Sreeja, Joytirmoy Rabha, KY Nagarjuna, Debasis Samanta, Pabitra Mitra and Monalisa Sarma. Motor imagery EEG signal processing and classification using machine learning approach. In *2017 International Conference on New Trends in Computing Sciences (ICTCS)*, pages 61–66. IEEE, 2017.

152 Jessica Rodrigues Brazète, Jean-François Gagnon, Ronald B Postuma, Josie-Anne Bertrand, Dominique Petit and Jacques Montplaisir. Electroencephalogram slowing predicts neurodegeneration in rapid eye movement sleep behavior disorder. *Neurobiology of aging*, 37:74–81, 2016.

153 Amin Khatami, Morteza Babaie, Hamid R Tizhoosh, Abbas Khosravi, Thanh Nguyen and Saeid Nahavandi. A sequential search-space shrinking using CNN transfer learning and a Radon projection pool for medical image retrieval. *Expert systems with applications*, 100:224–233, 2018.

154 Na Lu, Tengfei Li, Xiaodong Ren and Hongyu Miao. A deep learning scheme for motor imagery classification based on restricted Boltzmann machines. *IEEE transactions on neural systems and rehabilitation engineering*, 25(6):566–576, 2016.

155 Shiu Kumar, Alok Sharma, Kabir Mamun and Tatsuhiko Tsunoda. A deep learning approach for motor imagery EEG signal classification. In *2016 3rd Asia-Pacific World Congress on Computer Science and Engineering (APWC on CSE)*, pages 34–39. IEEE, 2016.

156 Nicolás I Tapia and Pablo A Estévez. Red: Deep recurrent neural networks for sleep EEG event detection. In *2020 International Joint Conference on Neural Networks (IJCNN)*, pages 1–8. IEEE, 2020.

157 Yann LeCun, Léon Bottou, Yoshua Bengio and Patrick Haffner. Gradient-based learning applied to document recognition. *Proceedings of the IEEE*, 86(11):2278–2324, 1998.

158 Sepp Hochreiter and Jürgen Schmidhuber. Long short-term memory. *Neural computation*, 9(8):1735–1780, 1997.

159 C. Lee Giles, Gary M. Kuhn and Ronald J. Williams. Dynamic recurrent neural networks: Theory and applications. *IEEE transactions on neural networks*, 5(2):153–156, 1994.

160 Mike Schuster and Kuldip K Paliwal. Bidirectional recurrent neural networks. *IEEE transactions on signal processing*, 45(11):2673–2681, 1997.

161 Ashish Vaswani, Noam Shazeer, Niki Parmar, Jakob Uszkoreit, Llion Jones, Aidan N Gomez, Łukasz Kaiser and Illia Polosukhin. Attention is all you need. *Advances in neural information processing systems*, 30, 2017.

162 Zhen Liang, Rushuang Zhou, Li Zhang, Linling Li, Gan Huang, Zhiguo Zhang and Shin Ishii. EEGFuseNet: Hybrid unsupervised deep feature characterization and fusion for high-dimensional EEG with an application to emotion recognition. *CoRR*, abs/2102.03777, 2021.

163 Xiaojin Zhu and Andrew B Goldberg. Introduction to semi-supervised learning. *Synthesis lectures on artificial intelligence and machine learning*, 3(1):1–130, 2009.

164 Xiangli Yang, Zixing Song, Irwin King and Zenglin Xu. A survey on deep semi-supervised learning. *arXiv preprint arXiv:2103.00550*, 2021.

165 Avital Oliver, Augustus Odena, Colin A Raffel, Ekin Dogus Cubuk and Ian Goodfellow. Realistic evaluation of deep semi-supervised learning algorithms. *Advances in neural information processing systems*, 31, 2018.

166 Xiaohua Zhai, Avital Oliver, Alexander Kolesnikov and Lucas Beyer. S4l: Self-supervised semi-supervised learning. In *Proceedings of the IEEE/CVF International Conference on Computer Vision*, pages 1476–1485, 2019.

167 Wade Barry, Sharanya Arcot Desai, Thomas K Tcheng and Martha J Morrell. A high accuracy electrographic seizure classifier trained using semi-supervised labeling applied to a large spectrogram dataset. *Frontiers in neuroscience*, 15: 697, 2021.

168 Subhrajit Roy, Kiran Kate and Martin Hirzel. A semi-supervised deep learning algorithm for abnormal EEG identification. *arXiv preprint arXiv:1903.07822*, 2019.

169 Huiqi Li, Yuanqing Li and Cuntai Guan. An effective BCI speller based on semi-supervised learning. In *2006 International Conference of the IEEE Engineering in Medicine and Biology Society*, pages 1161–1164. IEEE, 2006.

170 Haiyan Xu and Konstantinos N Plataniotis. Affective states classification using EEG and semi-supervised deep learning approaches. In *2016 IEEE 18th International Workshop on Multimedia Signal Processing (MMSP)*, pages 1–6. IEEE, 2016.

171 Carl Doersch, Abhinav Gupta and Alexei A Efros. Unsupervised visual representation learning by context prediction. In *Proceedings of the IEEE International Conference on Computer Vision*, pages 1422–1430, 2015.

172 Alexey Dosovitskiy, Jost Tobias Springenberg, Martin Riedmiller and Thomas Brox. Discriminative unsupervised feature learning with convolutional neural networks. *Advances in neural information processing systems*, 27, 2014.

173 Irene Sturm, Sebastian Lapuschkin, Wojciech Samek and Klaus-Robert Müller. Interpretable deep neural networks for single-trial EEG classification. *Journal of neuroscience methods*, 274:141–145, 2016.

174 Xiang Li, Zhigang Zhao, Dawei Song, Yazhou Zhang, Jingshan Pan, Lu Wu, Jidong Huo, Chunyang Niu and Di Wang. Latent factor decoding of multi-channel EEG for emotion recognition through autoencoder-like neural networks. *Frontiers in neuroscience*, 14:87, 2020.

175 Luis Perez and Jason Wang. The effectiveness of data augmentation in image classification using deep learning. *arXiv preprint arXiv:1712.04621*, 2017.

176 Kaiming He, Haoqi Fan, Yuxin Wu, Saining Xie and Ross Girshick. Momentum contrast for unsupervised visual representation learning. In *Proceedings of the IEEE/CVF Conference on Computer Vision and Pattern Recognition*, pages 9729–9738, 2020.

177 Ting Chen, Simon Kornblith, Mohammad Norouzi and Geoffrey Hinton. A simple framework for contrastive learning of visual representations. In *International Conference on Machine Learning*, pages 1597–1607. PMLR, 2020.

178 Jean-Bastien Grill, Florian Strub, Florent Altché, Corentin Tallec, Pierre Richemond, Elena Buchatskaya, Carl Doersch, Bernardo Avila Pires, Zhaohan Guo, Mohammad Gheshlaghi Azar, et al. Bootstrap your own latent-a new approach to self-supervised learning. *Advances in neural information processing systems*, 33:21271–21284, 2020.

179 Jiaming Song and Stefano Ermon. Multi-label contrastive predictive coding. *Advances in neural information processing systems*, 33:8161–8173, 2020.

180 Aaron van den Oord, Yazhe Li and Oriol Vinyals. Representation learning with contrastive predictive coding. *arXiv preprint arXiv:1807.03748*, 2018.

181 Petar Veličković, William Fedus, William L Hamilton, Pietro Liò, Yoshua Bengio and R Devon Hjelm. Deep graph infomax. *arXiv preprint arXiv:1809.10341*, 2018.

182 Yanqiao Zhu, Yichen Xu, Feng Yu, Qiang Liu, Shu Wu and Liang Wang. Deep graph contrastive representation learning. *arXiv preprint arXiv:2006.04131*, 2020.

183 Tom B. Brown, Benjamin Mann, Nick Ryder, Melanie Subbiah, Jared Kaplan, Prafulla Dhariwal, Arvind Neelakantan, Girish Sastry, Amanda Askell and Ilya Sutskever. Language models are few-shot learners. *Advances in neural information processing systems*, 33:1877–1901, 2020.

184 Jacob Devlin, Ming-Wei Chang, Kenton Lee and Kristina Toutanova. Bert: Pre-training of deep bidirectional transformers for language understanding. *arXiv preprint arXiv:1810.04805*, 2018.

185 Max Schwarzer, Ankesh Anand, Rishab Goel, R Devon Hjelm, Aaron Courville and Philip Bachman. Data-efficient reinforcement learning with self-predictive representations. *arXiv preprint arXiv:2007.05929*, 2020.

186 Zhaohan Daniel Guo, Bernardo Avila Pires, Bilal Piot, Jean-Bastien Grill, Florent Altché, Rémi Munos and Mohammad Gheshlaghi Azar. Bootstrap latent-predictive representations for multitask reinforcement learning. In *International Conference on Machine Learning*, pages 3875–3886. PMLR, 2020.

187 Yann LeCun and Ishan Misra. Self-supervised learning: The dark matter of intelligence. *Meta AI*, 23, 2021.

188 Alec Radford, Jeff Wu, Rewon Child, David Luan, Dario Amodei and Ilya Sutskever. Language models are unsupervised multitask learners. *OpenAI blog*, 2019.

189 Ran Liu, Mehdi Azabou, Max Dabagia, Chi-Heng Lin, Mohammad Gheshlaghi Azar, Keith Hengen, Michal Valko and Eva Dyer. Drop, swap, and generate: A self-supervised approach for generating neural activity. *Advances in neural information processing systems*, 34:10587–10599, 2021.

190 Mehdi Azabou, Mohammad Gheshlaghi Azar, Ran Liu, Chi-Heng Lin, Erik C Johnson, Kiran Bhaskaran-Nair, Max Dabagia, Bernardo Avila-Pires, Lindsey Kitchell, Keith B Hengen, et al. Mine your own view: Self-supervised learning through across-sample prediction. *arXiv preprint arXiv:2102.10106*, 2021.

191 Mehdi Azabou, Max Dabagia, Ran Liu, Chi-Heng Lin, Keith B. Hengen, WashU-St. Louis, and Eva L. Dyer. *Using self-supervision and augmentations to build insights into neural coding*. Proceedings of Workshop on Self-Supervised Learning—Theory and Practice on NeurIPS, *Proceedings of Machine Learning Research,* 1–7, 2021.

192 Joseph Y Cheng, Hanlin Goh, Kaan Dogrusoz, Oncel Tuzel and Erdrin Azemi. Subject-aware contrastive learning for biosignals. *arXiv preprint arXiv:2007.04871*, 2020.

193 Hubert Banville, Omar Chehab, Aapo Hyvärinen, Denis-Alexander Engemann and Alexandre Gramfort. Uncovering the structure of clinical EEG signals with self-supervised learning. *Journal of neural engineering*, 18(4):046020, 2021.

194 Steven Michael Peterson, Rajesh PN Rao and Bingni Wen Brunton. Learning neural decoders without labels using multiple data streams. *bioRxiv*, 2021.

195 Demetres Kostas, Stephane Aroca-Ouellette and Frank Rudzicz. BENDR: Using transformers and a contrastive self-supervised learning task to learn from massive amounts of EEG data. *Frontiers in human neuroscience*, 15: 253, 2021.

196 Alexei Baevski, Yuhao Zhou, Abdelrahman Mohamed and Michael Auli. wav2vec 2.0: A framework for self-supervised learning of speech representations. *Advances in neural information processing systems*, 33:12449–12460, 2020.

197 Richard S Sutton and Andrew G Barto. *Reinforcement Learning: An Introduction.* MIT press, 2018.

198 Duo Xu, Mohit Agarwal, Ekansh Gupta, Faramarz Fekri and Raghupathy Sivakumar. Accelerating reinforcement learning using EEG-based implicit human feedback. *Neurocomputing*, 460:139–153, 2021.

199 Esha Dutta, Ananya Bothra, Theodora Chaspari, Thomas Ioerger and Bobak J Mortazavi. Reinforcement learning using EEG signals for therapeutic use of music in emotion management. In *2020 42nd Annual International Conference of the IEEE Engineering in Medicine & Biology Society (EMBC)*, pages 5553–5556. IEEE, 2020.

200 Peter Kairouz, H Brendan McMahan, Brendan Avent, Aurélien Bellet, Mehdi Bennis, Arjun Nitin Bhagoji, Kallista Bonawitz, Zachary Charles, Graham Cormode, Rachel Cummings, et al. Advances and open problems in federated learning. *Foundations and trends® in machine learning*, 14(1–2):1–210, 2021.

201 Regulation (EU), 679, 2016 Complete: Protection Regulation. Regulation (EU) 2016/679 of the European parliament and of the council. *Regulation (EU)*, 679, 2016

202 Brendan McMahan, Eider Moore, Daniel Ramage, Seth Hampson and Blaise Aguera y Arcas. Communication-efficient learning of deep networks from decentralized data. In *Artificial Intelligence and Statistics*, pages 1273–1282. PMLR, 2017.

203 Qiang Yang, Yang Liu, Yong Cheng, Yan Kang, Tianjian Chen and Han Yu. Federated learning. *Synthesis lectures on artificial intelligence and machine learning*, 13(3):1–207, 2019.

204 Ce Ju, Dashan Gao, Ravikiran Mane, Ben Tan, Yang Liu and Cuntai Guan. Federated transfer learning for EEG signal classification. In *2020 42nd Annual International Conference of the IEEE Engineering in Medicine & Biology Society (EMBC)*, pages 3040–3045. IEEE, 2020.

205 Gerwin Schalk, Dennis J McFarland, Thilo Hinterberger, Niels Birbaumer and Jonathan R Wolpaw. Bci2000: A general-purpose brain-computer interface (BCI) system. *IEEE transactions on biomedical engineering*, 51(6):1034–1043, 2004.

206 Wenhui Cui, Woojae Jeong, Philipp Thölke, Takfarinas Medani, Karim Jerbi, Anand A. Joshi, and Richard M. Leahy. Neuro-GPT: *Towards a foundation model for EEG.* In *2024 IEEE International Symposium on Biomedical Imaging (ISBI)*, 1–5. IEEE, 2024.

207 Sheng Feng et al. Towards an end-to-end framework for invasive brain signal decoding with large language models. *arXiv preprint arXiv:2406.11568*, 2024.

208 Ujwal Chaudhary, Niels Birbaumer and Ander Ramos-Murguialday. Brain–computer interfaces for communication and rehabilitation. *Nature reviews neurology*, 12(9):513–525, 2016.

209 Aamir Arsalan, Muhammad Majid, Amna Rauf Butt and Syed Muhammad Anwar. Classification of perceived mental stress using a commercially available

EEG headband. *IEEE journal of biomedical and health informatics*, 23(6):2257–2264, 2019.

210 Iuliana Marin, Myssar Jabbar Hammood Al-Battbootti and Nicolae GOGA. Drone control based on mental commands and facial expressions. In *2020 12th International Conference on Electronics, Computers and Artificial Intelligence (ECAI)*, pages 1–4. IEEE, 2020.

211 Anirban Dutta. Brain–computer interface spellers for communication: Why we need to address their security and authenticity. *Brain sciences*, 10(3):139, 2020.

212 Sergio López Bernal, Alberto Huertas Celdrán, Gregorio Martínez Pérez, Michael Taynnan Barros and Sasitharan Balasubramaniam. Security in brain-computer interfaces: State-of-the-art, opportunities, and future challenges. *ACM computing surveys (CSUR)*, 54(1):1–35, 2021.

213 Mahmood Sharif, Sruti Bhagavatula, Lujo Bauer and Michael K Reiter. Accessorize to a crime: Real and stealthy attacks on state-of-the-art face recognition. In *Proceedings of the 2016 ACM SIGSAC Conference on Computer and Communications Security*, pages 1528–1540, 2016.

214 Ian J Goodfellow, Jonathon Shlens and Christian Szegedy. Explaining and harnessing adversarial examples. *arXiv preprint arXiv:1412.6572*, 2014.

215 Christian Szegedy, Wojciech Zaremba, Ilya Sutskever, Joan Bruna, Dumitru Erhan, Ian Goodfellow and Rob Fergus. Intriguing properties of neural networks. *arXiv preprint arXiv:1312.6199*, 2013.

216 Nicholas Carlini and David Wagner. Audio adversarial examples: Targeted attacks on speech-to-text. In *2018 IEEE Security and Privacy Workshops (SPW)*, pages 1–7. IEEE, 2018.

217 Kathrin Grosse, Nicolas Papernot, Praveen Manoharan, Michael Backes and Patrick McDaniel. Adversarial perturbations against deep neural networks for malware classification. *arXiv preprint arXiv:1606.04435*, 2016.

218 Jan Hendrik Metzen, Mummadi Chaithanya Kumar, Thomas Brox and Volker Fischer. Universal adversarial perturbations against semantic image segmentation. In *Proceedings of the IEEE International Conference on Computer Vision*, pages 2755–2764, 2017.

219 Nicholas Carlini and David Wagner. Towards evaluating the robustness of neural networks. In *2017 IEEE Symposium on Security and Privacy (SP)*, pages 39–57. IEEE, 2017.

220 Alexey Kurakin, Ian J Goodfellow and Samy Bengio. Adversarial examples in the physical world. In *Artificial Intelligence Safety and Security*, pages 99–112. Chapman and Hall/CRC, 2018.

221 Seyed-Mohsen Moosavi-Dezfooli, Alhussein Fawzi and Pascal Frossard. Deepfool: A simple and accurate method to fool deep neural networks. In *Proceedings of the IEEE Conference on Computer Vision and Pattern Recognition*, pages 2574–2582, 2016.

222 Nicolas Papernot, Patrick McDaniel, Ian Goodfellow, Somesh Jha, Z Berkay Celik and Ananthram Swami. Practical black-box attacks against machine learning. In *Proceedings of the 2017 ACM on Asia Conference on Computer and Communications Security*, pages 506–519, 2017.

223 Xiao Zhang and Dongrui Wu. On the vulnerability of CNN classifiers in EEG-based BCIs. *IEEE transactions on neural systems and rehabilitation engineering*, 27(5):814–825, 2019.

224 Xue Jiang, Xiao Zhang and Dongrui Wu. Active learning for black-box adversarial attacks in EEG-based brain-computer interfaces. In *2019 IEEE Symposium Series on Computational Intelligence (SSCI)*, pages 361–368. IEEE, 2019.

225 Lubin Meng, Jian Huang, Zhigang Zeng, Xue Jiang, Shan Yu, Tzyy-Ping Jung, Chin-Teng Lin, Ricardo Chavarriaga, and Dongrui Wu. *EEG-based*

brain-computer interfaces are vulnerable to backdoor attacks. IEEE Transactions on Neural Systems and Rehabilitation Engineering, 31:2224–2234, 2023.

226 National Institute of Mental Health. Brain stimulation therapies. https://www.nimh.nih.gov/health/topics/brain-stimulation-therapies/brain-stimulation-therapies. Accessed on 2024-01-10.

227 Yue Wang, Gaofeng Zhan, Ziwen Cai, Bo Jiao, Yilin Zhao, Shiyong Li and Ailin Luo. Vagus nerve stimulation in brain diseases: Therapeutic applications and biological mechanisms. *Neuroscience & biobehavioral reviews*, 127:37–53, 2021.

228 Mark S George, Sarah H Lisanby, David Avery, William M McDonald, Valerie Durkalski, Martina Pavlicova, Berry Anderson, Ziad Nahas, Peter Bulow, Paul Zarkowski, et al. Daily left prefrontal transcranial magnetic stimulation therapy for major depressive disorder: A sham-controlled randomized trial. *Archives of general psychiatry*, 67(5):507–516, 2010.

229 Matteo Bigoni, Lorenzo Priano, Alessandro Mauro and Paolo Capodaglio. Repetitive transcranial magnetic stimulation. *Rehabilitation interventions in the patient with obesity*, 205–215, 2020.

230 Bruce Luber, Shawn M McClintock and Sarah H Lisanby. Applications of transcranial magnetic stimulation and magnetic seizure therapy in the study and treatment of disorders related to cerebral aging. *Dialogues in clinical neuroscience*, 15(1): 2022.

231 Shervin Rahimpour, Musa Kiyani, Sarah E Hodges and Dennis A Turner. Deep brain stimulation and electromagnetic interference. *Clinical neurology and neurosurgery*, 203:106577, 2021.

232 Filippo Agnesi, Matthew D Johnson and Jerrold L Vitek. Deep brain stimulation: How does it work? *Handbook of clinical neurology*, 116:39–54, 2013.

233 Interfacing with the brain. https://neuralink.com/approach/. Accessed on 2023-08-10.

234 Neuralink. breakthrough technology for the brain. https://neuralink.com/. Accessed on 2009-08-10.

235 Sara Berger and Francesca Rossi. The future of AI ethics and the role of neurotechnology. In *Workshop on Adverse Impacts and Collateral Effects of Artificial Intelligence Technologies*. CEUR-WS, 2021.

236 Aswin Chari, Sanjay Budhdeo, Rachel Sparks, Damiano G Barone, Hani J Marcus, Erlick AC Pereira and Martin M Tisdall. Brain–machine interfaces: The role of the neurosurgeon. *World neurosurgery*, 146:140–147, 2021.

10

REAL-TIME HEALTHCARE APPLICATIONS

Exploring the Synergy of Generative AI and Edge Computing/5G

Mary Adedoyin

10.1 Introduction

The rapid advancement of healthcare technologies has paved the way for innovative solutions that significantly enhance patient care and system efficiency. Among these, Generative Artificial Intelligence (AI) and Edge computing/5G have emerged as pivotal technologies driving this transformation. Generative AI, known for its ability to create and synthesize data, offers unprecedented capabilities in automating and improving various aspects of healthcare. When combined with the ultra-low latency and high-speed connectivity of Edge computing and 5G networks, these technologies provide a robust framework for developing responsive and intelligent healthcare applications. Generative AI has revolutionized data processing and analysis in healthcare, enabling the creation of complex models that can predict patient outcomes, personalize treatment plans, and enhance diagnostic accuracy [1–3]. Edge computing, on the other hand, brings computational power closer to the data source, reducing latency and enabling real-time processing. The integration of 5G technology further amplifies these benefits by providing faster data transmission speeds and more reliable connectivity, essential for real-time applications [4]. The synergy between Generative AI and Edge computing/5G can lead to more responsive, accurate, and personalized healthcare solutions. For instance, real-time diagnostics can be significantly enhanced by the quick data processing capabilities of Edge/5G computing and the analytical prowess of Generative AI. This convergence not only promises to improve patient outcomes but also aims to optimize healthcare delivery, making it more efficient and effective.

DOI: 10.1201/9781003481959-10

This chapter aims to explore the synergy between Generative AI and Edge computing/5G and their combined impact on real-time healthcare applications. The rest of the chapter is organized as follows: Fundamentals of Generative (AI) and Edge computing/5G is presented in Section 10.2, highlighting the individual definition of these technologies, their key models, strengths, and applications. Section 10.3 provides a detailed overview of the importance of the synergy of these technologies and various real-time healthcare applications enabled by this synergy are outlined. It sets the foundation for understanding their integration. Section 10.4 presents technical challenges, proposed solutions, potential developments, and future opportunities through the synergy of Generative AI and Edge/5G. Section 10.5 concludes the chapter.

10.2 Fundamentals of Generative AI and Edge/5G computing

This section provides the fundamentals of Generative AI and Edge computing/ 5G, highlighting their individual definitions, key models, strengths, and applications in real-time healthcare settings.

10.2.1 Definition of Generative AI

Generative AI is a subset of AI that has the ability to create and synthesize data, enhance diagnostic accuracy, personalize treatment plans, and support advanced predictive analytics. These capabilities are pivotal in healthcare, where timely and precise data-driven decisions can significantly improve patient outcomes. It creates new data instances or contents that resemble a given dataset, often replicating existing forms like text, images, or audio. Unlike traditional AI, it is primarily concerned with recognizing patterns and making decisions based on existing data [1].

10.2.2 Key models in Generative AI

The Generative AI can be classified into text, audio, video, image, 3D visualization, and code as shown in Table 10.1. Large Language Models (LLMs) like GPT-4 have the ability to process vast amounts of medical data, including patient records, and real-time inputs from healthcare systems. LLMs are adept at analyzing patient queries, interpreting diagnostic information, and assisting clinicians in medical documentation. It also involves extracting meaningful insights from clinical data, which aids in decision-making for diagnostics, treatment plans, and medical research. It supports telemedicine by answering patient questions in real-time, providing basic health advice, and helping with symptom analysis. The key models in Generative AI

TABLE 10.1 Generative AI models

Text	Audio	Video	Image	3D visualization	Code
• GPT-4 (OpenAI) [1, 6]	• WaveNet (Deep Mind) [15]	• DALL-E 2 (OpenAI) [1, 25]	• DALL-E (OpenAI) [1, 25]	• NeRF (Google) [43]	• Codex (OpenAI) [53]
• BERT (Google) [1, 7]	• Tacotron (Google) [16]	• Cog-Video (BAAI) [26]	• BigGAN (DeepMind) [34]	• 3DGAN (DeepMind) [44]	• AlphaCode (DeepMind) [54]
• T5 (Google) [8]	• DeepVoice (Baidu) [17]	• VQVAE-2 (DeepMind) [27]	• Style-GAN [35]	• PointNet (Stanford) [45]	• CodeBERT (Microsoft Research) [55]
• RoBERTa (Facebook AI) [9]	• Jukebox (OpenAI) [18]	• VideoGPT (OpenAI) [28]	• CLIP (OpenAI) [36]	• Mesh R-CNN (Facebook AI) [46]	• GPT-3 Codex (OpenAI) [56]
• XLNet (Google/CMU) [5]	• WaveGlow (NVIDIA) [19]	• Vid2Vid (NVIDIA) [29]	• VQ-VAE (DeepMind) [37]	• Pix2Vox (Shanghai-Tech University) [47]	• CoPilot (GitHub & OpenAI) [57]
• Turing-NLG (Microsoft) [10]	• MelGAN (Facebook AI) [20]	• MoCoGAN (UC Berkeley) [30]	• Imagen (Google) [38]	• Occupancy Networks (MPI for Intelligent Systems) [48]	• PolyCoder (Microsoft) [58]
• Megatron-LM (NVIDIA) [11]	• FastSpeech (Microsoft) [21]	• TGAN (Tokyo University) [31]	• LDM (Stable Diffusion) [39]	• AtlasNet (Facebook AI) [49]	• CodeT5 (Salesforce) [59]
• PaLM (Google) [12]	• DeepSpeech (Mozilla) [22]	• StyleGAN-V (NVIDIA) [32]	• Mid-Journey [40]	• NVIDIA Instant NeRF [50]	• TabNine (TabNine) [60]
• GLaM (Google) [13]	• Vall-E (Microsoft) [23]	• MMV (Facebook AI) [33]	• DeepArt (DeepArt.io) [41]	• ConvONet (Autonomous Vision Group) [51]	• OpenAI API (OpenAI) [61]
• Gopher (Deep Mind) [14]	• TalkNet (NVIDIA) [24]		• Pix2Pix (Berkeley AI Research) [42]	• PointFlow (UIUC & Stanford) [52]	• PyTorch Lightning Code Model (PyTorch) [62]

include Generative Adversarial Networks (GANs), Variational Autoencoders (VAEs), transformer models, and diffusion models [2, 5].

- **GANs:** These consist of two neural networks, a generator and a discriminator, that are trained simultaneously. The generator creates fake data instances, while the discriminator evaluates their authenticity. The generator improves over time by learning to produce data that the discriminator cannot distinguish from real data [2].
- **VAEs:** These are probabilistic models that encode input data into a latent space and then decode it back to the original data format. VAEs are used for generating new data instances by sampling from the latent space.
- **Transformer Models:** Initially used for natural language processing, transformer models like GPT-3 can generate coherent text by predicting the next word in a sentence. These models have also been adapted for image and music generation [5].
- **Diffusion Models:** Diffusion models generate data by reversing a noise-adding process. They progressively add noise to data samples, then learn to denoise them step by step to create new data samples. The model adds noise gradually over many steps, converting data into random noise.

10.2.3   Strengths of Generative AI in real-time healthcare applications

Generative AI provides different strengths in real-time healthcare applications, which include:

- Personalized Care: This enables tailored treatment plans based on patient data.
- Improved Diagnostics: This enhances accuracy in disease detection through AI-generated imaging and predictive models.
- Faster Decision-Making: This assists clinicians with rapid, data-driven insights during critical care.
- Accelerated Drug Discovery: This speeds up the identification of new drugs and therapies by generating novel molecular structures.
- Efficient Data Utilization: This handles and processes large datasets in real-time for actionable healthcare insights.
- Innovation in Research: This creates synthetic medical data for research, training, and simulations without compromising patient privacy.

10.2.4   Applications of Generative AI in real-time healthcare

Generative AI is revolutionizing real-time healthcare by enabling different applications as summarized in Figure 10.1. Through advanced algorithms,

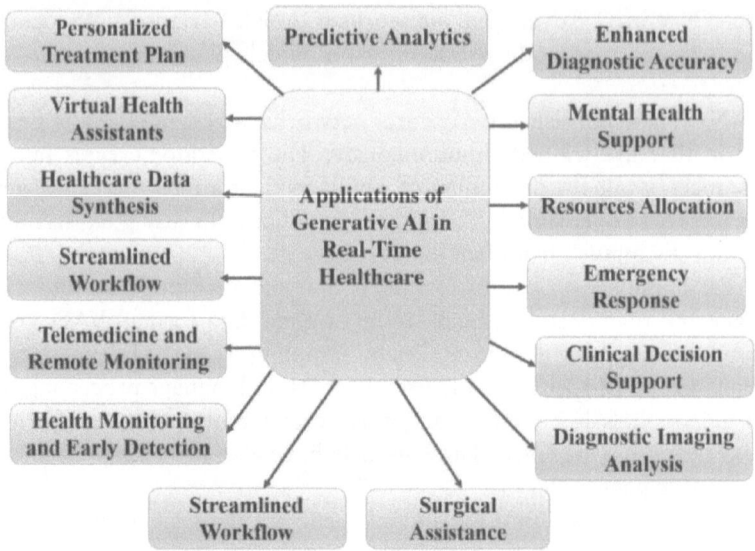

FIGURE 10.1 Applications of Generative AI in real-time healthcare.

it generates tailored insights, optimizes patient care, and facilitates efficient healthcare delivery, marking a transformative shift in medical practice. These applications include:

- Personalized Treatment Plans: Generative AI can create personalized treatment plans tailored to individual patient needs, improving the effectiveness of treatments and reducing adverse reactions by synthesizing patient data.
- Predictive Analytics: Generative AI can analyze vast amounts of patient data in real-time to predict disease outbreaks, patient deterioration, or potential complications. This enables proactive interventions and better patient management.
- Enhanced Diagnostic Accuracy: Generative AI models can assist in diagnosing conditions by analyzing medical images, lab results, and patient symptoms. They can highlight potential issues that might be overlooked by human practitioners, thereby improving diagnostic accuracy and speed.
- Virtual Health Assistants: Generative AI powers virtual health assistants that can interact with patients in real-time, providing medical advice, answering questions, and monitoring health conditions to ensure continuous care and support.
- Streamlined Workflow: In healthcare settings, Generative AI can automate routine administrative tasks such as data entry, appointment scheduling, and billing. This allows healthcare professionals to focus more on patient care rather than paperwork.

- Clinical Decision Support Systems: Integrating Generative AI into clinical decision support systems helps healthcare providers make informed decisions by generating and presenting relevant data insights, treatment recommendations, and diagnostic options.
- Drug Discovery and Development: Generative AI can accelerate the drug discovery process by simulating and generating potential drug candidates, predicting their efficacy and safety, and identifying new therapeutic uses for existing drugs.
- Telemedicine and Remote Monitoring: Generative AI enhances telemedicine by analyzing patient data in real-time, providing immediate feedback and recommendations to healthcare providers during virtual consultations, and supporting remote patient monitoring.
- Health Monitoring and Early Detection: Wearable devices and sensors can continuously monitor vital signs and health metrics. Generative AI can analyze this data in real-time to detect early signs of health issues, enabling timely medical interventions.
- Mental Health Support: Generative AI can create virtual therapeutic environments and tools that provide real-time support for mental health conditions, offering personalized coping strategies and monitoring patient progress.
- Resource Allocation: AI can optimize the allocation of healthcare resources by predicting patient admission rates, bed occupancy, and staff requirements. This ensures that hospitals and clinics are better prepared to handle patient loads efficiently.
- Emergency Response: In emergency situations, generative AI can analyze real-time data to prioritize patient care, manage emergency resources, and provide critical information to first responders, improving the overall response time and effectiveness.
- Clinical Decision Support: AI systems can provide clinical decision support by offering evidence-based recommendations for treatment options, alerting to potential drug interactions, and ensuring adherence to clinical guidelines.
- Diagnostic Imaging Analysis: Generative AI can enhance the interpretation of medical images, such as X-rays, MRIs, and CT scans.
- Healthcare Data Synthesis: Generative AI can synthesize new data from existing datasets, helping to fill gaps in medical records, enhance the quality of electronic health records (EHRs), and support research and development initiatives.
- Surgical Assistance: In surgical settings, Generative AI can assist by generating detailed surgical plans, simulating potential outcomes, and providing real-time guidance to surgeons based on patient-specific data.

10.2.5 Definition of Edge computing

Edge computing refers to a distributed computing paradigm, which involves processing data closer to the data source, at the "edge" of the network, rather than relying solely on centralized cloud servers. The components of Edge computing include edge devices, edge servers, gateways, and cloud integration. The summary of the components of Edge computing is presented in Table 10.2.

TABLE 10.2 Components of Edge computing

Components of Edge computing	Explanation	Examples	Functions
Edge Devices	They are the end points where data is generated and initially processed	Sensors, wearables, smart cameras, Internet of Things (IoT) devices, and local servers	• They collect and preprocess data locally • They reduce the amount of data sent to edge servers or the cloud by performing initial filtering and analysis
Edge Servers	These are intermediate servers located near the edge devices. They handle more complex processing tasks that are too resource-intensive for edge devices	Local data centers, network edge servers	• They aggregate and process data from multiple edge devices • They perform real-time analytics and decision-making • They provide faster response times compared to centralized cloud servers
Gateways	They act as bridges between edge devices and edge servers or cloud services. They manage data traffic and ensure secure communication	Intel® Health Application Platform, Cisco IOx-enabled router	• They collect and route data from edge devices to edge servers or the cloud • They translate different protocols and formats for compatibility • They enhance data security through encryption and authentication

(Continued)

TABLE 10.2 (Continued)

Components of Edge computing	Explanation	Examples	Functions
Cloud Integration	It connects Edge computing infrastructure with centralized cloud services	Cloud storage services (e.g., AWS, Google Cloud) Cloud-based analytics and machine learning platforms	• They store large volumes of data that are not time-sensitive • They provide additional processing power and advanced analytics capabilities • They ensure long-term data storage and backup

10.2.6 Strengths of Edge computing in real-time healthcare applications

Edge computing offers several strengths in real-time healthcare applications by processing data closer to where it is generated. The strengths include:

- Reduced Latency: Edge computing minimizes the delay between data generation and processing by processing data at the edge of the network. This is crucial for time-sensitive healthcare applications such as remote patient monitoring, emergency response, and real-time diagnostic support.
- Enhanced Privacy and Security: Edge computing keeps sensitive patient data closer to its source, reducing the need to transmit it over potentially insecure networks. This enhances data privacy and security, which is critical in healthcare where patient confidentiality is paramount.
- Reliability and Resilience: Edge computing can continue to function independently of central servers, providing greater reliability and resilience. This is particularly important in healthcare settings where uninterrupted access to patient data and applications is critical.
- Scalability: Edge computing can scale efficiently by adding more edge devices as needed. This is useful in large healthcare systems with multiple facilities or in scenarios where there is a need to process vast amounts of data from numerous Internet of Things (IoT) devices and sensors.
- Bandwidth Optimization: Edge computing optimizes bandwidth usage by processing data locally and only sending relevant information to the central cloud. This is especially beneficial in environments with limited network capacity or high data volume, such as hospitals with numerous connected devices.

- Real-Time Monitoring and Alerts: Edge computing enables real-time monitoring and immediate alerts for patient conditions. For example, wearable health devices can continuously monitor vital signs and trigger instant alerts to healthcare providers if abnormalities are detected, allowing for rapid intervention.
- Local Data Processing and Storage: Edge devices can store and process data locally, which is useful in remote or rural healthcare settings with limited or intermittent internet connectivity. This ensures continuous operation and access to critical patient data regardless of network status.
- Improved Patient Care: Healthcare providers can offer more immediate and personalized care by enabling real-time data analysis and decision-making at the edge. This can lead to better patient outcomes, especially in critical care and emergency situations.
- Support for Advanced Technologies: Edge computing supports the implementation of AI and ML at the point of care. This allows for real-time analytics and insights without the need for constant cloud connectivity.
- Cost Efficiency: Edge computing can reduce costs associated with data transmission and cloud storage by processing data locally. This is beneficial for healthcare organizations looking to manage operational expenses while still leveraging advanced computing capabilities.
- Interoperability and Integration: Edge computing can facilitate the integration of various healthcare devices and systems, ensuring seamless data exchange and interoperability. This is essential for creating a cohesive healthcare ecosystem where different devices and applications work together efficiently.
- Environmental Adaptability: Edge computing can be adapted to various environmental conditions and requirements, making it suitable for diverse healthcare settings, from urban hospitals to rural clinics and mobile health units.

10.2.7 Applications of Edge computing in real-time healthcare

Edge computing in real-time healthcare offers several applications as summarized in Figure 10.2, which enhances patient monitoring, improves response times, reduces latency, and supports real-time decision-making in critical care environments, leading to more efficient and effective healthcare delivery. These applications include:

- Wearable Devices: Devices such as smartwatches and fitness trackers can monitor vital signs (e.g., heart rate, blood pressure) and detect anomalies in real-time. The data is processed at the edge, allowing for immediate alerts to healthcare providers.

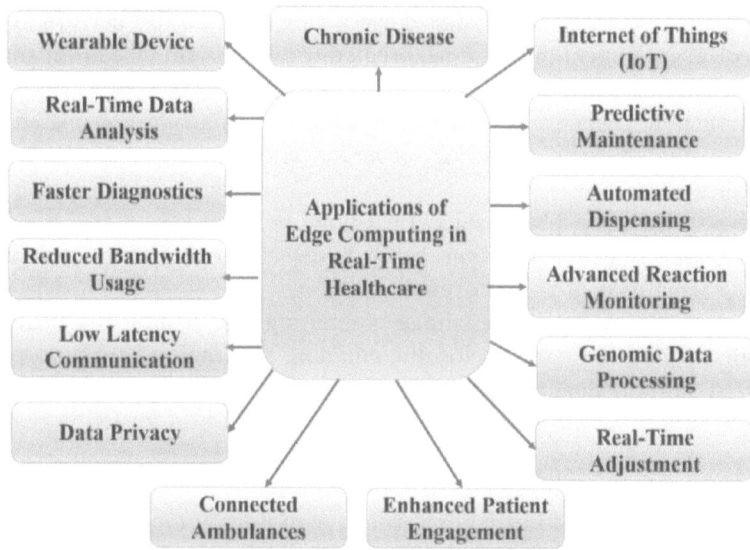

FIGURE 10.2 Applications of Edge computing in real-time healthcare.

- Chronic Disease Management: Patients with chronic conditions (e.g., diabetes, hypertension) can use Edge computing devices to continuously monitor their health parameters and receive timely interventions.
- Real-Time Data Analysis: Edge computing enables the real-time analysis of data from various sources (e.g., ambulances, emergency rooms) to provide immediate insights and improve response times.
- Connected Ambulances: Equipped with edge devices, ambulances can transmit patient data to hospitals, allowing for better preparation and faster treatment upon arrival.
- Faster Diagnostics: Edge computing can process medical images (e.g., X-rays, MRIs) on-site, providing quicker results and enabling faster decision-making.
- Reduced Bandwidth Usage: Only relevant information is sent to central servers, reducing the amount of data transmitted and improving efficiency by processing and filtering data at the edge.
- Low Latency Communication: Edge computing ensures low-latency communication between patients and healthcare providers during virtual consultations, enhancing the quality of interaction and decision-making.
- Data Privacy: Sensitive patient data can be processed locally at the edge, minimizing the risk of data breaches and ensuring compliance with privacy regulations.
- IoT Integration: Edge computing integrates various IoT devices (e.g., smart beds, monitoring systems) within hospitals to optimize operations and patient care.

- Predictive Maintenance: Edge devices can monitor the performance of medical equipment in real-time, predicting failures and scheduling maintenance to avoid downtime.
- Automated Dispensing: Edge computing can manage automated drug dispensing systems, ensuring accurate and timely administration of medications.
- Adverse Reaction Monitoring: Real-time monitoring and analysis of patient responses to medications can help detect adverse reactions early and adjust treatment plans accordingly.
- Genomic Data Processing: Edge computing can handle the processing of large genomic datasets locally, enabling personalized treatment plans based on individual genetic profiles.
- Real-Time Adjustments: Treatment regimens can be adjusted in real-time based on continuous monitoring and analysis of patient data.
- Enhanced Patient Engagement: Patients can benefit from more responsive and interactive healthcare applications with Edge computing.

10.2.8 Definition of 5G

5G wireless technology provides higher capacity, faster-speed, and low-latency communication capabilities that support the proliferation of connected devices and advanced applications [5]. 5G networks provide the high bandwidth and low latency required for real-time data processing at the edge. They achieve this through features like network slicing, which allows for the creation of virtual networks tailored to specific applications.

10.2.9 Strengths of 5G in real-time healthcare applications

5G technology offers numerous strengths in real-time healthcare applications, fundamentally transforming the way healthcare services are delivered. These strengths include:

- Ultra-Low Latency: 5G networks provide ultra-low latency, which is essential for real-time healthcare applications. This allows for immediate transmission and processing of data, enabling critical applications like remote surgery, real-time monitoring, and rapid response to medical emergencies.
- High Bandwidth: 5G offers significantly higher bandwidth compared to previous generations of mobile networks. This enables the transmission of large amounts of data, such as high-resolution medical imaging, quickly and efficiently. It also supports the use of advanced technologies like virtual reality (VR) and augmented reality (AR) in medical training and telemedicine.

- Enhanced Connectivity: 5G can connect a vast number of devices simultaneously, supporting the Internet of Medical Things (IoMT). This means that wearable devices, sensors, and other medical equipment can continuously collect and share patient data in real-time, facilitating comprehensive monitoring and timely interventions.
- Remote Patient Monitoring: 5G enables continuous, real-time remote monitoring of patients through connected devices. This is particularly beneficial for managing chronic diseases, post-operative care, and elderly patients, allowing healthcare providers to track health metrics and respond quickly to any abnormalities.
- Telemedicine and Telehealth: The high-speed connectivity of 5G enhances telemedicine services, providing high-quality video consultations with minimal lag. This improves patient access to healthcare, especially in remote or underserved areas, and ensures that consultations are as close to in-person experiences as possible.
- Mobile and Portable Medical Devices: With 5G, portable and mobile medical devices can function more effectively and reliably. This enables healthcare professionals to provide high-quality care in various settings, including at patients' homes, in rural clinics, or during emergency situations.
- Advanced Diagnostics and Imaging: The high-speed and low-latency capabilities of 5G facilitate the rapid transfer of large diagnostic images and datasets to specialists, regardless of their location. These speed up the diagnostic process and ensure timely treatment decisions.
- Support for AI and ML: 5G networks can support the high data throughput required for AI and ML applications in healthcare. This includes real-time analytics for predictive diagnostics, personalized treatment plans, and automated clinical decision support systems.
- Improved Patient Experience: With 5G, patients can benefit from a more seamless and interactive healthcare experience. Real-time health tracking, instant access to medical records, and high-quality virtual consultations contribute to better patient engagement and satisfaction.
- Enhanced Data Security: While 5G introduces new security challenges, it also offers advanced security features that can be leveraged to protect sensitive healthcare data. Network slicing, for instance, can create isolated, secure channels for transmitting medical information.
- AR and VR: 5G supports the use of AR and VR in healthcare for purposes such as surgical training, patient education, and treatment planning. These technologies can provide immersive, real-time experiences that enhance learning and improve patient outcomes.
- Scalable Health Networks: 5G can support the creation of scalable health networks that can adapt to varying demands and conditions. This is particularly useful during health crises, pandemics, or natural disasters when healthcare resources need to be rapidly deployed and managed.

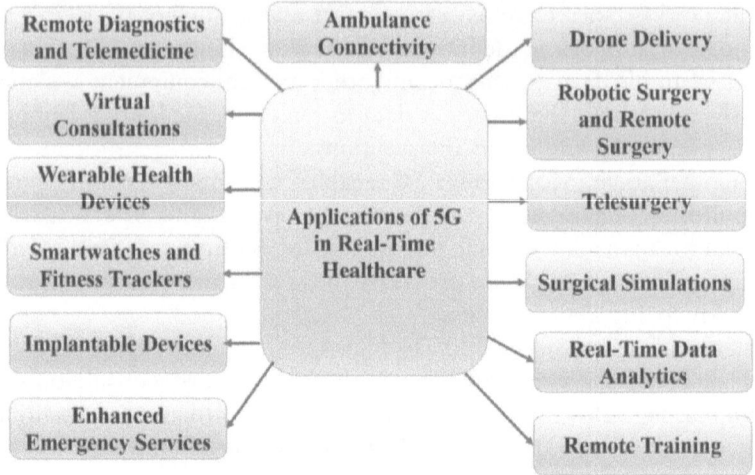

FIGURE 10.3 Applications of 5G in real-time healthcare.

10.2.10 Applications of 5G in real-time healthcare

5G revolutionizes real-time healthcare by enabling different applications as summarized in Figure 10.3, with ultra-fast data transfer, low latency, and reliable connectivity. These applications include:

- Remote Diagnostics and Telemedicine: 5G facilitates high-definition video conferencing and real-time data transmission, making remote consultations and diagnostics more effective. Doctors can remotely examine patients, view high-resolution images, and provide immediate medical advice.
- Virtual Consultations: High-quality video calls allow physicians to conduct thorough examinations, monitor patient conditions, and provide diagnoses without geographical constraints.
- Wearable Health Devices and Continuous Monitoring: 5G supports the connectivity of numerous wearable health devices that monitor vital signs and other health metrics continuously. The data collected is transmitted in real-time to healthcare providers, enabling continuous patient monitoring and timely interventions.
- Smartwatches and Fitness Trackers: Devices that monitor heart rate, oxygen levels, and other vitals can send alerts to healthcare providers if abnormalities are detected.
- Implantable Devices: Pacemakers and glucose monitors that transmit real-time data to healthcare providers, allowing for immediate response to critical health changes.
- Enhanced Emergency Services: 5G can improve emergency response services by enabling faster communication and data sharing between emergency responders, hospitals, and healthcare providers. Real-time data

from the field can be transmitted to emergency rooms, preparing them for incoming patients and improving patient outcomes.

- Ambulance Connectivity: Real-time transmission of patient data from ambulances to emergency rooms, allowing hospital staff to prepare in advance.
- Drone Delivery: Use of drones to deliver medical supplies, such as blood or medications, to emergency sites quickly and efficiently.
- Robotic Surgery and Remote Surgery: Low latency and high reliability of 5G enable surgeons to perform robotic and remote surgeries with high precision. Surgeons can control robotic instruments in real-time, even from distant locations.
- Telesurgery: Surgeons in different locations can collaborate on surgeries, providing expertise that may not be locally available.
- Surgical Simulations: Trainees can practice surgeries in a virtual environment, gaining hands-on experience without risks to patients.
- Remote Training: Medical professionals can participate in real-time training sessions and seminars from anywhere, accessing expert knowledge and guidance.
- Real-Time Data Analytics: 5G enables the real-time collection and analysis of vast amounts of health data, facilitating advanced analytics and AI-driven insights for personalized medicine and predictive healthcare.

10.3 Synergy of Generative AI and Edge computing/5G in healthcare

The convergence of Generative AI and Edge computing/5G as shown in Figure 10.4 marks a pivotal advancement in healthcare technology. The capability of Generative AI to synthesize and analyze vast amounts of data, when combined with the high-speed, low-latency, and localized processing power of Edge computing/5G, creates a robust platform for real-time healthcare applications. This convergence allows for more efficient and effective healthcare delivery, leveraging the strengths of the technologies to address the growing demands of modern healthcare systems.

A study by the authors in [63] describes a system that detects gestures using ultrasonic signals and edge devices. Seven gestures, plus idle, can be recognized and combined. Ultrasonic transceivers detect 2D gestures, processed entirely on the edge device. The system achieves 84.18–98.4% accuracy using optimized preprocessing and specific firmware design. The system utilizes a Generative AI to create synthetic training data for the analysis algorithm. 5G ensures seamless communication between the edge device and a central server for model updates and additional processing power when needed. The AI model can learn to identify subtle abnormalities more effectively by using synthetic data for training, leading to improved diagnostic accuracy. Edge computing enables real-time analysis, eliminating the need to send data to the cloud for processing, thus reducing response times and allowing for

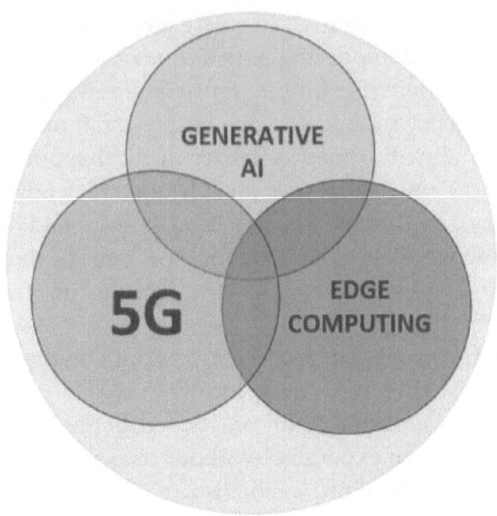

FIGURE 10.4 Convergence of Generative AI, Edge computing and 5G.

faster diagnosis. The authors in [64] identified barriers to implementing AI in Dutch clinical radiology using a qualitative case study of seven hospitals. The key facilitators included cost containment pressure, high expectations for AI, innovative strategies, and local champions. Hindrances include inconsistent AI performance, unstructured implementation, uncertain clinical value, and varying acceptance. Hence, structured implementation and clinical evidence are needed for the effective use of AI. The AI algorithms detect anomalies and potential issues with higher accuracy than traditional methods, highlighting areas of concern for radiologists. The local processing with Edge computing reduces the time needed for image analysis, providing near-instant results. 5G connectivity ensures that radiologists can access and review images in real-time, even from remote locations. Some clinics have implemented an advanced telemedicine platform enhanced with AI-driven diagnostic tools, Edge computing, and 5G. During virtual consultations, patient data is processed on-site using edge devices, and AI algorithms provide diagnostic support. High-quality video consultations are facilitated by 5G connectivity. AI assists doctors by analyzing patient data and suggesting possible diagnoses, improving accuracy. The immediate data processing and AI analysis during consultations speed up decision-making. The high-quality, low-latency video consultations expand access to healthcare, especially for patients in remote areas. Google plays a role in healthcare communication, developing smart devices like the Fitbit tracker for health monitoring. Fitbit measures blood oxygen levels with optical sensors, using low-power LEDs that shut down if there is an issue. AI algorithms analyze data to optimize resource allocation and predict patient needs [65]. The real-time data processing at the edge enhances operational efficiency. The continuous monitoring of patient vitals with Edge computing ensures immediate detection of any issues. 5G connectivity facilitates seamless communication.

The importance of the synergy of Generative AI and Edge computing/5G in real-time healthcare applications is presented in Table 10.3. The synergy between these technologies enables the deployment of intelligent healthcare solutions that can process and analyze data at unprecedented speeds, providing immediate insights and actions.

TABLE 10.3 Importance of the synergy of Generative AI and Edge computing/5G in real-time healthcare applications

Applications	Generative AI	Edge computing	5G
Enhanced Real-Time Data Processing and Analysis	• It provides advanced data analysis and predictive insights by processing large volumes of medical data	• It processes data locally, ensuring immediate analysis and response	• It facilitates rapid data transfer with minimal latency, enabling real-time interactions and updates
Improved Patient Monitoring and Response	• It predicts patient conditions and potential health risks using continuous data analysis	• It allows for real-time monitoring of patients through wearable devices and sensors, providing immediate feedback and alerts	• It ensures that data from monitoring devices is transmitted instantaneously, allowing for swift medical interventions
Remote and Mobile Healthcare	• It supports telemedicine by analyzing patient data and providing diagnostic support during virtual consultations	• It enables portable and mobile medical devices to function effectively, allowing healthcare providers to offer care in diverse settings	• It enhances telemedicine by providing high-quality video and data transmission with low latency, ensuring seamless virtual care
Advanced Diagnostic and Imaging Capabilities	• It analyzes medical images and diagnostic data to provide accurate and fast results	• It processes images locally, reducing the time needed for analysis and diagnosis	• It facilitates the rapid transfer of large imaging files and diagnostic data, ensuring that specialists can access and analyze information quickly

(Continued)

TABLE 10.3 (Continued)

Applications	Generative AI	Edge computing	5G
Real-Time Surgical Applications	• It assists in planning and guiding surgical procedures through advanced analytics and simulations.	• It provides real-time data processing and feedback during surgeries, ensuring precision and responsiveness.	• It enables reliable, low-latency communication between surgical robots and surgeons, supporting complex remote and robotic surgeries
Optimized Resource Management	• It predicts patient admissions, resource needs, and staff requirements, optimizing resource allocation	• It manages local data to ensure that resources are allocated efficiently within healthcare facilities	• It facilitates seamless communication and coordination among healthcare teams, improving operational efficiency
Enhanced Patient Engagement and Experience	• It personalizes patient care plans and provides tailored health recommendations	• It delivers real-time health insights and interactive applications directly to patients through their devices	• It ensures fast and reliable connectivity for patient-facing applications, improving engagement and satisfaction

The healthcare setting is undergoing a rapid transformation powered by the adoption of cutting-edge technologies. This section explores several applications that are revolutionizing healthcare. The summary of these real-time applications for convergence of generative AI, Edge computing, and 5G is presented in Table 10.4.

10.4 Technical challenges, proposed solutions, potential developments, and future opportunities

The synergy between Generative AI and Edge computing/5G holds immense promise for advancing real-time healthcare applications. Figure 10.5 presents the summary of the technical challenges, proposed solutions, potential development, and future opportunities for further revolutionizing healthcare services to ensure the secure, efficient, and reliable implementation of these technologies. Table 10.5 summarizes the implementation concerns, technical challenges, and proposed solutions that can be employed.

TABLE 10.4 Real-time healthcare applications for the convergence of Generative AI, Edge computing, and 5G

Applications	Generative AI	Edge computing	5G	Examples
Remote Diagnosis	• It provides advanced diagnostic tools that can analyze medical images and patient data with high accuracy	• It processes data locally to reduce latency and ensure quick diagnostic results	• It facilitates fast, reliable data transmission from remote locations to central healthcare facilities	• Real-time analysis of X-rays, MRIs, and CT scans • Immediate feedback on patient conditions in remote areas
Telemedicine	• It enhances virtual consultations with AI-powered decision support tools	• It ensures smooth video conferencing and data processing at the edge to minimize delays	• It provides the necessary bandwidth and low latency for high-quality video and audio communication	• Virtual consultations with specialists • Remote patient monitoring and follow-up care
Personalized Treatment Plans	• It analyzes patient data to create personalized treatment plans based on individual health profiles	• It processes data in real-time at the point of care, enabling immediate adjustments to treatment	• It ensures seamless data integration from various sources, such as wearable devices and electronic health records (EHRs)	• Tailored medication regimens and therapy plans • Dynamic adjustment of treatment protocols based on real-time data
Predictive Analytics and Patient Monitoring	• It predicts potential health issues by analyzing trends in patient data	• It continuously monitors patients' vital signs and other health indicators, providing real-time alerts	• It supports continuous data streaming from patient monitoring devices to healthcare providers	• Early detection of chronic conditions, such as diabetes and heart disease • Real-time monitoring of critical patients in hospitals or at home

(Continued)

TABLE 10.4 (Continued)

Applications	Generative AI	Edge computing	5G	Examples
Emergency Response Systems	• It assists in triaging and prioritizing emergency cases based on the severity and available resources	• It processes critical data locally to ensure rapid decision-making during emergencies	• It enables fast communication between emergency responders and healthcare facilities	• Automated triage systems in emergency rooms • Real-time coordination of ambulances and medical teams
Robotic Surgery and Automation	• It provides precision and control in robotic-assisted surgeries	• It ensures low-latency control of surgical robots, enhancing precision and safety	• It facilitates real-time video feeds and communication between surgeons and robotic systems	• Remote-controlled robotic surgeries • Automation of routine surgical procedures
AR and VR in Healthcare	• It enhances AR/VR experiences with intelligent simulations and real-time data overlays	• It processes AR/VR data locally to reduce latency and improve user experience	• It provides the necessary bandwidth and low latency for seamless AR/VR applications	• AR-guided surgeries and medical training • VR-based rehabilitation programs for patients
Medication Management and Adherence	• It analyzes patient behavior and medication data to optimize adherence strategies	• It processes adherence data locally to provide immediate feedback and reminders	• It ensures continuous connectivity for real-time monitoring of medication intake	• Smart pill dispensers that alert patients to take their medication • Real-time adherence tracking and feedback systems

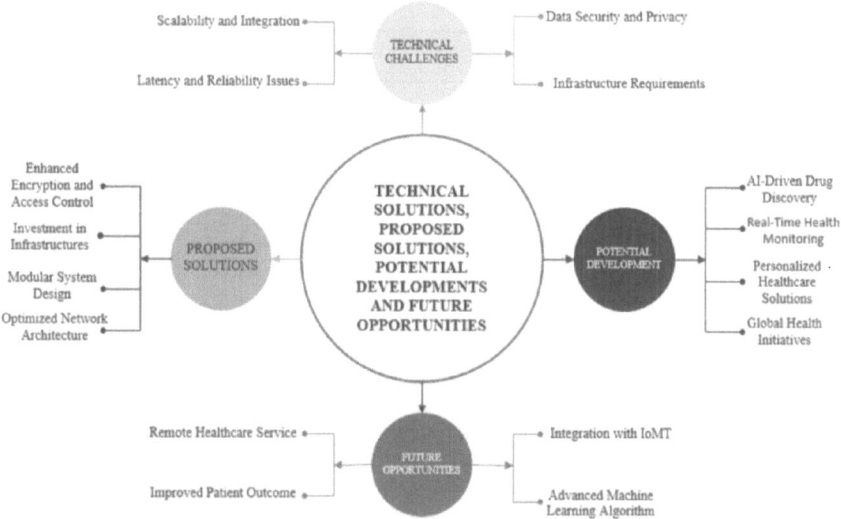

FIGURE 10.5 Implementation concerns, technical challenges, and proposed solutions.

TABLE 10.5 Implementation concerns, technical challenges, and proposed solutions

Implementation concerns	Challenges	Proposed solutions
Data Security and Privacy [66]	• The decentralized nature of Edge computing can increase the risk of data breaches. Each edge device becomes a potential point of vulnerability • Healthcare data must comply with regulations. Ensuring that all devices and data handling processes meet these stringent requirements is challenging • Ensuring end-to-end encryption of data transmitted over 5G networks is essential to protect patient privacy	• Implement robust encryption protocols for data in transit and at rest • Regularly update and patch edge devices to protect against vulnerabilities • Employ AI-based security solutions to detect and mitigate potential threats in real-time

(Continued)

TABLE 10.5 (Continued)

Implementation concerns	Challenges	Proposed solutions
Infrastructure Requirements [67]	• The initial setup cost for edge devices, 5G infrastructure, and AI systems can be substantial • Continuous maintenance and upgrades are required to ensure optimal performance and security • Integrating new technologies with existing healthcare systems and ensuring they work seamlessly together can be difficult	• Develop a phased implementation plan to manage costs and ensure smooth integration with existing systems • Invest in scalable infrastructure that can be expanded as needed • Establish partnerships with technology providers to leverage their expertise and resources
Scalability [68]	• As healthcare applications generate vast amounts of data, systems must be scalable to process and analyze this data efficiently • Integrating diverse healthcare applications and ensuring they work together seamlessly is complex • Efficiently allocating resources to handle varying workloads is crucial for maintaining performance	• Employ scalable cloud and Edge computing solutions that can dynamically allocate resources based on demand • Use open standards and APIs to facilitate interoperability between different healthcare systems and devices • Implement AI-driven resource management solutions to optimize the allocation of computing resources
Latency and Reliability [69]	• Despite the low latency of 5G networks, there can still be delays due to network congestion or data processing at edge devices • Ensuring continuous availability and reliability of edge devices and AI systems is challenging, particularly in remote or underserved areas • Achieving real-time data processing and decision-making requires highly efficient and reliable systems	• Optimize network architecture to reduce latency and ensure reliable data transmission • Implement redundancy and failover mechanisms to maintain system reliability • Use advanced algorithms and high-performance computing resources to achieve real-time data processing

10.4.1 Proposed solutions

The proposed solutions for the implementation concerns include:

i Enhanced Encryption and Access Control: These are critical solutions in the synergy of Generative AI, Edge computing, and 5G for real-time healthcare applications due to the sensitive nature of medical data and the distributed nature of Edge environments. The following are the enhanced encryption and access control techniques:

- Implementing strong encryption techniques ensures that healthcare data remains protected while in transit and at rest within Edge computing environments. This prevents unauthorized access and safeguards patient privacy.
- Encrypting data from its origin to its destination ensures that only authorized parties can decrypt and access sensitive information, maintaining confidentiality throughout data transmission and storage.
- Robust access control mechanisms authenticate users and devices before granting them access to healthcare data. This ensures that only authorized personnel can interact with sensitive patient information.
- Implementing role-based access control (RBAC) ensures that individuals only have access to the specific data and functionalities necessary for their roles, minimizing the risk of unauthorized data exposure.
- Logging and monitoring access attempts and actions taken on healthcare data provides accountability and transparency, enabling quick detection and response to potential security breaches.

ii Investment in Infrastructure: This is a crucial solution to address technical challenges in the synergy of Generative AI, Edge computing, and 5G for real-time healthcare applications. The following are the techniques which can be adopted:

- Deploying edge nodes, servers, and gateways closer to healthcare facilities and patient locations. This proximity reduces latency for real-time data processing and enhances the responsiveness of healthcare applications.
- Deploying scalable infrastructure allows healthcare providers to accommodate increasing data volumes generated by Generative AI applications and IoT devices, ensuring reliable performance and responsiveness.
- Expanding coverage, deploying small cells, and upgrading network equipment to support higher bandwidth and lower latency. This enables seamless connectivity for real-time healthcare applications across diverse geographic areas.

iii Modular System Design: This is a solution to the technical challenges in the synergy of Generative AI, Edge computing, and 5G for real-time healthcare applications. The following are the measures that can be utilized:

- Component Interchangeability: Modular design allows components (such as AI models, Edge devices, and 5G modules) to be easily replaced or upgraded without disrupting the entire system. This flexibility supports scalability as healthcare needs evolve and technologies advance.
- Tailored Configurations: Systems can be customized by assembling modules that best fit specific healthcare tasks, optimizing performance for applications like patient monitoring, diagnostics, or telemedicine.
- Efficient Resource Utilization: Each module can focus on its specialized function, maximizing computational resources and energy efficiency, which is crucial for Edge devices with limited processing capabilities.
- Standardized Interfaces: Modular systems often use standardized interfaces and protocols, facilitating seamless integration across diverse healthcare environments, including different Edge devices and 5G networks.
- Data Exchange: Integration supports efficient data exchange between modules, enabling real-time communication and collaboration among AI algorithms, Edge nodes, and centralized healthcare systems.
- Simplified Maintenance: Modular designs simplify maintenance and troubleshooting processes, as malfunctioning modules can be isolated and replaced without affecting the overall system functionality.
- Continuous Improvement: Upgrades and enhancements to individual modules can be implemented incrementally, ensuring the system stays current with technological advancements and regulatory requirements.

iv Optimized Network Architecture: This is a crucial proposed solution to the technical challenges in the synergy of Generative AI, Edge computing, and 5G for real-time healthcare applications. The following techniques can be adopted:

- Placing Edge computing nodes closer to data sources (e.g., medical devices, patient monitors) minimizes the distance data needs to travel, significantly reducing latency and enabling real-time data processing and decision-making.
- Optimizing routing algorithms to ensure data takes the quickest path between devices, Edge nodes, and central servers, further minimizing delays.
- Dedicating specific bandwidth and resources to different healthcare applications based on priority and necessity. This ensures critical healthcare tasks receive the necessary bandwidth, avoiding congestion and ensuring smooth operation.

- Dynamically allocating resources based on current demand, optimizing network performance, and ensuring that high-priority applications maintain optimal functionality.

10.4.2   Future directions

The future directions include:

- Integration with IoMT: IoMT refers to the interconnected network of medical devices and applications that collect and share data in real-time. IoMT devices, such as wearable sensors, smart implants, and remote monitoring tools, continuously collect health data. Integrating these devices with Edge computing allows real-time data processing, enabling immediate analysis and response. The data collected from IoMT devices can be fed into Generative AI models to generate insights, detect anomalies, and predict health events, enhancing proactive patient care. Healthcare providers can receive real-time alerts and insights from IoMT devices by processing data at the Edge, allowing for timely medical interventions and reducing the risk of complications. Generative AI can analyze the data from IoMT devices to tailor treatment plans to individual patients, improving the efficacy of healthcare delivery. 5G provides the high-speed, low-latency connectivity required to support a large number of IoMT devices, ensuring seamless and reliable data transmission across the healthcare network. Integrating IoMT devices with secure Edge and 5G infrastructure enhances data protection, as data can be encrypted and securely transmitted within the healthcare network.
- Development of Advanced ML Algorithm: The development of advanced ML algorithms, including deep learning and reinforcement learning, will further enhance healthcare applications.
- Provision of Remote Healthcare Services: This leverages the synergy of Generative AI, Edge computing, and 5G technology to deliver efficient, real-time medical care outside traditional clinical settings.

10.5   Conclusion

The integration of Generative AI with Edge computing/5G represents a transformative shift in the healthcare sector, driving the future of real-time healthcare applications. This synergy enhances the capability to process vast amounts of data at unprecedented speeds, offering immediate insights and enabling proactive patient care. Generative AI brings advanced data analysis and predictive capabilities, allowing for more accurate diagnostics, personalized treatment plans, and innovative medical solutions. When combined with Edge computing, the data processing is decentralized, reducing latency and ensuring that critical healthcare services are not disrupted by network issues. This local processing capability ensures that healthcare providers can make timely and informed decisions, enhancing patient outcomes and operational efficiency. The adoption of 5G technology further amplifies these benefits by providing the high-speed, low-latency connectivity necessary for seamless data transmission and real-time application performance. This connectivity supports a range of healthcare applications, from remote diagnostics and telemedicine to continuous patient monitoring and emergency response systems, all operating with enhanced reliability and efficiency. Together, Generative AI, Edge computing, and 5G create a robust framework that addresses the pressing challenges of modern healthcare. Healthcare providers can offer more precise, efficient, and accessible care by leveraging this technological triad, ultimately improving patient outcomes and advancing the medical field. This synergy not only enhances the capabilities of healthcare systems but also sets the stage for future innovations that will continue to improve the quality and accessibility of medical care worldwide. As these technologies evolve and become more integrated into healthcare infrastructures, they hold the promise of delivering smarter, faster, and more effective healthcare solutions, paving the way for a new era of medical advancements.

References

1 S. Sai, A. Gaur, R. Sai, V. Chamola, M. Guizani and J. Rodrigues, "Generative AI for transformative healthcare: a comprehensive study of emerging models, applications, case studies, and limitations," vol. 12, *IEEE Access*, 2024.

2 I. Goodfellow, J. Pouget-Abadie, M. Mirza, B. Xu, D. Warde-Farley, S. Ozair and Y. Bengio, "Generative adversarial nets," *Advances in Neural Information Processing Systems*, vol. 27, pp. 2672–2680, 2014.

3 Y. Y. Ghadi, S. F. A. Shah, T. Mazhar, T. Shahzad and H. Hamam, "Enhancing patient healthcare with mobile edge computing and 5G: challenges and solutions for secure online health tools," *Journal Cloud Computing*, vol. 13, no. 93, 2024.

4 M. A. Adedoyin and O. E. Falowo, "Combination of ultra-dense network and other 5G enabling technologies: a survey," *IEEE Access*, vol. 8, pp. 22893–22932, 2020.

5 P. Evangelatos, C. Iliou, T. Mavropoulos, K. Apostolou, T. Tsikrika, S. Vrochidis and I. Kompatsiaris, "Named entity recognition in cyber threat intelligence using transformer-based models," in *2021 IEEE International Conference on Cyber Security and Resilience* (CSR), July 2021, pp. 348–353.

6 I. A. Zahid, S. S. Joudar, A. S. Albahri, O. S. Albahri, A. H. Alamoodi, J. Santamaría and L. Alzubaidi, "Unmasking large language models by means of OpenAI GPT-4 and Google AI: a deep instruction-based analysis," *Intelligent Systems with Applications*, vol. 200431, 2024.

7 J. Kenton and L. Toutanova, "BERT: Pre-training of deep bidirectional transformers for language understanding," in *Proceedings of NAACL-HLT*, vol. 1, p. 2, June 2019.

8 J. Ni, G. H. Abrego, N. Constant, J. Ma, K. B. Hall, D. Cer and Y. Yang, "Sentence-T5: Scalable sentence encoders from pre-trained text-to-text models," arXiv:2108.08877, 2021.

9 E. J. M. Arcilla, P. M. A. Samson, R. M. Dioses, F. V. Contreras Jr., R. C. Regala, J. C. Morano and J. S. Guialil, "Enhancement of Support Vector Machine Utilizing RoBERTa Applied to Sentiment Analysis of Facebook Data," *IRE Journals*, vol. 7, pp. 386–391, 2024.

10 S. Smith, M. Patwary, B. Norick, P. LeGresley, S. Rajbhandari, J. Casper and B. Catanzaro, "Using DeepSpeed and Megatron to train Megatron-Turing NLG 530B, a large-scale generative language model," arXiv:2201.11990, 2022.

11 D. Narayanan, M. Shoeybi, J. Casper, P. LeGresley, M. Patwary, V. Korthikanti and M. Zaharia, "Efficient large-scale language model training on GPU clusters using Megatron-LM," in *Proceedings of the International Conference for High Performance Computing, Networking, Storage and Analysis*, pp. 1–15, Nov. 2021.

12 A. Chowdhery, S. Narang, J. Devlin, M. Bosma, G. Mishra, A. Roberts and N. Fiedel, "PaLM: scaling language modeling with pathways," *Journal of Machine Learning Research*, vol. 24, no. 240, pp. 1–113, 2023.

13 A. Lih, "What Are Galleries, Libraries, Archives, and Museums (GLAM) to the Wikimedia Community," in *Leveraging Wikipedia: Connecting Communities of Knowledge*, ALA Editions, 2018, pp. 7–16.

14 W. Rae, S. Borgeaud, T. Cai, K. Millican, J. Hoffmann, F. Song and G. Irving, "Scaling language models: Methods, analysis & insights from training gopher," arXiv preprint arXiv:2112.11446, 2021.

15 A. Van Den Oord, S. Dieleman, H. Zen, K. Simonyan, O. Vinyals, A. Graves and K. Kavukcuoglu, "WaveNet: A generative model for raw audio," arXiv preprint arXiv:1609.03499, vol. 12, 2016.

16 R. J. Weiss, R. J. Skerry-Ryan, E. Battenberg, S. Mariooryad and D. P. Kingma, "Wave-Tacotron: spectrogram-free end-to-end text-to-speech synthesis," in *ICASSP 2021-2021 IEEE International Conference on Acoustics, Speech and Signal Processing (ICASSP)*, 2021, pp. 5679–5683.

17 A. Gibiansky, S. Arik, G. Diamos, J. Miller, K. Peng, W. Ping, J. Raiman, and Y. Zhou, "Deep voice 2: multi-speaker neural text-to-speech," *Advances in Neural Information Processing Systems*, vol. 30, 2017.

18 M. J. Jeon and J. Kim, "A study on the production of real-time algorithmic composition system using the VQ-VAE algorithm of OpenAI Jukebox," *Journal of Digital Contents Society*, vol. 22, no. 3, pp. 375–381, 2021.

19 R. Prenger, R. Valle and B. Catanzaro, "Waveglow: A flow-based generative network for speech synthesis," in *2019 IEEE International Conference on Acoustics, Speech and Signal Processing (ICASSP)*, pp. 3617–3621, May 2019.

20 L. Bonde and S. Dembele, "A unified generative artificial intelligence approach for converting social media content," in *2024 International Conference on Artificial Intelligence, Big Data, Computing and Data Communication Systems (icABCD)*, pp. 1–5, Aug. 2024.

21 Y. Ren, Y. Ruan, X. Tan, T. Qin, S. Zhao, Z. Zhao and T. Y. Liu, "Fastspeech: fast, robust and controllable text to speech," *Advances in Neural Information Processing Systems*, vol. 32, 2019.

22 E. Nacimiento-García, C. S. González-González and F. L. Gutiérrez-Vela, "Automatic captions on video calls, a must for the elderly: Using Mozilla DeepSpeech for the STT," in *Proceedings of the XXI International Conference on Human Computer Interaction*, pp. 1–7, Sep. 2021.

23 S. Chen, S. Liu, L. Zhou, Y. Liu, X. Tan and J. Li and F. Wei, "VALL-E 2: Neural codec language models are human parity zero-shot text to speech synthesizers," pp. 1–21, arXiv preprint:2406.05370, 2024.

24 S. Beliaev, Y. Rebryk and B. Ginsburg, "TalkNet: Fully-convolutional non-autoregressive speech synthesis model," arXiv preprint arXiv:2005.05514, 2020.

25 G. Marcus, E. Davis and S. Aaronson, "A very preliminary analysis of DALL-E 2," arXiv preprint arXiv:2204.13807, 2022.

26 W. Hong, M. Ding, W. Zheng, X. Liu and J. Tang, "Cogvideo: Large-scale pretraining for text-to-video generation via transformers," arXiv preprint arXiv:2205.15868, 2022.

27 A. Razavi, A. van den Oord and O. Vinyals, "Generating diverse high-fidelity images with VQ-VAE-2," *Advances in Neural Information Processing Systems*, vol. 32, 2019.

28 E. Karaarslan and Ö Aydın, "Generate Impressive Videos with Text Instructions: A Review of OpenAI Sora," *Stable Diffusion, Lumiere and Comparable Models*, pp. 1–16, 2024.

29 L. Zhuo, G. Wang, S. Li, W. Wu and Z. Liu, "Fast-vid2vid: Spatial-temporal compression for video-to-video synthesis," in *European Conference on Computer Vision*, pp. 289–305, Oct. 2022. Cham: Springer Nature Switzerland.

30 T. Brooks, J. Hellsten, M. Aittala, T. C. Wang, T. Aila, J. Lehtinen and T. Karras, "Generating long videos of dynamic scenes," *Advances in Neural Information Processing Systems*, vol. 35, pp. 31769–31781, 2022.

31 K. Ohnishi, S. Yamamoto, Y. Ushiku and T. Harada, "Hierarchical video generation from orthogonal information: optical flow and texture," *Proceedings of the AAAI Conference on Artificial Intelligence*, vol. 32, no. 1, 2018.

32 I. Skorokhodov, S. Tulyakov and M. Elhoseiny, "StyleGAN-V: A continuous video generator with the price, image quality and perks of StyleGAN2," in *Proceedings of the IEEE/CVF Conference on Computer Vision and Pattern Recognition*, pp. 3626–3636, 2022.

33 W. Wei, K. Wang, S. Qiu and H. He, "A multimodal vigilance (MMV) dataset during RSVP and SSVEP brain-computer interface tasks," *Scientific Data*, vol. 11, no. 1, p. 867, 2024.

34 G. Song and Y. Men, and M. Long, "Efficient large scale image synthesis through adversarial learning," in *ResearchGate*, pp. 1–10, 2022.

35 T. Karras, S. Laine, M. Aittala, J. Hellsten, J. Lehtinen and T. Aila, "Analyzing and improving the image quality of StyleGAN," in *Proceedings of the IEEE/CVF Conference on Computer Vision and Pattern Recognition (CVPR)*, pp. 8110–8119, 2020.

36 F. Carlsson, P. Eisen, F. Rekathati and M. Sahlgren, "Cross-lingual and multilingual CLIP," in *Proceedings of the Thirteenth Language Resources and Evaluation Conference (LREC)*, pp. 6848–6854, June 2022.

37 A. Razavi, A. van den Oord and O. Vinyals, "Generating diverse high-fidelity images with VQ-VAE-2," *Advances in Neural Information Processing Systems*, vol. 32, 2019.

38 R. M. Luque Revuelto, "The use of cartography and digital imagery as a didactic resource in secondary education: Some precisions regarding Google Earth." *BAGE*, no. 55, pp. 183–210, 2011.

39 S. W. Kim, B. Brown, K. Yin, K. Kreis, K. Schwarz, D. Li and S. Fidler, "NeuralField-LDM: Scene generation with hierarchical latent diffusion models," in *Proceedings of the IEEE/CVF Conference on Computer Vision and Pattern Recognition*, pp. 8496–8506, 2023.

40 S. Mansour, "Intelligent graphic design: the effectiveness of midjourney as a participant in a creative brainstorming session," *International Design Journal*, vol. 13, no. 5, pp. 501–512, 2023.

41 D. K. Vishwakarma, "A state-of-the-arts and prospective in neural style transfer," in *2019 6th International Conference on Signal Processing and Integrated Networks (SPIN)*, pp. 244–247, Mar. 2019. IEEE.

42 F. Dellaert and L. Yen-Chen, "Neural volume rendering: NeRF and beyond," arXiv preprint arXiv:2101.05204, 2020.

43 A. Rodriguez, *Deep Learning Systems: Algorithms, Compilers, and Processors for Large-Scale Production*, Springer Nature, 2022.

44 C. R. Qi, H. Su, K. Mo and L. J. Guibas, "PointNet: Deep learning on point sets for 3D classification and segmentation," in *Proceedings of the IEEE Conference on Computer Vision and Pattern Recognition (CVPR)*, pp. 652–660, 2017.

45 C. R. Qi, H. Su, K. Mo and L. J. Guibas, "PointNet: Deep learning on point sets for 3D classification and segmentation," in *Proceedings of the IEEE Conference on Computer Vision and Pattern Recognition*, pp. 652–660, 2017.

46 G. Gkioxari, J. Malik and J. Johnson, "Mesh R-CNN," in *Proceedings of the IEEE/CVF International Conference on Computer Vision (ICCV)*, pp. 9785–9795, 2019.

47 Y. Wang, Q. Zhang, J. Kim and H. Li, "Encoder-decoder based neural network for perspective estimation," in *Proceedings of the 2021 3rd International Conference on Image Processing and Machine Vision*, pp. 42–46, May 2021.

48 S. Peng, M. Niemeyer, L. Mescheder, M. Pollefeys and A. Geiger, "Convolutional occupancy networks," in *Computer Vision–ECCV 2020: 16th European Conference, Glasgow, UK, August 23–28, 2020, Proceedings, Part III*, vol. 16, pp. 523–540. Springer International Publishing, 2020.

49 S. Peng, M. Niemeyer, L. Mescheder, M. Pollefeys and A. Geiger, "Convolutional occupancy networks," in *Computer Vision–ECCV 2020: 16th European Conference on Computer Vision, Glasgow, UK, August 23–28, 2020, Proceedings, Part III*, vol. 16, pp. 523–540. Springer International Publishing, 2020.

50 D. Hartman, *A Living Covenant: The Innovative Spirit in Traditional Judaism*, Turner Publishing Company, 2013.

51 J. Finnie-Ansley, P. Denny, B. A. Becker, A. Luxton-Reilly and J. Prather, "The robots are coming: Exploring the implications of OpenAI Codex on introductory programming," in *Proceedings of the 24th Australasian Computing Education Conference*, pp. 10–19, Feb. 2022.

52 M. J. Benson, A. J. Banko, C. J. Elkins, D. G. An, S. Song, M. Bruschewski and J. K. Eaton, "MRV challenge 2: phase locked turbulent measurements in a roughness array," *Experiments in Fluids*, vol. 64, no. 2, p. 28, 2023.

53 R. W. Brennan and J. Lesage, "Exploring the Implications of OpenAI Codex on Education for Industry 4.0," in *International Workshop on Service Orientation in Holonic and Multi-Agent Manufacturing*, Cham: Springer International Publishing, 2022, pp. 254–266.

54 Y. Li, D. Choi, J. Chung, N. Kushman, J. Schrittwieser, R. Leblond and O. Vinyals, "Competition-level code generation with AlphaCode," *Science*, vol. 378, no. 6624, pp. 1092–1097, 2022.

55 Z. Feng, D. Guo, D. Tang, N. Duan, X. Feng, M. Gong and M. Zhou, "CodeBERT: A pre-trained model for programming and natural languages," arXiv preprint arXiv:2002.08155, 2020.

56 Trummer, "CodexDB: Generating code for processing SQL queries using GPT-3 Codex," arXiv preprint arXiv:2204.08941, 2022.

57 M. Wermelinger, "Using GitHub Copilot to solve simple programming problems," in *Proceedings of the 54th ACM Technical Symposium on Computer Science Education (SIGCSE)*, vol. 1, pp. 172–178, Mar. 2023.

58 F. Cassano, J. Gouwar, D. Nguyen, S. Nguyen, L. Phipps-Costin, D. Pinckney and A. Jangda, "MultiPL-E: a scalable and polyglot approach to benchmarking neural code generation," *IEEE Transactions on Software Engineering*, vol. 49, no. 7, pp. 3675–3691, 2023.

59 Y. Wang, W. Wang, S. Joty and S. C. Hoi, "CodeT5: Identifier-aware unified pre-trained encoder-decoder models for code understanding and generation," arXiv preprint arXiv:2109.00859, 2021.

60 H. Toledo, A. Baly, O. Castro, S. Resik, J. Laferté, F. Rolo and C. A. Duarte, "A phase I clinical trial of a multi-epitope polypeptide TAB9 combined with Montanide ISA 720 adjuvant in non-HIV-1 infected human volunteers," *Vaccine*, vol. 19, no. 30, pp. 4328–4336, 2001.

61 S. Tingiris and B. Kinsella, *Exploring GPT-3: An Unofficial First Look at the General-Purpose Language Processing API from OpenAI*, Packt Publishing Ltd, 2021.

62 M. Joseph, "PyTorch Tabular: A framework for deep learning with tabular data," arXiv preprint arXiv:2104.13638, 2021.

63 B. Saez, J. Mendez, M. Molina, E. Castillo, M. Pegalajar and D. P. Morales, "Gesture recognition with ultrasounds and edge computing," *IEEE Access*, vol. 9, pp. 38999–39008, 2021.

64 L. Strohm, C. Hehakaya, E. R. Ranschaert, W. P. Boon and E. H. Moors, "Implementation of artificial intelligence (AI) applications in radiology: hindering and facilitating factors," *European Radiology*, vol. 30, pp. 5525–5532, 2020.

65 D. H. Devi, K. Duraisamy, A. Armghan, M. Alsharari, K. Aliqab, V. Sorathiya and N. Rashid, "5G technology in healthcare and wearable devices: a review," *Sensors*, vol. 23, no. 5, pp. 2519, 2023.

66 P. Gupta, B. Ding, C. Guan and D. Ding, "Generative AI: a systematic review using topic modelling techniques," *Data and Information Management*, vol. 100066, 2024.

67 L. Militano, A. Zafeiropoulos, E. Fotopoulou, R. Bruschi, C. Lombardo, A. Edmonds and S. Papavassiliou, "AI-powered infrastructures for intelligence and automation in beyond-5G systems," in *2021 IEEE Globecom Workshops (GC Wkshps)*, pp. 1–6, Dec. 2021.

68 B. Pradhan, S. Das, D. S. Roy, S. Routray, F. Benedetto and R. H. Jhaveri, "An AI-assisted smart healthcare system using 5G communication," *IEEE Access*, vol. 11, pp. 108339–108355, 2023.

69 D. Rico and P. Merino, "A survey of end-to-end solutions for reliable low-latency communications in 5G networks," *IEEE Access*, vol. 8, pp. 192808–192834, 2020.

11

HEALTHSYNCC: AN AI-POWERED MOBILE APPLICATION FOR HEALTH MANAGEMENT

*Ebenezer Juliet Selwyn, Anmol Tiwari,
Gadewar Gayatri Pandurang, Sweta Soundarya Das,
and Raj Vardhan*

11.1 Introduction

The healthcare industry is changing a lot due to the latest advances in modern technologies. This includes artificial intelligence (AI), computer vision, and robotics. All of these are at the forefront and have greatly contributed toward improvements in patient outcomes as well as operational effectiveness. HealthSyncc is a comprehensive mobile application that embodies this shift since it integrates advanced technologies for enhancing user power over their health information and interacting with medical services.

AI revolutionizes different sectors including healthcare by offering advanced data analysis, predictive capabilities, and automation, among others (Jiang et al., 2017). In medicine, AI algorithms can analyze big datasets to detect patterns and provide diagnostic support leading to better patient outcomes (Esteva et al., 2017). AI's subset, computer vision, allows machines to interpret and act on visual data. Computer vision is employed in healthcare for diagnostic imaging, patient monitoring, and automating administrative tasks (Litjens et al., 2017). Robotic process automation (RPA) comprises the use of software robots to automate rule-based and repetitive tasks. In the health industry, RPA is used to enhance operational efficiency by automating processes like appointment scheduling, patient record management, and billing (Lacity & Willcocks, 2016).

11.2 Literature review

There is a lot of research that supports the merging of AI, computer vision, and robotics in healthcare. Research has shown that AI can be used for diagnostic imaging with machine learning models matching human experts in

DOI: 10.1201/9781003481959-11

their accuracy (Gulshan et al., 2016). They have also been used effectively for real-time patient monitoring which helps reduce the workload on healthcare givers (Greenspan et al., 2016). RPA has also proved to speed up administrative processes, reducing costs significantly while ensuring efficiency improves (Aguirre & Rodriguez, 2017). The most recent development in AI focuses on predictive modeling strategies that can predict outbreaks of diseases, develop personalized treatment plans, and improve patients' adherence to medication (Rajkomar et al., 2018). Similarly, the use of AI-powered bots in healthcare environments has enhanced patient engagement and satisfaction as they are always present to offer help at any time (Miner et al., 2016).

For instance, in healthcare, computer vision is used in surgical assistance as well as diagnostics such that robots with visual sensors can perform minimally invasive surgery with a high degree of accuracy (Hager et al., 2016). This approach has reduced administrative errors and improved patient records' accuracy through automation of document management using computer vision (Liu et al., 2019). Various medical institutions have resorted to RPA to automate tasks such as inventory management, claims processing, and patient registration, among others (Willcocks et al., 2015). Moreover, the integration of RPA with other technologies like AI and computer vision makes it even more powerful in transforming healthcare services.

The adoption of AI in healthcare is expected to grow, with advancements in predictive analytics, personalized medicine, and automated diagnostics leading the way. AI algorithms will continue to refine their ability to analyze vast amounts of data, providing clinicians with deeper insights and more accurate diagnoses (Topol, 2019). Furthermore, the integration of AI with other emerging technologies such as blockchain could enhance the security and interoperability of healthcare data (Zhang et al., 2018). Computer vision will likely expand its role in healthcare, not only in diagnostic imaging but also in areas such as robotic-assisted surgery and telemedicine. The ability of computer vision systems to process and interpret visual data in real-time will support more precise and minimally invasive surgical procedures, improving patient outcomes and reducing recovery times (Murphy et al., 2019). RPA continues to streamline administrative processes, reducing the workload on healthcare professionals and allowing them to focus more on patient care. As RPA technologies become more sophisticated, they will be able to handle increasingly complex tasks, further enhancing operational efficiencies (Lacity & Willcocks, 2016).

Top eight mobile applications for doctor consultation in India were reviewed based on the services provided by them and concluded with their challenges (Agarwal & Biswas, 2020). Pal et al. (2023) presented the analysis of nine lively healthcare applications in India, namely, PharmEasy, Tata 1 MG, Apollo 24 × 7, Practo, Netmeds, Medibuddy, MFine, DocsApp, and Tata Health, in the aspect of user review. They also gave suggestions and strategic solutions to improve the user satisfaction rate. Their findings help the business model developers to understand the basic requirements of developing a user-centric app and help the researchers by providing them with a methodological guideline for determining new factors in the future as the mHealth industry evolves with time. Nowadays, in the health domain, large language models (LLMs) along with AI algorithms provide great support in patient care by means of effective communication between patients and the medical practitioner. Also, LLMs help in easy and accurate report generation, impact medical research in accessing scientific findings, and create a breakthrough in medical education (Clusmann et al., 2023). The complete survey of the state-of-the-art LLMs, especially open-source LLMs, utilization in the healthcare domain was presented. The various healthcare use cases, performance metrics, and challenges in the LLMs for healthcare apps were also explored (Nazi & Peng, 2024). The integration of LLMs in the health industry has caused a great revolution in administrative tasks, such as clinical documentation, medical research, and patient care. LLM-powered AI assistants can enhance telemedicine by understanding and responding to patient queries, providing medication reminders, offering general health information, and helping with medical question answering to improve patient engagement. LLMs help in summarizing extensive patient notes, reports, and medical histories and assisting healthcare professionals in quickly extracting relevant information and insights. Finally, LLMs support the practitioner in diagnosing the disease in an accurate manner. So, the integration of LLMs in the proposed HealthSyncc apps has demonstrated outstanding performance in disease diagnosis, medical document summarization, personalized patient care, and appointment booking.

11.3   Features and functionalities

HealthSync is an innovative comprehensive app designed to empower users to manage their healthcare in the digital age efficiently. It comprises AI-powered functionalities, document management computer vision, and RPA tools to simplify different health processes. This multifunctional app seamlessly integrates various features to ensure that people affordably obtain essential healthcare. The app will save all the prescription and test results in a safe, protected platform for easier access. To ensure the privacy of each patient, an adult can choose to protect their medical information with their family members if they wish to do so. We explore the architectural design of the portal and discuss how various modules are implemented and deployed. We also discuss a use case illustrating the authentication mechanism of the portal. Figure 11.1 shows the use case diagram of the HealthSyncc.

1 User Management: This module manages all user activities related to their accounts. It encompasses the following:

Registration: Provides data and credentials for login used by freshers to register.

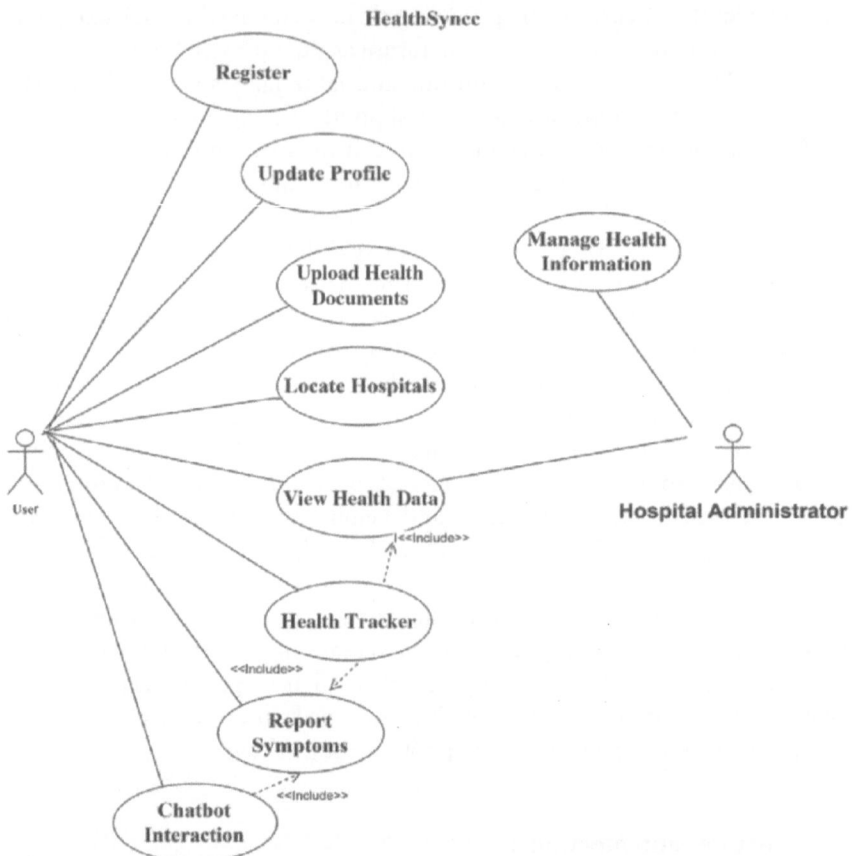

FIGURE 11.1 Use case diagram of the HealthSyncc App depicting the functionalities.

Login: This enables existing users to use the application by logging in with a registered username and password.

Reset password: Allows users to restore a forgotten password or change it for security purposes.

Profile management: This allows users to change their contact details, preferences, app settings, and other personal information through the app, etc.

2 Appointment Scheduling: One can easily schedule an appointment with a provider of healthcare through this application. This functionality allows for simple booking, rescheduling, or cancellation of appointments and hence effective time management and access to health services.

3 Medical Record Management: HealthSyncc helps users organize and store their medical records in a safe environment. Therefore, all important

documents like lab reports, prescriptions, and vaccination records can be uploaded here too making it easier for shared care and decision-making process.

4 Document Management: Apart from handling medical records, Health-Syncc also handles other documents related to health insurance policies, identification, and other personal records. With this feature in place, one can conveniently get various documents when required, hence reducing the need for manual paperwork as well as document retrieval.

5 Hospital Location Services: Location services that come with Health-Syncc are used by patients to find hospitals near them; they can look for hospitals within their locale with ease. The availability of information about location, contact details, and services provided by these medical practitioners makes it easier to find quick help from your proximity area.

6 Chatbot Support: The chatbot support feature gives instant assistance and information on health-related issues. The health chatbot is designed with AI to give users customized responses, help, and prompts about various health issues which will encourage interaction with patients and the availability of healthcare information.

7 Health Tracking Tools: It allows you to measure physical activity, diet, sleep patterns, and vital signs. Additionally, users can input their health data and keep track over time for purposes of disease tracking; setting health goals; and making informed lifestyle choices toward better overall health status.

8 Personalized Alert Mechanisms: To remind a patient about things like scheduled appointments, medication schedules, or even annual check-ups, HealthSyncc has personalized alert mechanisms. These alerts make it easier for people to plan their daily routines around them so they can follow all instructions provided by doctors without any problem.

11.4   Methodology

In this section, we will explore the methodologies that have been used in the creation of HealthSync from the designing and developing sides. Methodological considerations are very important as they guarantee that the application is efficient, usable, and secure. There is also a user-centered design approach that we will discuss here in terms of iterative prototyping, usability testing methods, and user feedback. We would like to deliver an intuitive and innovative user experience by giving priority to users' needs and choices.

11.4.1   Overall architecture

To design the structure of HealthSyncc, we've taken into account not only our use of AI but also other advanced technologies such as computer vision

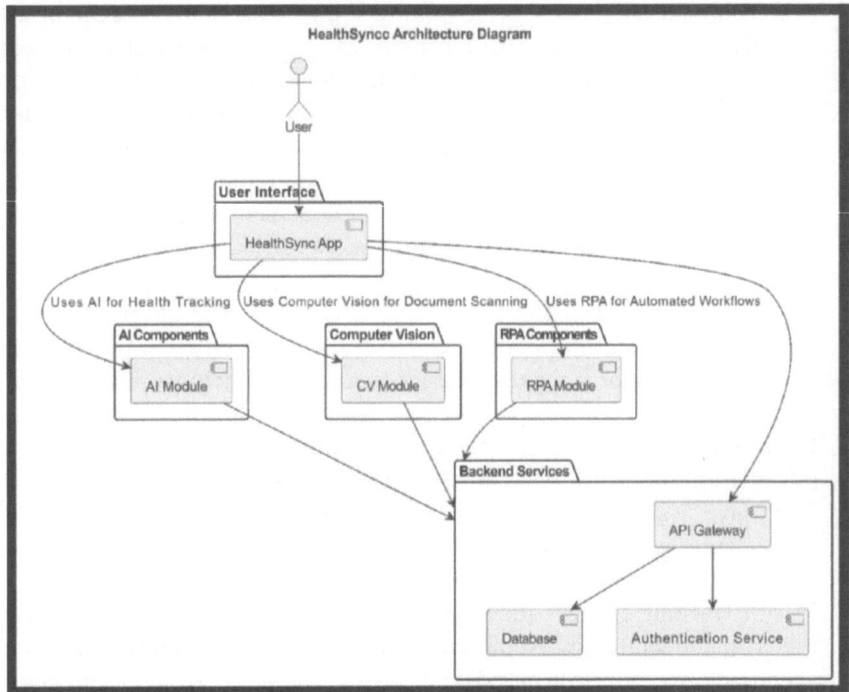

FIGURE 11.2   Overall architecture of the HealthSyncc App.

and RPA. This means that by applying it, HealthSyncc becomes a holistic, safe, and user-friendly system for handling health data, thereby allowing users to obtain useful ideas and streamline regular healthcare management duties. Figure 11.2 shows the overall architecture of the HealthSyncc application.

11.4.2   Usage and role of LLMs in the proposed HealthSyncc

There are several reasons for using LLMs in healthcare applications. They are listed below.

1 In the healthcare sector, useful information extraction from voluminous data generation plays a vital role, and hence the LLMs are trained on massive datasets of biological and medical texts to provide medical care and support for patients. It also assists the medical practitioner in taking good clinical decisions.

2 Like other domains, the demand for personalized services is increasing in the health sector. LLMs can be used to tailor medications, treatment plans,

and recommendations for individual patients, which can help to improve patient healthcare.

3 LLMs have the potential to improve efficiency and accuracy by automating a variety of tasks in healthcare, such as scheduling appointments and generating reports. This can free up healthcare professionals to focus on providing care to patients.

The proposed healthcare app has been empowered with AI components to perform services such as patient healthcare recommendations, automatic medical record management through summarization and organizing the records based on keywords or topics, chatbot support for instant assistance of patients, and a personalized alert mechanism. All these services use LLMs to identify potential health issues, generate treatment plans, recommend medications, effective document summary and classification, and bot services for query answering. By automating healthcare services, improving diagnosis and treatment, and supporting research, LLMs can help to make healthcare more efficient, effective, and accessible.

Figure 11.3 shows the role of AI in healthcare management by providing valuable insights to the patients through LLMs called Chat GPT-4-based recommendation systems. This module comprises functionality for the automatic creation of notes based on the conversation between the medical practitioner and the patients, summarization of notes, and extraction of key points from the summary for an effective recommendation. This LLM has been already trained or fine-tuned to recognize and extract important entities such as patient names, dates, medical conditions, medications, and other relevant information from patient notes. Also, it has been equipped to categorize the patients based on the content of the notes. Also, GPT-4 has been employed to analyze voluminous healthcare data and understand electronic health records by extracting valuable information. LLMs assist healthcare professionals by summarizing complex medical literature, staying updated on the latest research, and generating patient-specific recommendations. LLMs play a vital role in the healthcare domain by offering benefits such as betterment of diagnosis and treatment, personalized learning experiences, automation of administrative tasks, and support for medical education and research. In summary, the integration of LLMs in healthcare has the potential to revolutionize the industry, fostering efficiency, effectiveness, and accessibility.

Figure 11.4 illustrates how computer vision technology is utilized in HealthSyncc for processing health documents. Through the app, users can upload health documents that are scanned using optical character recognition to change images into text. The data extracted is checked for correctness prior to being saved in the database. The app provides users with easy access

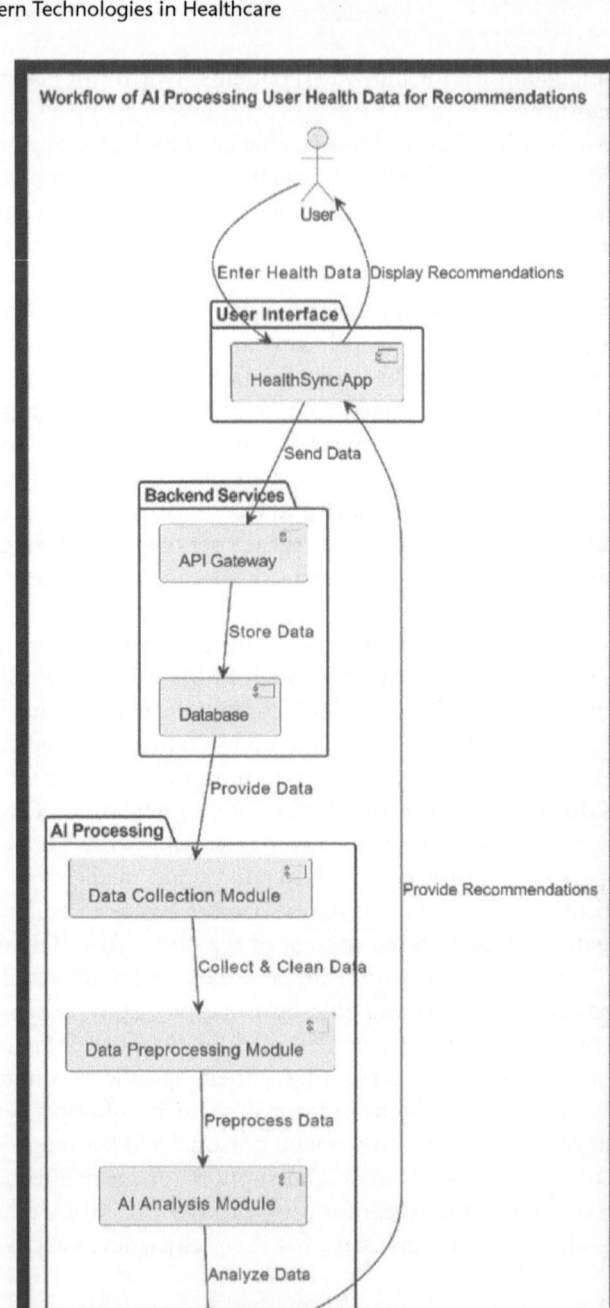

FIGURE 11.3 AI-driven health recommendations workflow.

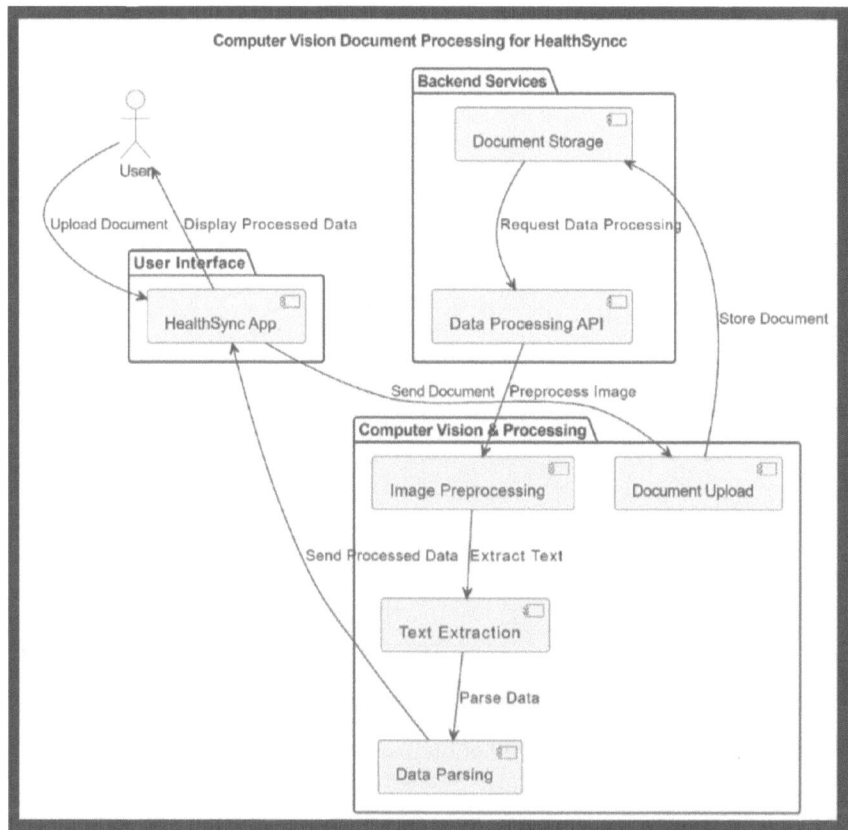

FIGURE 11.4   Computer vision document processing.

to their health records by making the processed data available for retrieval and management.

The flowchart in Figure 11.5 shows how RPA is used in HealthSyncc for automating the appointment scheduling process. The app is used by users to schedule appointments, while the RPA bot verifies open slots in hospital databases. After locating an appropriate time slot, the bot schedules the appointment and also notifies the user with a confirmation. This automation lessens the need for manual work and guarantees a seamless and effective scheduling process, enhancing user satisfaction and operational productivity.

11.4.3   Design perspective

App objectives must be clear before designing a prototype and creating storyboards for it. This phase also involves establishing the app's functionality, which is informed by its user interface (UI). It defines how people will engage

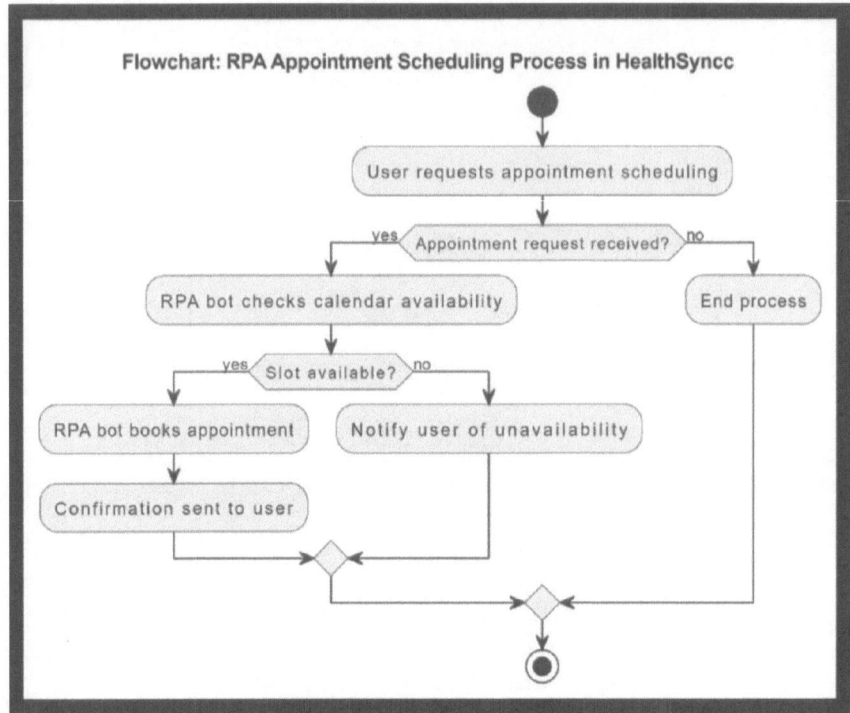

Flowchart: RPA Appointment Scheduling Process in HealthSyncc

User requests appointment scheduling

Appointment request received?

RPA bot checks calendar availability

End process

Slot available?

RPA bot books appointment

Notify user of unavailability

Confirmation sent to user

FIGURE 11.5 Robotic process automation in appointment scheduling.

with it. Wireframing is one common practice in this work where an app must be created in a skeletal form. It performs two main functions: enabling developers to understand the app's functionality and helping designers conceive UI design.

Wireframing is widely used. Before beginning, it is always recommended to have a short understanding of what it is. Wireframing is a fundamental part of the design process and can serve as a digital project foundation for mobile apps or websites. Wireframes help provide early clarity of vision by providing visual representations that show the layout, structure, or even functional requirements. This facilitates understanding of the scope of work by both designers and stakeholders to align on objective points. They also help in iterative design processes, allowing ideas and concepts to be refined based on feedback received. Since wireframes are low fidelity representations, they can easily be changed by making them an effective medium for exploring different design options as they are highly adjustable; plus, they work well as a communication tool facilitating efficient collaboration among designers, developers, and clients who may not share same location but can speed up the development process.

Figure 11.6 shows the process flowchart of the HealthSyncc. Health-Syncc is a platform that offers various functionalities aimed at transforming health management. These encompass appointment fixing, medical records

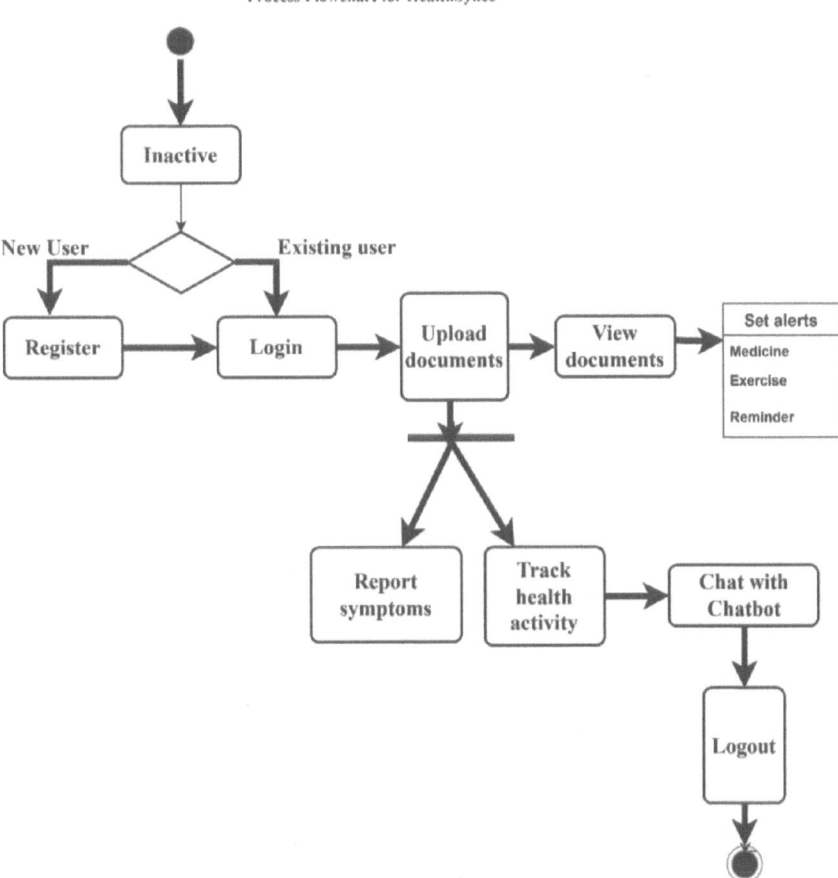

Process Flowchart for HealthSyncc

FIGURE 11.6 Process flowchart of the HealthSyncc.

handling, wellness tracking, filing system and document management, hospital finder services, chatbot support, tools for keeping track of one's well-being, and personalized notification systems. All these traits are meant to improve the user experience and enable patients to manage their conditions proactively. The next part will explain each functionality in detail by examining its implementation method as well as how it influences user engagement to have an impact on health outcomes.

To start with, the right color palette for a health-related app is vital as it can significantly impact user experience and perception of such an app. First, emotions are triggered by colors and can affect our moods, so it is necessary to select shades that allow for calmness, trust, and positivity toward health promotion. Second, colors serve to convey information efficiently. For example, using green for wellness features and red for alerts or notifications.

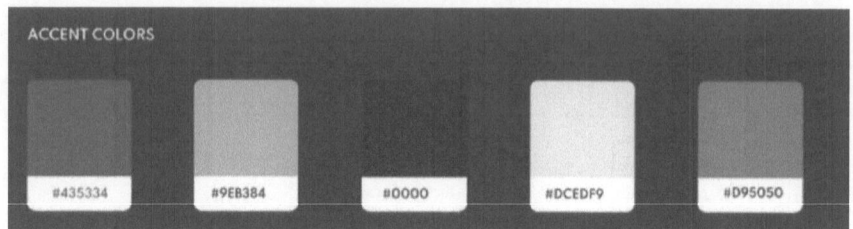

FIGURE 11.7 The color palette of the HealthSyncc.

Additionally, brand recognition is improved while maintaining uniformity in the color scheme and creating visually cohesive experience for users. Lastly, thinking about accessibility guidelines helps to ensure color choices meet the needs of visually impaired users. Thus, properly selecting a color palette contributes to better engagement, trust, and satisfaction among app users in healthcare sector. Figure 11.7 shows the color palette of the HealthSyncc App.

UI/UX design for apps is a field that has a variety of tools designed for the needs of designers. Popular choices include Adobe XD, Sketch, Invision, and Figma. However, Figma stands out as the most preferred tool by many designers and teams among others. Figma is popular because it uses cloud technology that allows real-time collaboration, and hence the team members can work on projects regardless of their locations. This helps to streamline the design process making it possible to have continuous feedback and iteration loops.

Furthermore, Figma comes with robust prototyping features, comprehensive design libraries, and an easy-to-use interface, and thus it is suitable for individual designers and large-scale teams. It is versatile enough to be used across various platforms such as web, desktop, or mobile so that it can be accessed by people through different devices.

Additionally, its intuitive design tools enable users to effortlessly create complex UI/UX elements that are also interactive. Consequently, many designers prefer it because of its efficiency, time taken to complete projects, collaborative attributes, and flexibility in handling diverse project needs. Figure 11.8 shows how the HealthSyncc App's user-centric interfaces were created using Figma in a UX/UI design manner while showing off the platform's capabilities in creating engaging digital experiences.

11.4.4 Development perspective

If the design stage is implemented efficiently, there will be a clear understanding of what is required and how it should be done. Next comes building the app using lessons learned during initial planning, design, and development. After that, the developer/company can decide which development environment they want to develop in.

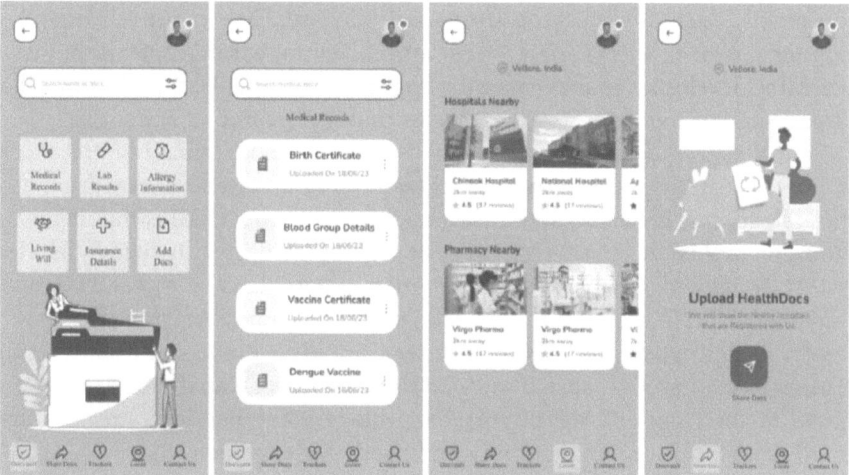

FIGURE 11.8   Screenshots of user interface of the HealthSyncc.

This stage takes the longest of all, thereby creating a number of practical difficulties in getting a particular functionality or even new ideas coming up that were not addressed in the previous two stages. This is where the Business Logic of the App Development becomes one of the major role players which must be written by this time. This section delves into the technical aspects of building the HealthSyncc, highlighting the development of front-end and back-end categories.

11.4.4.1   Front-end development perspective

Front-end development gives a plethora of alternatives for constructing user interfaces and interactive experiences on mobile applications. Some of the prevalent options are native development, cross-platform solutions, and hybrid frameworks. Native development involves using platform-specific languages and tools such as Swift or Objective-C for iOS, Java, or Kotlin for Android with the aim of creating applications that are customized to each operating system. Hybrid frameworks such as Ionic and Cordova enable developers to use web technologies like HTML, CSS, and JavaScript to make their applications run on various platforms with one code base. Such solutions include React Native and Xamarin which enable programmers to write code once (JavaScript or C#) which will have a native look and feel when deployed across different platforms.

Flutter is one of the most popular choices among developers due to its distinctiveness and several benefits. Flutter, an open-source UI toolkit developed by Google, provides a fast and productive way for building native apps on mobile, web, and desktop from one codebase. One major advantage of Flutter is that it allows for a "write once, run anywhere" approach, hence enabling developers to make visually appealing high-quality applications that are assured of uniform execution across multiple operating systems.

The most frequently asked question is why do we use flutter? Flutter incorporates a reactive framework as well as layered architecture that facilitates hot reload, fast iteration, and the ease of customization of UI components. In addition to this, there is a wide range of pre-built widgets provided by Flutter, which come with extensive documentation and are backed by solid community backing that makes it an ideal choice for developers striving for productivity, flexibility, and performance in their app development efforts. Overall, Flutter's adaptability, speed, and developer-oriented capabilities make it a good fit for front-end development especially when handling projects that need cross-platform compatibility and good user experience.

Device compatibility is an important area to consider while developing HealthSync so that the application runs smoothly on different devices. HealthSync, however, can work with some mobile devices including smartphones and tablets with various operating systems like Android and iOS. The interface as well as the content of HealthSync could be changed by using responsive design principles, thus providing adaptive layouts so it can fit diverse screen sizes, aspect ratios, and resolutions dynamically. It therefore guarantees that, irrespective of the device they are using, their users will be able to realize any functionalities or features associated with HealthSync, thereby making it easily accessible and usable.

Additionally, HealthSync is optimized toward leveraging the capabilities of modern mobile devices such as touch screens, cameras, GPS sensors, and so on to deliver a better user experience. Other advanced functions that could be achieved through employing this optimization include capturing medical documents via the phone's camera, accessing health-related location-based services for hospital navigation, and wellness tracking in connection with health monitoring sensors. To increase its usefulness and effectiveness, HealthSync has been made more powerful by exploiting the full potential of these equipped gadgets.

11.4.5 Hardware requirements

- Mobile Device: HealthSync is compatible with smartphones and tablets.
- Processor: A modern processor capable of handling mobile applications efficiently.
- Memory (RAM): At least 2 GB of RAM is recommended for smooth performance.
- Storage: Sufficient internal storage space to install the HealthSync application and store user data.

- Camera: While not mandatory, a camera enables users to capture medical documents and images for record-keeping purposes.
- Internet Connectivity: Access to a stable internet connection is required for certain features, such as syncing data with the cloud and accessing online resources.

11.4.6 Software requirements

- Operating System: Android and iOS platforms are both supported by HealthSync.

  - For Android: Android version 5.0 (Lollipop) or later is recommended.
  - For iOS: iOS version 11 or later is recommended.

- Web Browser: Sometimes access to a web browser may be required by HealthSync to use certain features like online resources or viewing electronic health records.
- Permissions: In this case, users will have to let HealthSync get through location services, camera, storage, contacts, and so on.

11.4.6.1 Back-end development perspective

The back end of HealthSync acts as the application's mainstay, which stores, retrieves, and processes data to support its numerous functionalities. There are various choices available when developing the back-end infrastructure, each with its own advantages and considerations. Traditional back-end solutions include the installation of custom servers, serverless architectures, or the use of cloud platforms. While custom servers allow complete control over infrastructure, they demand extensive maintenance and scalability management. Conversely, developers can focus just on code implementation since serverless architectures abstract away any server management complexities. Scalable and reliable infrastructure services suitable for a wide range of applications are offered by cloud platforms like AWS, Google Cloud, or Microsoft Azure.

However, for HealthSync, Firebase is a preferred back-end solution because of its easy integration with Flutter framework and the array of mobile application development features it has. Firebase is comprehensive in terms of back-end services which include real-time database, authentication, cloud storage, and hosting, all managed through a single console. It comes in a serverless architecture that automatically scales and ensures high availability; hence, no manual infrastructure management is needed. Moreover, Firebase possesses secure attributes such as user identification, data confidentiality controls, and regulatory compliance with privacy policies. The real-time database capability enables live data synchronization across devices, thereby allowing immediate updates and close cooperation among users. In the end, it speeds up the process of HealthSync back-end development through quick prototyping, smooth deployment, and scalability within a reliable secure base for the functionality of the application.

Application Programming Interfaces (APIs) are essential in connecting HealthSync mobile applications to external databases or services. Therefore, by using APIs, HealthSync can integrate into various healthcare providers' systems, medical database centers, and third-party service providers that offer these health-related data, thus improving the system's usability. The API serves as a connection between several software applications allowing them to communicate with each other. API refers to the set of rules and protocols that define how two software applications should interact with each other. They do not expose this web of technologies but provide a standard way for programmers to use them to access external services or platforms or retrieve information from it.

APIs enable HealthSync to access medical records, appointment schedules, and wellness information, among others that are made available through healthcare providers like hospitals, clinics, and even private practice establishments besides medical databases as well as third party services that offer these health-related data. Through APIs, HealthSync can obtain real-time patient data updates and synchronization such that whenever users need their details, they can find the latest ones. It does so by allowing customers to connect directly with the company's database without involving any intermediaries like stock brokers or investment banks in case they want to know about their balance sheets for instance.

Furthermore, with the API, HealthSync can be integrated with external services and platforms to increase its functionality as well as offer other features and abilities. As an example of this, HealthSync can make use of APIs from fitness trackers, wearable health monitors, or telemedicine platforms to allow users to monitor their health vitals, track their fitness metrics, or even talk to healthcare experts from some miles away. By so doing, the APIs have enabled HealthSync to provide a complete range of healthcare services and improve user experience by linking them smoothly with pertinent healthcare resources and utilities.

11.4.7 Dependencies

External APIs: The project relies on external APIs for access to real-time data, information, resources, and services concerning health documents; these are a few of the things that could change or be disrupted leading to poor functioning or any other aspect of the app.

Integration with Authentication Services: User account management and security in third-party authentication services is expected to work seamlessly with this project, which it largely depends on. Dependence on the availability and compatibility of these services may influence user registration, login details, and data security features.

Compliance with Regulatory Requirements: These are conditions that must be met by the project in terms of adhering to various regulations such as HIPAA and GDPD concerning patient privacy and security. This reliance on legal and regulatory issues affects the design, development, and rollout of the app.

Availability of Development Resources: The availability of skilled developers, i.e., software engineers, UX/UI designers, or data scientists, will determine whether this project succeeds or not.

11.5   Data security and privacy measures

To guarantee that robust data security measures are in place and privacy is maintained, it is necessary to include these features in the development and use of Healthsync, a comprehensive mobile health application. In an era marked by increasing digitalization and data breaches, securing sensitive health information (SHI) has become less of a legal requirement than it is a moral responsibility. Healthsync contains personal health data like medical records, diagnostic reports, and wellness metrics that necessitate implementing tight security measures aimed at safeguarding privacy and confidentiality. Regarding unauthorized access to healthcare data, various consequences arise like theft of identity and financial fraudulence leading to reputation damage and compromised patient care.

Henceforth, prioritizing the security of data and privacy should be vital to establish trust among users as well as caregivers confirming HealthSync's position as a dependable working platform for handling personal health information securely. By following the below policies and encryption techniques, we ensure that our user database is protected from cyber-attacks.

11.5.1   Encryption techniques

HealthSync utilizes strong encryption algorithms like AES-256 to safeguard data both in transit (during transmission between the app and servers) and at rest (when stored on servers). This encryption scrambles data into an unreadable format, rendering it indecipherable without the appropriate decryption key (Singh et al., 2020).

11.5.2   Authentication and authorization

Multi-factor authentication (MFA) is employed to strengthen user login security. In addition to usernames and passwords, MFA may involve one-time passwords received via SMS, fingerprint recognition, or facial recognition for an extra layer of verification (Al-Janabi et al., 2019).

11.5.3 Access management techniques

Role-based access control (RBAC) restricts data access based on user roles within the app. For instance, patients might only access their health data, while healthcare providers might have access to a wider range of information based on their specific roles and permissions (Institute for Information Systems Security, 2023).

11.5.4 Secure communication with user

HTTP or Hypertext Transfer Protocol is a protocol used by the Internet to transmit data. The operating mode is such that a client sends a request to the server and receives the required information in return. HTTP enables browsers and servers to communicate with each other, transferring different types of files such as text, images, and multimedia.

Therefore, including HTTP in HealthSync means using it for secure transmission of data among its front-end, back-end, and external servers or services. There are several key advantages to incorporating HTTP protocols into HealthSync:

- Enhanced Security: HTTPS keeps private user information secure by the way of encrypting transmitted data.
- Seamless Integration: RESTful APIs facilitate simple attachment of external services and devices.
- Scalability: Efficient management of growing user bases and data volumes is enabled by the architecture of HTTP.
- Cross-Platform Compatibility: HealthSync will work across different platforms and devices with ease.
- Improved User Experience: Users will be satisfied overall due to fast retrieval of data and real-time updating.
- Standardized Communication: Interoperability and industry standards are encouraged by HTTP protocols in communication.

11.5.5 Regulatory policies and guidelines

HealthSync adheres to various rules and guiding principles to be in line with data protection and privacy standards in India. These policies are important for the preservation of user health information secrecy, authenticity, and accessibility.

Some regulations followed by HealthSync within India consist of:

- Information Technology Act, 2000 (IT Act): The Information Technology Act is a legislation that touches on different aspects of electronic governance in India as well as cybersecurity. HealthSync follows IT Act guidelines, especially those pertaining to data security, privacy, and protection.
- Personal Data Protection Bill (PDPB): PDPB helps to regulate how personal data is processed and handled; it is done by individual organizations. Therefore, HealthSync ensures that its internal procedures align with the provisions of PDPB to ensure legitimate and fair handling of customer details.
- Health Insurance Portability and Accountability Act (HIPAA): Though not strictly applicable within India, HIPAA sets the standard for safeguarding SHI in America. HealthSync implements HIPAA compliant measures that help keep personal health information confidential, thus meeting international standards.
- EHR norms: HealthSync adheres to EHR norms stipulated by regulatory bodies such as MoHFW and NDHM. These govern the interoperability, privacy, and security of EHRs.
- Consent Mechanism: HealthSync implements a strong consent mechanism that ensures that users give informed consent for the collection, processing, and sharing of their health data. This involves explicit consent for specific purposes and user's control over their granular data sharing preferences.
- Data Localization: If any India-based authority requires it, HealthSync goes along with the localized data storage requirements. It means keeping user data within Indian borders to guarantee data sovereignty as well as enable regulatory oversight for completeness' sake.

11.6   Revenue generation model

For HealthSync and any venture to succeed in the long run, a strong revenue model is essential. This importance comes from its capacity to elaborate on how the project will change its goods into permanent income streams. To begin with, a sound revenue model guarantees the project's financial sustainability by covering operational expenses and enabling further growth. In addition, financial stability allows for effective resource allocation so that activities and investments can be prioritized based on their potential to generate revenues.

Additionally, a well-defined revenue model makes the project attractive to potential investors and partners indicating its profitability as well as strategic foresight that was considered during the formulation stage. It also enables scalability and growth by providing resources required for expansion and innovation. As a way of reducing risks of market fluctuations as well as economic uncertainties, diversification of revenue sources strengthens the project's resilience. Of greatest importance is ensuring that such efforts generate users' value while at the same time building up stakeholder value by making sure that it fits in well with what matters most to users in terms of a value proposition for any given project.

There are different business models that can be adopted for revenue generation, each of which is unique. In the case of HealthSync, a mobile health app, the choice of revenue model depends on user behavior, market dynamics, and long-term goals of the project.

The subscription-based approach is one of the models, where customers must make recurring payments at regular intervals such as monthly or annually to access the offering. Another popular model is freemium, which offers basic features for free but charges for premium features or content. Conversely, pay-per-use enables customers to pay according to their usage of a product or service. In-app advertising also serves as a revenue model whereby income is made through ads shown within an application. However, because it focuses on the management of people's health and well-being where a distraction-free environment is especially essential during emergencies, HealthSync may not be best suited for in-app advertising despite the potential financial benefits associated with it.

Transaction fees are another common means of making money in this market space; here companies usually charge some percentage cut or flat fee per transaction that takes place on their platform. This can also include licensing and royalty revenues acquired when others utilize intellectual property in return for fees or royalties. These models have various benefits and may vary depending on factors like target markets, products' nature, services offered, and overall business approach.

HealthSync can earn its revenue by selling its comprehensive digital solutions to hospitals as a way of managing in-house patient records, thus significantly reducing their workload of paper-based administration. Our platform serves subscribing hospitals through efficient operations and the delivery of healthcare services that are better improved. Our platform prioritizes and promotes these subscribed hospitals within the "Nearby Hospitals" feature, increasing their visibility to users seeking medical services in their vicinity.

A subscription-based system where hospitals pay an annual fee for using our services is the best revenue model for HealthSync. This kind of subscription ensures a reliable source of income for HealthSync while giving hospitals continued access to the benefits of our platform. Subscribing allows facilities to have access to features like patient records management, appointment scheduling, and data analytics which enable them to offer quality healthcare effectively.

Aligning the incentives of HealthSync with those of hospitals, this revenue model ensures that both parties profit from the platform's efficacy and efficiency when it comes to healthcare management. Additionally, a subscription-based approach gives hospitals an affordable alternative to traditional paper-based record-keeping methods which makes it an appealing investment for them. Eventually, this approach nurtures a symbiotic relationship between HealthSync and its partner hospitals by spurring mutual growth and prosperity in the healthcare ecosystem.

11.7 Comparison of the proposed HealthSyncc with the conventional healthcare platforms

The user reviews and general information of nine mHealth apps from India, namely, PharmEasy, Tata 1 MG, Apollo 24 × 7, Practo, Netmeds, Medibuddy, MFine, DocsApp, and Tata Health, and their features are tabulated in Table 11.1. Healthcare Ecosystem (https://healthsynconnect.com/) contains a healthcare web application with features such as Electronic Medical Records, Lab Management System, Pharmacy Management System, and Hospital Management System, offering a holistic solution for healthcare management. It also provides a secure and scalable database infrastructure that stores and manages healthcare files in a centralized storage, ensuring data integrity and availability. They usually provide services like consulting doctors online, booking doctor appointments, booking lab tests, online pharmacy, medicine delivery, online consultation, and health records keeping. However, the proposed HealthSyncc App has been developed using AI algorithms to provide significant patient care services with intelligence and automation.

The comparison presented in Table 11.2 highlights the proposed HealthSyncc's advanced features such as AI-powered document handling, and user interaction, showcasing a significant improvement compared to conventional online health platforms.

11.8 Challenges

11.8.1 Design challenges

- Complexity of User Interface: Making a HealthSync user-friendly interface suitable for people with differing levels of ability in using technology can be difficult. Striking the balance between simplicity and functionality with accessibility as well as inclusivity is a significant design challenge.
- Visualization of Data: A design problem lies in visualizing complex health data and insights effectively in a way that can be understood. However, this entails the need for carefully choosing data visualization techniques to represent such things as medical records, test results, or health trends in a simple yet exhaustive manner.

TABLE 11.1 Features of the conventional healthcare apps and the proposed HealthSyncc

Sl. No.	Name of healthcare app	Features
1	PharmEasy [31]	• Home delivery • Diagnostic tests • Teleconsultations
2	Tata 1 MG [32]	• E-Pharmacy • Online Consultations • Online booking of lab tests and reporting • Authentic Information
3	Apollo 24 X 7 [33]	• E-Pharmacy • Online consultations • Online booking of lab tests and reporting • Accessing Health records in real time • Diabetics management • Buy insurance
4	Practo [34]	• Online doctor consultation • Online booking of doctors for in-clinic consultation • Offers comprehensive telemedicine solutions
5	Netmeds [35]	• Online ordering of medicines and home delivery • Online doctors consultation • Scheduling regular health checkup • Free access to a wealth of healthcare articles and video • Query responses from experienced pharmacists
6	Medibuddy [36]	• Online doctor consultations • Online lab test bookings • Medicine delivery • Corporate health and wellness services
7	MFine[37]	• Online doctor consultations • Medicine delivery • Lab test bookings • Long-term care taker program
8	DocsApp [38]	• Online doctor consultation • E-Pharmacy • Online booking of lab tests and reporting
9	Proposed HealthSyncc app	In addition to the above features, it possesses • AI powered • Healthcare recommendation using LLM • Computer vision based improved diagnosis • Automatic scheduling of appointments • Chatbots for query answering

TABLE 11.2 Comparison of the proposed HealthSyncc app with conventional healthcare apps

Features	Proposed HealthSyncc	Conventional E-Health portals
User Management	Mobile app, secure encryption	Mostly web-based, some mobile apps
Appointment Scheduling	Automated, AI-enhanced	Manual, basic automation
Medical Record Management	Integrated, computer vision-enhanced	Basic digital storage
Document Management	Advanced with AI and computer vision	Simple digital document storage
Hospital Location Services	Geolocation features	Limited to search functions
Chatbot Support	AI-powered, 24/7 assistance	Limited or no chatbot support
Health Tracking Tools	Comprehensive, personalized	Basic tracking
Personalized Alert Mechanisms	Advanced, AI-driven	Basic reminders
Security and Privacy	Strong encryption, role-based control	Varies, often basic security

- Compatibility across Platforms: It may not be easy to ensure that users have similar experiences irrespective of devices and platforms such as smartphones, tablets, and web browsers. Optimal user engagement will require adaptable interfaces that can move seamlessly among different screen sizes as well as resolutions.

11.8.2   Development challenges

- Complexity of Integration: It is a difficult task to develop a system that combines functions like scheduling appointments, keeping medical records, and facilitating real-time communication. For modules from different software packages to function together and maintain their interactivity yet keep the entire system stable and efficient, there must be planning.
- Security Concerns: It is not easy but essential to implement strong security measures to protect user's sensitive data. With thorough scrutiny regarding the appropriate encryption, authentication, and access control techniques, this will enable HealthSync to deal with its vulnerability from

hacking due to breaches of data as well as unauthorized entry into its systems.

- Scalability and Performance: Scalability and performance become critical development issues as HealthSync expands in terms of user base and features. The developers must consider things such as caching mechanisms, database optimization, and back-end architecture when devising strategies that will guarantee almost no downtime or any form of latency.

11.9 Conclusion

HealthSyncc is a disruptive innovation that can change the way health maintenance and management is done as it represents a paradigm shift in healthcare. HealthSync empowers people through comprehensive planning and user-oriented design. This means that they make things simple for clients in setting up appointments, keeping medical reports, and messaging instantly by encouraging proactive patient care. Apart from the significant value it offers to its users, HealthSyncc presents a sustainable business model for hospitals and other healthcare providers based on subscription revenue models. As such, medical centers digitize patients' records to facilitate efficient operations, leading to cost reductions in the administrative sector while improving the quality of care available. AI-powered HealthSyncc is in a strong position to take charge of this technological revolution. Its wide range of capabilities, including AI-powered health suggestions and document organization based on computer vision, tackles present obstacles and capitalizes on upcoming progressions. As the HealthSyncc App advances with these technologies, it will establish fresh benchmarks in healthcare delivery and patient involvement, molding the future of customized health maintenance with a focus on user experience, security, and scalability.

References

Agarwal, N., & Biswas, B. (2020). Doctor consultation through mobile applications in India: An overview, challenges and the way forward. Healthcare Informatics Research, 26(2), 153–158.

Al-Janabi, S., Gupta, B., & Irwin, D. (2019, September). Multi-Factor Authentication for Mobile Health Applications: A Survey. In 2019 IEEE International Conference on Systems, Man, and Cybernetics (SMC) (pp. 2142–2147). IEEE.

Amble, A., Pedersen, O. I., & Hervik, S. (2019). Machine learning for personalized medicine: A survey of data-driven approaches to improve diagnosis, treatment and patient safety. Journal of Internal Medicine, 286(6), 580–602.

Aguirre, S., & Rodriguez, A. (2017). Automation in Financial Services: Robotic Process Automation. In 2017 IEEE Conference on Emerging Technologies and Factory Automation (ETFA) (pp. 1–8). IEEE.

Clusmann, J., Kolbinger, F. R., Muti, H. S., Carrero, Z. I., Eckardt, J. N., Laleh, N. G., ... & Kather, J. N. (2023). The future landscape of large language models in medicine. Communications Medicine, 3(1), 141.

Esteva, A., Kuprel, B., Novoa, R. A., Ko, J., Swetter, S. M., Blau, H. M., & Thrun, S. (2017). Dermatologist-level classification of skin cancer with deep neural networks. Nature, 542(7639), 115–118.

Greenspan, H., van Ginneken, B., & Summers, R. M. (2016). Guest editorial deep learning in medical imaging: Overview and future promise of an exciting new technique. IEEE Transactions on Medical Imaging, 35(5), 1153–1159.

Gulshan, V., Peng, L., Coram, M., Stumpe, M. C., Wu, D., Narayanaswamy, A., ... & Webster, D. R. (2016). Development and validation of a deep learning algorithm for detection of diabetic retinopathy in retinal fundus photographs. JAMA, 316(22), 2402–2410.

Hager, G. D., Okamura, A. M., & Kazanzides, P. (2016). Surgical robotics: Systems integration and validation. Annual Review of Control, Robotics, and Autonomous Systems, 1, 363–392.

Institute for Information Systems Security (2023, February 15). RBAC: Role-Based Access Control. https://thorteaches.com/cissp-certification-rbac/

Jiang, F., Jiang, Y., Zhi, H., Dong, Y., Li, H., Ma, S., ... & Wang, Y. (2017). Artificial intelligence in healthcare: Past, present and future. Stroke and Vascular Neurology, 2(4), 230–243.

Lacity, M. C., & Willcocks, L. P. (2016). Robotic process automation: The next transformation lever for shared services. Journal of Information Technology Teaching Cases, 6(2), 1–11.

Li, Y., Li, Z., Ren, K., & Zhan, Z. (2021). Federated learning with enhanced privacy protection for health care applications. Journal of Medical Systems, 45(1), 1–12.

Litjens, G., Kooi, T., Bejnordi, B. E., Setio, A. A. A., Ciompi, F., Ghafoorian, M., ... & van der Laak, J. A. (2017). A survey on deep learning in medical image analysis. Medical Image Analysis, 42, 60–88.

Liu, Y., Gadepalli, K., Norouzi, M., Dahl, G. E., Kohlberger, T., Boyko, A., ... & Stumpe, M. C. (2019). Detecting cancer metastases on gigapixel pathology images. Medical Image Analysis, 59, 101567.

Lu, Y., Chen, S., Yang, J., Tang, Y., & Lv, J. (2020). Wearable sensors for health monitoring: Current trends and challenges. Sensors (Switzerland), 20(3), 805. https://www.ncbi.nlm.nih.gov/pmc/articles/PMC7028514/

Miner, A. S., Milstein, A., Schueller, S., Hegde, R., Mangurian, C., Linos, E., & Mahoney, M. (2016). Smartphone-based conversational agents and responses to questions about mental health, interpersonal violence, and physical health. JAMA Internal Medicine, 176(5), 619–625.

Murphy, K. P., Di Resta, C., & Segal, A. (2019). Computer Vision and Image Processing in Health Informatics. In Health Informatics: A Computational Perspective in Healthcare (pp. 171–201). Springer.

Nazi, Z. A., & Peng, W. (2024, August). Large language models in healthcare and medical domain: A review. In Informatics (Vol. 11, No. 3, p. 57). MDPI.

Pal, S., Biswas, B., Gupta, R., Kumar, A., & Gupta, S. (2023). Exploring the factors that affect user experience in mobile-health applications: A text-mining and machine-learning approach. Journal of Business Research, 156, 113484.

Rajkomar, A., Dean, J., & Kohane, I. (2018). Machine learning in medicine. New England Journal of Medicine, 378(6), 574–584.

Singh, S., Singh, V., & Singh, M. (2020). A novel secure healthcare data transmission model using AES-256 encryption and digital signature algorithm. International Journal of Advanced Science and Technology, 125(7), 867–878.

Topol, E. (2019). Deep Medicine: How Artificial Intelligence Can Make Healthcare Human Again. Basic Books.

Willcocks, L. P., Lacity, M. C., & Craig, A. (2015). Robotic process automation: The next transformation lever for shared services. Journal of Information Technology Teaching Cases, 5(2), 1–11.

Zhang, P., White, J., Schmidt, D. C., Lenz, G., & Rosenbloom, S. T. (2018). FHIRChain: Applying blockchain to securely and scalably share clinical data. Computational and Structural Biotechnology Journal, 16, 267–278.

12

CHALLENGES AND FUTURE TRENDS IN IMPLEMENTING AI IN HEALTHCARE

Adanze Nge Cynthia

12.1 Introduction

A wave of promising applications in healthcare has emerged due to recent advancements in artificial intelligence (AI). These advancements aim to transform how medical services are delivered, diagnosed, and administered. AI systems have the impressive capability to analyse large volumes of data, identify complex patterns, and offer valuable insights that can enhance decision-making, improve patient outcomes, and optimise healthcare operations (Alowais et al., 2023). Additionally, AI-powered chatbots can function as virtual health assistants, providing patients with 24/7 access to information and basic care guidance (Clark & Bailey, 2024).

However, despite the numerous advantages and potential of AI in healthcare, its integration presents a multitude of challenges that require resolution to ensure successful and ethical implementation. Data privacy and security remain paramount. Robust security measures must be implemented to safeguard sensitive patient data and mitigate the risk of breaches and unauthorised access (Batko & Ślęzak, 2022).

Furthermore, the potential for bias within AI algorithms, if left unchecked, can exacerbate existing healthcare disparities (Chen et al., 2023). Additionally, ethical considerations regarding the potential displacement of healthcare professionals by AI automation necessitate careful evaluation (Elendu et al., 2023).

Moving forward, addressing these challenges is crucial to fully harnessing AI's capabilities in healthcare. Establishing robust data governance frameworks can ensure responsible data collection and utilisation. Transparency in AI algorithms and a focus on fairness in their design will be pivotal in

DOI: 10.1201/9781003481959-12

mitigating bias and promoting equitable access to healthcare. Furthermore, fostering collaboration between AI developers, healthcare professionals, and policymakers will pave the way for the ethical and conscientious integration of AI within healthcare systems.

This chapter will delve deeply into these challenges and trends, providing a comprehensive overview of AI in healthcare today and charting a course for its future development. It will examine the ethical, legal, and socio-economic barriers that hinder the seamless deployment of AI solutions, shedding light on the complexities of realising the full potential of these cutting-edge technologies.

Additionally, the chapter will explore the regulatory and legal frameworks governing AI in healthcare, highlighting the importance of establishing clear guidelines and standards to ensure patient safety, data protection, and accountability (Mennella et al., 2024). It will delve into the complexities of developing and validating AI algorithms for high-stakes medical applications, underscoring the need for rigorous testing, monitoring, and evaluation processes.

The ethical considerations surrounding the implementation of AI in healthcare are of paramount importance. This chapter will also explore the potential risks and challenges arising from issues such as algorithmic bias, transparency, and the effects on the roles and decision-making processes of healthcare professionals (Naik et al., 2022). The text will further explore the socio-economic consequences of adopting AI, such as concerns regarding healthcare availability, disruptions in the workforce, and the disparity in access to digital resources.

Last but not least, the chapter will explore forthcoming trends and emerging technologies that have the potential to influence the field of AI in healthcare. It will offer insights into potential avenues for innovation and progress, ranging from the integration of AI with other advanced technologies such as the Internet of Things (IoT), big data analytics, and blockchain, to the development of explainable AI and human-AI collaborative systems.

12.2   Challenges of AI in healthcare

This section examines the obstacles that must be overcome to fully realise the transformative potential of AI technology in healthcare. It sheds light on the difficulties faced by healthcare professionals and healthcare organisations in utilising AI to its fullest potential.

Let us delve into some of the key challenges that arise when utilising these cutting-edge technologies in healthcare settings. It is important to remember that these are just a few of the existing challenges and not an exhaustive list, and some of them may overlap.

12.2.1 *Data privacy, security, and transparency*

The widespread implementation of AI in healthcare is significantly impeded by concerns surrounding privacy and security. Integrating AI raises privacy issues due to the need to manage large amounts of sensitive patient data (Khan et al., 2023).

The highly sensitive and confidential nature of patient data makes safeguarding patient identities during handling and storage a major concern. When using patient data for AI applications, clear and informed consent guidelines must be provided (Wang et al., 2022). Lack of transparency in data collection, handling, and application is a significant barrier to data privacy (Rossi & Lenzini, 2020).

Individuals may sometimes be unaware that their data is being collected, let alone how it is being used. This lack of transparency hinders their ability to manage their data effectively and make informed decisions about its use. Therefore, it is crucial to protect patients' information regarding the use of their data for AI development and ensure they can revoke consent as needed (Biswas, 2023).

To effectively address questions regarding data ownership and control, clear and concise answers are needed that explicitly identify those responsible for managing each category of data and its intended purpose.

Concerns arise regarding the accessibility and use of confidential patient information because AI is often developed by private companies (Quach et al., 2022). Additionally, there's a significant challenge in achieving a balance between healthcare innovation and privacy. We need to safeguard patient privacy while effectively leveraging data for AI advancement (Jeyaraman et al., 2023).

Recent partnerships between public and private entities aiming to implement AI have raised concerns about inadequate privacy safeguards. These situations have led to a growing demand for improved oversight of comprehensive health data research to protect patient autonomy and privacy (Murdoch, 2021).

This study by Murdoch (2021) supports the notion that addressing these concerns is crucial. The study also emphasises the importance of private data custodians taking appropriate measures to prioritise data protection and prevent unauthorised access. It's also worth noting that some existing privacy laws globally are facing scrutiny regarding the collection and processing of personal data by AI and automation technologies (Almeida et al., 2022). These laws may not be sufficient to effectively safeguard individuals from potential risks associated with these technologies.

The lack of transparency and accountability in AI systems can result in significant decisions with far-reaching consequences for individuals (Menash, 2023). Furthermore, using personal data to train AI algorithms can lead to biased and unfair results, as evidenced by cases like Amazon's AI recruitment tool exhibiting gender bias in 2018 (Dastin, 2022).

Moreover, the collection and storage of patient data through AI systems are highly susceptible to cyberattacks, including hacking, which poses a potential risk of compromising sensitive patient information (Seh et al., 2020). This vulnerability is exacerbated when healthcare providers and researchers share data, increasing the likelihood of breaches without sufficient security measures (Karen Cabuyao, 2023).

Therefore, protocols and guidelines must prioritise the adoption of sophisticated methodologies for anonymising and safeguarding patient data, while placing significant importance on upholding patient autonomy and obtaining informed consent.

12.2.2   Cost and infrastructure

Despite the considerable potential of AI in healthcare, several challenges must be addressed before its widespread adoption and utilisation. These obstacles encompass issues related to infrastructure and cost limitations. To ensure the successful integration of AI for improved healthcare outcomes, it's imperative to employ strategic planning, secure funding, and foster teamwork.

The costs associated with procuring AI software, hardware, and robotic systems, along with regular maintenance and updates, can be prohibitive (Reilly, 2024). Furthermore, integrating AI in healthcare presents significant challenges for low- and middle-income countries (LMICs) due to resource constraints. This is often due to a lack of advanced IT infrastructure in many healthcare facilities. These facilities may also lack the processing power, data storage, and reliable internet access required for AI systems to operate effectively (Petersson et al., 2022).

Another significant cost-related obstacle, particularly in LMICs, is the ongoing need for system upgrades. Even if AI projects are initiated, their long-term sustainability is jeopardised by limited access to funding and the allocation of restricted budgets to these innovative technologies (Thwaites et al., 2020).

12.2.3   Ethical issues

Undoubtedly, the emergence of AI, particularly in healthcare, has given rise to numerous ethical concerns that demand prompt and effective solutions. One prominent issue is the presence of bias in data and AI algorithms. These biases can stem from societal factors, with a significant portion originating from influences related to race, socio-economic status, environment, and gender (Rajkomar et al., 2018). Another ethical concern is confidentiality and protection of sensitive medical information. AI systems used in healthcare often rely on extensive datasets containing personal health information. This dependence raises concerns about data privacy, consent, and the potential for misuse or unauthorised access to this highly sensitive data (Naik et al., 2022).

To safeguard patient privacy and maintain trust in AI-driven healthcare solutions, it's imperative to establish robust data governance frameworks, employ anonymisation techniques, and enforce stringent security measures. Ensuring transparency and explainability of AI models is paramount from an ethical standpoint. Several AI algorithms, particularly those employing deep learning, can be opaque and difficult to interpret, making it challenging to understand the rationale behind a specific decision or recommendation (Ali et al., 2023).

This lack of transparency can lead to concerns regarding accountability, especially in consequential medical decisions where understanding and scrutinising the reasoning behind the AI's results is crucial. Ethical concerns also arise regarding the distribution of responsibility and liability in situations where AI systems, particularly healthcare robots, contribute to negative consequences or medical errors. Can healthcare robots demonstrate intelligent decision-making capabilities in emergency or complex scenarios, considering their lack of emotional intelligence (Deo & Anjankar, 2023)?

A major drawback of robots is their inability to fully comprehend the inner mental processes of patients. This contrasts with the advantages of a morally conscious human doctor who can draw on personal experiences (Gibelli et al., 2021).

Furthermore, an entity lacking emotions and humanness is inadequate in understanding a patient's emotions. Prioritising virtues and emotional intelligence, alongside the conventional emphasis on knowledge, technical expertise, and adherence to ethical principles, is of utmost importance. Possessing these qualities is essential for delivering exceptional clinical care (Gelhaus, 2011).

In the medical field, robots should therefore take on a supportive role, assisting medical staff rather than supervisory roles. Robots can assist surgeons in performing minimally invasive surgeries with greater control and precision.

One such example is the Da Vinci Surgical System, a robotic system approved by the U.S. Food and Drug Administration (FDA) for surgical procedures (Bryant et al., 2018). Here, the robot assists the surgeon by performing tasks such as adjusting motion scaling, filtering out hand tremors, and manipulating the camera view.

The robot does not operate autonomously or make independent clinical decisions; instead, it enhances the surgeon's capabilities by providing greater dexterity, visibility, and precision during complex operations.

12.2.4 *Regulatory landscape*

The rapid development, deployment, and use of AI in healthcare are not adequately addressed by clear and specific regulations, creating uncertainty and hindering innovation. Without stringent regulatory landscapes, ensuring ethical and responsible implementation becomes extremely difficult.

In the healthcare sector, numerous stringent codes of conduct govern daily practice, ensuring every actor is accountable to those they serve. However, there is currently no global law or regulation specifically addressing the application of AI in healthcare (Mitchell & Ploem, 2018).

Moving forward, a comprehensive legal framework should undoubtedly be created for the entire AI process, from laboratory research to clinical application, based on the "do no harm" principle. These guidelines should be rigorous yet sensible.

The legal system should collaborate effectively with healthcare stakeholders and policymakers to create adaptable laws that don't impede AI advancement (Kayaalp, 2018).

One of the main obstacles is the dynamic and ever-evolving nature of AI systems, particularly those built on machine learning algorithms. Unlike traditional medical devices with static functionality, AI models can adapt and change their behaviour in response to new data inputs or retraining.

This raises concerns about choosing suitable validation and monitoring procedures, as well as how to guarantee the continued safety, effectiveness, and performance of AI systems throughout their lifespan (Sloane & Silva, 2020).

Another challenge for regulators is the absence of standardised testing and evaluation frameworks for AI-based medical technologies. Since AI systems can continuously adapt and change, traditional clinical trial methodologies might not be the best option for evaluating their effectiveness and safety (Mennella et al., 2024). Robust and reliable testing protocols must be developed by regulatory oversight bodies to keep pace with the rapid speed of AI innovation.

Finally, healthcare AI regulation is fragmented across regions and jurisdictions, with different guidance and requirements. To develop and deploy AI-based medical technologies globally while maintaining oversight and patient safety, regulations and international cooperation must be harmonised (Palaniappan et al., 2024).

Therefore, it is imperative that AI developers, healthcare professionals, regulatory bodies, policymakers, and stakeholders collaborate to address these regulatory issues. Agile and adaptive regulatory frameworks that prioritise patient safety, transparency, and ethics are crucial for AI to transform and improve healthcare worldwide, keeping pace with rapid AI advancements.

12.2.5 *Workforce*

The integration of AI into healthcare presents challenges for the workforce, demanding new skills and competencies among healthcare professionals. One concern is that automation and AI-powered systems may displace some human jobs.

While AI is unlikely to entirely replace healthcare professionals, it may alter their responsibilities and skill sets. Healthcare workers may need to adapt to new workflows involving collaboration with AI systems, interpreting AI insights, and using AI for decision support (Braganza et al., 2021).

However, pioneers in the field of AI have organised numerous conferences and disseminated materials emphasising the genuine benefits AI offers to medical practitioners. AI and medical personnel need to collaborate to achieve better outcomes because it enhances productivity and reduces stress.

Instead of opposing the use of AI in healthcare, these professionals advise other healthcare professionals to work together for the benefit of the patients they are dedicated to serving (O'Neill, 2017). Another challenge is the current skills gap and the need for reskilling for the majority of healthcare professionals to keep pace with the rapidly evolving and new AI developments in the healthcare sector (Li, 2022). Using these new technologies, robots, and other AI interventions requires knowledge and experience in specific fields, such as data analysis and operating robotic and AI machinery. The difficulty lies in educating current employees about these cutting-edge technologies.

This is often a costly undertaking, and most healthcare professionals may be resistant to AI performing tasks they have been doing flawlessly for so long with their hands and minds.

The incorporation of AI into healthcare also raises concerns about the potential deskilling of medical professionals and the exacerbation of existing workforce disparities (Yan, 2024). Reliance on AI-powered systems for tasks like diagnosis, treatment recommendations, and clinical decision-making may erode critical thinking skills and reduce healthcare practitioners' ability to exercise independent judgement. This over-reliance on AI may have negative consequences for patient care. Furthermore, if AI-powered tools and technologies are primarily developed and deployed in well-resourced healthcare settings, the gap between underserved communities and those with advanced AI capabilities may widen, exacerbating healthcare disparities and workforce shortages (World Health Organization, 2021). These concerns highlight the importance of a comprehensive approach to mitigating the potential negative effects of AI on the healthcare workforce. This includes implementing robust training programmes, interdisciplinary collaboration, and policies to ensure the responsible and ethical use of AI in medical practice (Asan et al., 2020). Figure 12.1 presents a schematic representation of the challenges of AI in the healthcare sector.

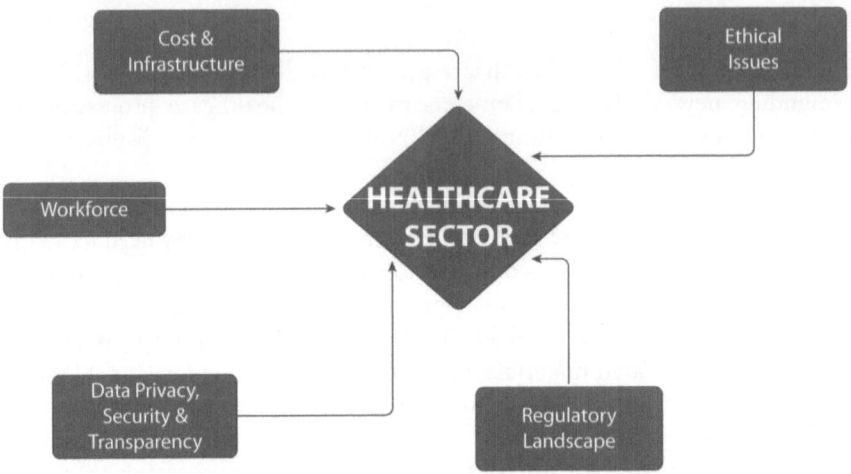

FIGURE 12.1 Challenges of AI application in the healthcare sector.

12.3 Future trends of AI in the healthcare sector

There are so many future trends that are feasible with the implementation of AI in the healthcare industry.

12.3.1 Precision medicine and personalised care

Precision medicine and personalised care represent significant paradigm shifts in the healthcare field, capitalising on advancements in AI to customise medical treatments and interventions for each individual patient (Johnson et al., 2021).

This emerging trend holds great potential to transform healthcare delivery by moving away from the conventional standardised model towards a more patient-centred and data-driven approach.

One of the key advantages of AI is its ability to identify patterns and provide personalised treatment recommendations based on vast amounts of genetic, clinical, and environmental data while minimising negative effects (Schork, 2019).

AI-powered precision medicine platforms can assist clinicians in customising treatment plans that are both more efficacious and less likely to cause harm or adverse reactions. This is achieved by identifying genetic markers or biomarkers linked to specific diseases or drug responses.

The customised approach is particularly important in the context of chronic illnesses such as cancer (Liao et al., 2023), where treatment outcomes can vary significantly between individuals.

Furthermore, precision medicine extends beyond just treatments, encompassing wellness programmes, lifestyle changes, and preventative care. Predictive analytics powered by AI allows doctors to identify individuals with a higher genetic predisposition to certain diseases (Arafah et al., 2023). This enables proactive measures, such as lifestyle modifications, targeted screenings, or early-stage treatments, to slow disease onset or progression.

12.3.2   Medical imaging and diagnostics

The increasing sophistication and widespread adoption of AI-powered medical imaging and diagnostic tools are anticipated. AI algorithms can enhance the precision of disease detection and diagnosis for radiologists and pathologists by analysing medical images, such as X-rays, ultrasounds, CT scans, and MRI scans. This can lead to earlier identification and improved diagnostic accuracy (Hosny et al., 2018).

This transformation is primarily driven by AI's ability to analyse complex imaging data and identify subtle patterns or anomalies that may be missed by the human eye. AI algorithms can leverage deep learning techniques and extensive datasets to develop the ability to identify disease markers, tissue abnormalities, and structural irregularities with a degree of precision and reliability that is comparable to, or even surpasses, that of human experts (Mehta, 2023). This leads to enhanced diagnostic accuracy, minimises diagnostic errors, and facilitates earlier disease identification. Furthermore, incorporating AI into medical imaging and diagnostics creates new opportunities for personalised healthcare. AI algorithms can analyse imaging data alongside other clinical and genomic information to help tailor treatment strategies to individual patients, predict treatment responses, and optimise therapeutic outcomes (Sahu et al., 2022).

This patient-centred approach holds promise for increasing treatment effectiveness, reducing side effects, and improving overall patient satisfaction.

12.3.3   Pharmaceutical research advancement and drug discovery

AI has the potential to expedite the process of drug discovery and development by analysing extensive datasets derived from biological, chemical, and clinical sources. AI can assist in identifying promising drug candidates, predicting their potential effectiveness and adverse effects, and optimising the design of clinical trials (Qureshi et al., 2023). This could significantly reduce the time and expense associated with bringing new medications to market. One of AI's most significant contributions to pharmaceutical research is its ability to facilitate target identification and validation. By analysing genomic data and biological pathways, AI algorithms can identify potential therapeutic targets linked to specific diseases.

This allows researchers to prioritise candidates with the greatest chance of success (Vidhya et al., 2023). Furthermore, AI-driven predictive modelling can simulate drug-target interactions, predict potential side effects, and optimise drug design. This accelerates the drug discovery process and reduces the time and cost of bringing new therapies to market (Paul et al., 2021).

Another potential approach to speeding up the development of novel treatments for existing diseases is AI-enabled drug repurposing. AI systems can discover underused or neglected medications that could be repurposed for different uses by analysing extensive biomedical datasets, such as electronic health records, clinical trial databases, and academic articles (Yadav et al., 2024). Moreover, AI-driven data analytics can assemble valuable information from clinical trial data, revealing trends, correlations, and patterns that can inform regulatory submissions and treatment choices (Niazi, 2023).

12.3.4 Chatbots and virtual assistants

AI-powered chatbots and virtual assistants in healthcare hold promise for facilitating easier access to individualised health records, sorting symptoms by severity, and providing self-care and illness management advice. These AI assistants can also help healthcare providers improve patient engagement and adherence to treatment plans (Al Kuwaiti et al., 2023).

Patients can take charge of their health in a multitude of ways, including seeking medical advice, monitoring chronic conditions, and accessing educational resources. The COVID-19 pandemic has further highlighted the importance of chatbots and virtual assistants in telemedicine and remote patient monitoring.

These AI-powered technologies allow healthcare providers to remotely monitor patient vitals, track symptoms, and offer real-time support and guidance, improving the delivery of virtual care services and increasing access to healthcare for underserved populations (Wosik et al., 2020).

However, the widespread use of chatbots and virtual assistants in healthcare presents both advantages and disadvantages. A key concern lies in the area of privacy and security surrounding AI-driven decision-making. This includes protecting patient data, complying with regulations, and ensuring ethical considerations are addressed. Additionally, thorough training, validation, and continuous monitoring are essential to guarantee the accuracy, reliability, and credibility of chatbot suggestions and responses (Li, 2023).

12.3.5 Remote patient monitoring

The implementation of AI will facilitate enhanced functionalities for remote patient monitoring. This will enable healthcare providers to continuously monitor patients' vital signs, activity levels, and other health-related information beyond the confines of clinical settings. This intervention has the potential to facilitate timely interventions, mitigate complications, and reduce the need for hospitalisation (Dubey & Tiwari, 2023). Patients with chronic conditions, such as heart disease, diabetes, or respiratory disorders, can benefit greatly from remote patient monitoring. AI-powered systems can monitor vital signs, medication adherence, and lifestyle factors.

This provides healthcare providers with valuable insights and facilitates prompt modifications to treatment plans (Peyroteo et al., 2021), potentially avoiding hospital admissions or complications.

Furthermore, utilising AI-powered remote patient monitoring has the potential to enhance post-operative care and rehabilitation. This technology allows healthcare professionals to closely observe patients' recovery progress and offer necessary guidance or interventions, eliminating the need for frequent face-to-face appointments (Haleem et al., 2021).

Overall, integrating remote patient monitoring and AI holds promise for improving patient outcomes, expanding access to healthcare services, reducing healthcare costs, and empowering individuals to actively participate in their health management.

12.3.6   AI enabled robotics and surgical advancements

AI-driven robotic systems will continue to improve, allowing surgeons to perform complex operations with greater accuracy and precision. AI algorithms can analyse real-time data and offer guidance and decision support during surgery (Mithany et al., 2023). This has the potential to pave the way for autonomous surgical tasks in the future. The schematic diagram in Figure 12.2 illustrates the application of AI in the healthcare sector.

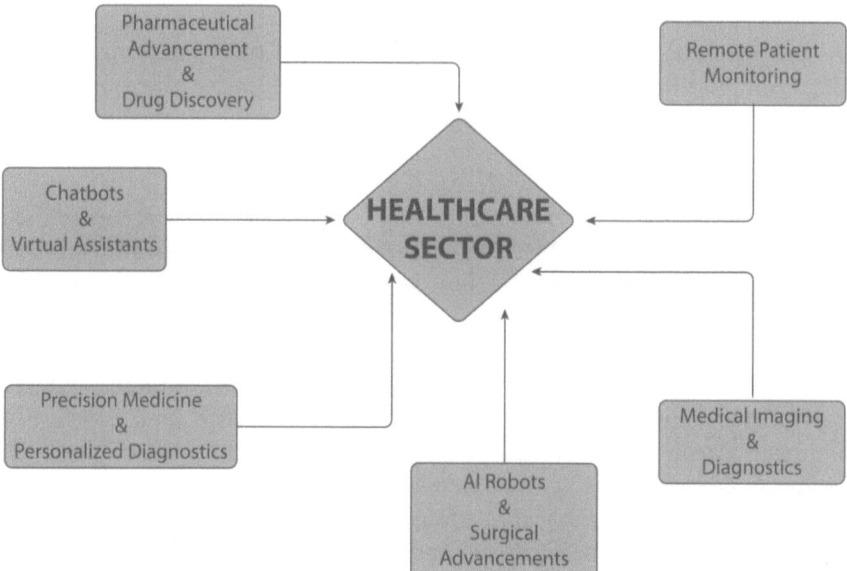

FIGURE 12.2   Future trends of AI application in the healthcare sector.

12.3.6.1 Advances in surgical robots

Surgical robots have become increasingly sophisticated and prevalent in healthcare, offering the promise of minimally invasive procedures, increased precision, and quicker patient recovery times.

Minimally invasive surgery (MIS) describes procedures that can be carried out with a minimal number of incisions, greatly benefiting the patient by potentially reducing trauma and shortening recovery times compared to traditional surgery (Ranev & Teixeira, 2020).

Progress in computing power, related technologies, and the introduction of imaging modalities like computed tomography (CT), magnetic resonance imaging (MRI), and ultrasound (US) have significantly benefitted robot-assisted surgery. This cutting-edge technology, known as computer-integrated surgery (CIS), combines robotic assistance, pre- and intra-operative imaging, and patient-specific data, completely changing the way surgeries are planned and performed (Takács et al., 2016). An example is the Stryker robotic system, approved by the FDA for assisting surgeons in total hip, knee, and partial knee replacements. The system comprises a robotic arm, camera stand, and guidance module. Software and attachments, such as cutting tools, are adaptable to specific procedures. Surgeons plan the procedure using preoperative images, and the robotic arm creates a virtual boundary to guide orthopaedic tools during surgery, with an optical tracker facilitating position tracking (Biswas et al., 2023).

12.3.6.2 Advances in diagnostic robots

AI-powered diagnostic robots have the potential to revolutionise disease detection and health monitoring. Sophisticated AI algorithms, integrated with robotic hardware, can analyse complex medical data including medical images, bio signals, and genomic information. These AI-enabled diagnostic robots can effectively detect patterns and anomalies that may be difficult for human experts, facilitating earlier and more accurate diagnoses (Habuza et al., 2021). For example, robotic systems equipped with computer vision and deep learning can analyse X-rays, CT scans, and MRI images, enabling them to accurately detect tumours, fractures, or other abnormalities.

Additionally, diagnostic robots equipped with AI can continuously monitor patients' vital signs, activity levels, and other biometric data, allowing for immediate health monitoring and timely intervention for potential problems (Mustafa & Nsour, 2023). As these diagnostic robots become more advanced and integrated into healthcare settings, they will have a significant impact on improving diagnostic accuracy, optimising workflows, and ultimately improving patient outcomes.

12.3.6.3 Advances in rehabilitation robots

The use of AI-driven rehabilitation robots is transforming physical therapy, facilitating a more personalised and efficient recovery process for patients. Equipped with machine learning algorithms, these advanced robotic systems can analyse a patient's movements, gait patterns, and progress over time to create customised rehabilitation plans (Lanotte et al., 2023). Rehabilitation robots can deliver accurate and repetitive movements and exercises, providing unwavering and continuous assistance during recovery. Additionally, these robots can incorporate gamification into therapy sessions, thereby enhancing patient engagement and motivation (Gassert & Dietz, 2018).

With continued progress in AI, rehabilitation robots will become more intelligent, enabling them to predict recovery paths, detect potential obstacles, and adapt treatment strategies accordingly. The incorporation of AI into rehabilitation robotics presents significant opportunities for improving patient outcomes, alleviating the workload of therapists and facilitating the provision of more efficient and accessible rehabilitation services.

12.3.6.4 Advances in elderly care robots

AI-driven robots are increasingly being developed and used to assist in elderly care, with the aim of improving their quality of life, promoting independence, and reducing the burden on carers. These advanced robotic systems can perform a variety of tasks specifically designed to meet the needs of elderly individuals, including physical assistance, cognitive support, and social interaction (Sawik et al., 2023).

12.3.6.5 Assistive robots

A particular area of focus is the development of assistive robots designed to aid with mobility, activities of daily living (ADLs), and fall prevention. AI algorithms enable these robots to learn and adapt to the specific needs of each patient, offering tailored assistance and supervision for activities such as transferring from bed, dressing, and moving safely (Abarca & Elias, 2023).

12.3.6.6 Health monitoring robots

Furthermore, AI-driven robots can monitor the health and well-being of elderly people. These robots use sensors and data analysis to monitor vital signs, identify health problems, and alert carers or healthcare professionals when assistance is needed. AI algorithms can identify patterns and predict risks, enabling proactive healthcare and prevention (Padhan et al., 2023).

12.3.6.7 Advances in telepresence robots

AI-powered telepresence robots are making remote healthcare delivery more accessible and convenient. These advanced robotic systems allow doctors to virtually treat patients from remote locations, bridging geographical gaps and expanding access to high-quality medical care (Leoste et al., 2024). These robots use AI to personalise patient care, make recommendations, and notify healthcare providers of potential issues.

Additionally, AI-enabled telepresence robots can help healthcare professionals schedule appointments, update medical records, and access patient data in real-time. This improves efficiency, reduces human error, and equips healthcare providers with the information they need during remote consultations (Sarker et al., 2021).

12.3.6.8 AI capabilities of telepresence robots

Telepresence robots use advanced AI algorithms for communication, navigation, and data analysis. Natural language processing (NLP) allows robots to have natural conversations, understand patient questions, and provide relevant information or instructions. Robots use computer vision and machine learning to navigate, recognise people, and collect and analyse visual data for diagnostic or monitoring purposes (Hung et al., 2023). Robots are significantly transforming the healthcare sector in numerous ways. This should serve as a foundation for further research, identifying areas where robots face challenges and require improvement, while also recognising their strengths and exploring ways to enhance their performance and maintain efficiency.

12.4 Way Forward

The successful future use of AI in healthcare hinges largely on public education and engagement. By educating the public about AI in healthcare, transparency, trust, and public acceptance of these technologies can be improved, including among healthcare professionals. This communication can inform ethical decisions when designing and implementing AI interventions to align with public social, cultural, and religious values (Dlugatch et al., 2023).

Furthermore, to ensure the effective implementation and adoption of AI-based tools and technologies, it is essential to develop them with a comprehensive understanding of the local context, infrastructure, resources, and cultural nuances. A potentially fruitful strategy involves fostering collaboration between healthcare professionals in the diaspora, who possess global expertise and familiarity with cutting-edge AI technologies, and their indigenous counterparts (Parag et al., 2023). This collaboration can facilitate significant transformations within healthcare systems, particularly in developing countries.

Such a partnership can leverage the knowledge and perspectives of diaspora experts while guaranteeing that solutions are grounded in local realities and tailored to address the specific challenges faced by communities. Moreover, it is essential to utilise local resources when tackling healthcare challenges through AI implementation. One possible approach is to train AI models using readily available data sources in the local area, such as community health records or traditional knowledge systems (Chomutare et al., 2022). Additionally, this may involve utilising existing infrastructure and community networks to streamline the implementation and acceptance of AI-driven solutions, as well as reduce the cost burden associated with using AI in low-resource countries. This approach not only addresses the distinct challenges faced by different communities but also ensures the sustainability, cultural appropriateness, and significant impact of AI-based solutions in improving healthcare accessibility.

12.5   Recommendations

12.5.1   Data privacy and security

12.5.1.1   Interactive consent documents

Instead of static consent forms, consider allowing people to manage their health data dynamically. Design AI systems that respect their choices and adapt data access based on their preferences. This empowers patients to stay informed and in control, fostering trust and transparency in healthcare AI.

12.5.1.2   Blockchain technology integration

Further exploration is warranted regarding the integration of blockchain technology into AI and robotics applications to enhance data security and transparency. By leveraging its decentralised and tamper-resistant characteristics, blockchain offers a secure framework for storing and managing health data. This ensures transparency and traceability while minimising the risk of unauthorised access.

12.5.1.3   Continuous research

Promote continuous research on anonymisation techniques and alternative data-driven approaches. The field of AI and robotics in healthcare is constantly evolving, necessitating ongoing research efforts.

12.5.2 Cost and infrastructure

12.5.2.1 Standardised, open-source AI platforms and infrastructure

Explore cloud-based, open-source tools and partnerships to make healthcare AI more affordable. Public-private funding can further unlock access. This approach would facilitate wider adoption, collaboration, and cost-sharing among healthcare institutions, reducing the burden of individual investment in proprietary solutions.

12.5.2.2 Public-private partnerships and funding initiatives

Encourage collaboration (through grants, tax breaks, and partnerships) between public and private entities to invest in sustainable research, development, and infrastructure. This will lower costs and accelerate progress in AI and robotics for healthcare.

12.5.2.3 Capacity building and training

Train healthcare workers to optimise existing infrastructure and maximise the value of AI and robotics. This ensures institutions get the most out of their current investments.

12.5.3 Ethical issues

12.5.3.1 Ethical AI guidelines and training

To ensure the responsible use of AI and robotics in healthcare, clear ethical guidelines are essential. Specialised training for developers, engineers, and healthcare workers, combined with dedicated ethical review boards, will promote understanding and responsible implementation. These boards, comprising ethicists, doctors, and patients, should address bias, fairness, transparency, and accountability in AI algorithms and systems throughout their design, development, and use.

12.5.3.2 Demystifying AI in healthcare

Engage patients and the public through education and platforms for informed choices about their data. Provide platforms where people can openly express concerns about the benefits, risks, and ethics, empowering everyone to shape a responsible future for AI in healthcare.

12.5.4 Regulatory landscape

12.5.4.1 Harmonised regulatory frameworks

Promote the creation of global regulatory frameworks that will standardise requirements across jurisdictions, thereby streamlining the approval processes for robotics and AI in healthcare.

12.5.4.2   Interdisciplinary regulatory committees

Establish multidisciplinary regulatory committees comprising professionals from the fields of ethics, law, technology, and medicine to collaborate on evaluating AI and robotics healthcare solutions. This will guarantee a thorough assessment that takes ethical concerns and technological advancements into account.

12.5.4.3   Ethical impact assessments

When approving AI and robotics healthcare technologies, include ethical impact assessments that evaluate potential biases, privacy concerns, and ethical considerations. This ensures adherence to moral principles and protection of patient rights in authorised technologies.

12.5.5   Workforce

12.5.5.1   Upskilling and reskilling programmes

Establish comprehensive training programmes to equip healthcare workers with the skills and know-how required to operate robots and AI effectively. This includes classes on ethical issues, interacting with AI systems, and interpreting data.

12.5.5.2   Foster interdisciplinary collaboration

To ensure a workforce with a diverse range of skills, promote collaboration among educators, technologists, and healthcare professionals. This will enable the sharing of knowledge and experience.

12.5.5.3   Support well-being initiatives

Adopt strategies to address how AI and robotics will affect healthcare workers' well-being, such as measures to allay concerns about job displacement and provide mental health support. Develop explicit plans for the workforce transition to reduce job displacement, such as early retirement initiatives, upskilling, and redeployment programmes.

12.5.5.4   Attracting and retaining talent

Implement plans for competitive compensation, work-life balance support, and a nurturing environment to attract and retain skilled healthcare professionals, fostering adaptability in the dynamic healthcare landscape.

12.6 Conclusion

The use of AI in healthcare holds immense potential to revolutionise patient care, diagnosis, and treatment. However, successful integration necessitates addressing challenges such as data privacy, security, and ethical considerations. Building trust among patients and healthcare professionals requires careful navigation of these issues. Additionally, cost and infrastructure limitations, particularly in LMICs, necessitate innovative solutions and collaborative efforts. Regulations, public education, and technological advancements will play a key role in shaping the future of AI in healthcare. Despite these hurdles, the transformative potential of these technologies lies in their ability to increase efficiency, precision, and ultimately improve patient outcomes. Stakeholders across the healthcare industry must collaborate to overcome current challenges and embrace evolving trends to fully unlock the potential of AI in shaping the future of healthcare.

References

Abarca, V. E., & Elias, D. A. (2023). A review of parallel robots: Rehabilitation, assistance, and humanoid applications for neck, shoulder, wrist, hip, and ankle joints. *Robotics, 12*(5), 131. https://doi.org/10.3390/robotics12050131

Al Kuwaiti, A., Nazer, K., Al-Reedy, A., Al-Shehri, S., Al-Muhanna, A., Subbarayalu, A. V., Al Muhanna, D., & Al-Muhanna, F. A. (2023). A review of the role of artificial intelligence in healthcare. *Journal of Personalized Medicine, 13*(6), 951. https://doi.org/10.3390/jpm13060951

Ali, S., Abuhmed, T., El-Sappagh, S., Muhammad, K., Alonso-Moral, J. M., Confalonieri, R., Guidotti, R., Del Ser, J., Díaz-Rodríguez, N., & Herrera, F. (2023). Explainable artificial intelligence (XAI): What we know and what is left to attain trustworthy artificial intelligence. *Information Fusion, 99*, 101805. https://doi.org/10.1016/J.INFFUS.2023.101805

Almeida, D., Shmarko, K., & Lomas, E. (2022). The ethics of facial recognition technologies, surveillance, and accountability in an age of artificial intelligence: A comparative analysis of US, EU, and UK regulatory frameworks. *AI and Ethics, 2*(3), 377. https://doi.org/10.1007/S43681-021-00077-W

Alowais, S. A., Alghamdi, S. S., Alsuhebany, N., Alqahtani, T., Alshaya, A. I., Almohareb, S. N., Aldairem, A., Alrashed, M., Bin Saleh, K., Badreldin, H. A., Al Yami, M. S., Al Harbi, S., & Albekairy, A. M. (2023). Revolutionizing healthcare: The role of artificial intelligence in clinical practice. *BMC Medical Education, 23*(1), 1–15. https://doi.org/10.1186/S12909-023-04698-Z

Arafah, A., Khatoon, S., Rasool, I., Khan, A., Rather, M. A., Abujabal, K. A., Faqih, Y. A. H., Rashid, H., Rashid, S. M., Bilal Ahmad, S., Alexiou, A., & Rehman, M. U. (2023). The future of precision medicine in the cure of Alzheimer's disease. *Biomedicines, 11*(2). https://doi.org/10.3390/BIOMEDICINES11020335

Asan, O., Bayrak, A. E., & Choudhury, A. (2020). Artificial intelligence and human trust in healthcare: Focus on clinicians. *Journal of Medical Internet Research, 22*(6). https://doi.org/10.2196/15154

Batko, K., & Ślęzak, A. (2022). The use of big data analytics in healthcare. *Journal of Big Data, 9*(1), 1–24. https://doi.org/10.1186/s40537-021-00553-4

Biswas, S. (2023). Impacts of AI, Robotics, and Automation on Data Privacy and Privacy Laws to Adhere: A Global Perspective. https://www.linkedin.com/pulse/impacts-ai-robotics-automation-data-privacy-laws-adhere-biswas/

Biswas, P., Sikander, S., & Kulkarni, P. (2023). Recent advances in robot-assisted surgical systems. *Biomedical Engineering Advances*, 6, 100109. https://doi.org/10.1016/J.BEA.2023.100109

Braganza, A., Chen, W., Canhoto, A., & Sap, S. (2021). Productive employment and decent work: The impact of AI adoption on psychological contracts, job engagement and employee trust. *Journal of Business Research*, 131, 485–494. https://doi.org/10.1016/J.JBUSRES.2020.08.018

Bryant, A., Wei, B., Veronesi, G., & Cerfolio, R. (2018). Robotic surgery: Techniques and results for resection of lung cancer. In Harvey I. Pass, David Ball, & Giorgio V. Scagliotti (eds.), *IASLC Thoracic Oncology* (pp. 283–288.e1). Elsevier. https://doi.org/10.1016/B978-0-323-52357-8.00028-7

Cabuyao, K. (2023). Artificial Intelligence and Cybersecurity – CEPS [International Hospital Federation]. https://www.ceps.eu/ceps-publications/artificial-intelligence-and-cybersecurity-2/

Chen, R. J., Wang, J. J., Williamson, D. F. K., Chen, T. Y., Lipkova, J., Lu, M. Y., Sahai, S., & Mahmood, F. (2023). Algorithm fairness in artificial intelligence for medicine and healthcare. *Nature Biomedical Engineering*, 7(6), 719. https://doi.org/10.1038/S41551-023-01056-8

Chomutare, T., Tejedor, M., Svenning, T. O., Marco-Ruiz, L., Tayefi, M., Lind, K., Godtliebsen, F., Moen, A., Ismail, L., Makhlysheva, A., & Ngo, P. D. (2022). Artificial intelligence implementation in healthcare: A theory-based scoping review of barriers and facilitators. *International Journal of Environmental Research and Public Health*, 19(23), 16359.

Clark, M., & Bailey, S. (2024). Chatbots in health care: Connecting patients to information. In *Emerging Health Technologies*. National Institutes of Health. https://www.ncbi.nlm.nih.gov/books/NBK602381/

Dastin, J. (2022). Amazon scraps secret AI recruiting tool that showed bias against women. *Ethics of Data and Analytics*, 296–299. https://doi.org/10.1201/9781003278290-44

Deo, N., & Anjankar, A. (2023). Artificial intelligence with robotics in healthcare: A narrative review of its viability in India. *Cureus*. https://doi.org/10.7759/CUREUS.39416

Dlugatch, R., Georgieva, A., & Kerasidou, A. (2023). Trustworthy artificial intelligence and ethical design: Public perceptions of trustworthiness of an AI-based decision-support tool in the context of intrapartum care. *BMC Medical Ethics*, 24(1). https://doi.org/10.1186/S12910-023-00917-W

Dubey, A., & Tiwari, A. (2023). Artificial intelligence and remote patient monitoring in US healthcare market: A literature review. *Journal of Market Access & Health Policy*, 11(1). https://doi.org/10.1080/20016689.2023.2205618

Elendu, C., Amaechi, D. C., Elendu, T. C., Jingwa, K. A., Okoye, O. K., Okah, M. J., Ladele, J. A., Farah, A. H., & Alimi, H. A. (2023). Ethical implications of AI and robotics in healthcare: A review. *Medicine (Baltimore)*, 102(50), E36671. https://doi.org/10.1097/MD.0000000000036671

Gassert, R., & Dietz, V. (2018). Rehabilitation robots for the treatment of sensorimotor deficits: A neurophysiological perspective. *Journal of NeuroEngineering and Rehabilitation*, 15(1), 1–15. https://doi.org/10.1186/S12984-018-0383-X

Gelhaus, P. (2011). Robot decisions: On the importance of virtuous judgment in clinical decision making. *Journal of Evaluation in Clinical Practice*, 17(5), 883–887. https://doi.org/10.1111/J.1365-2753.2011.01720.X

Gibelli, F., Ricci, G., Sirignano, A., Turrina, S., & De Leo, D. (2021). The increasing centrality of robotic technology in the context of nursing care: Bioethical implications analyzed through a scoping review approach. *Journal of Healthcare Engineering*, 2021, 1478025. https://doi.org/10.1155/2021/1478025

Habuza, T., Navaz, A. N., Hashim, F., Alnajjar, F., Zaki, N., Serhani, M. A., & Statsenko, Y. (2021). AI applications in robotics, diagnostic image analysis and precision medicine: Current limitations, future trends, guidelines on CAD systems for medicine. *Informatics in Medicine Unlocked*, 24, 100596. https://doi.org/10.1016/J.IMU.2021.100596

Haleem, A., Javaid, M., Singh, R. P., & Suman, R. (2021). Telemedicine for healthcare: Capabilities, features, barriers, and applications. *Sensors (Switzerland)*, 2(3), 100117. https://doi.org/10.1016/J.SINTL.2021.100117

Hosny, A., Parmar, C., Quackenbush, J., Schwartz, L. H., & Aerts, H. J. W. L. (2018). Artificial intelligence in radiology. *Nature Reviews Cancer*, 18(8), 500–501. https://doi.org/10.1038/S41568-018-0016-5

Hung, L., Lake, C., Hussein, A., Wong, J., & Mann, J. (2023). Using telepresence robots as a tool to engage patient and family partners in dementia research during COVID-19 pandemic: A qualitative participatory study. *Research Involvement and Engagement*, 9(1), 12. https://doi.org/10.1186/s40900-023-00421-w

Jeyaraman, M., Balaji, S., Jeyaraman, N., & Yadav, S. (2023). Unraveling the ethical enigma: Artificial intelligence in healthcare. *Cureus*, 15(8), e43262. https://doi.org/10.7759/cureus.43262

Johnson, K. B., Wei, W. Q., Weeraratne, D., Frisse, M. E., Misulis, K., Rhee, K., Zhao, J., & Snowdon, J. L. (2021). Precision medicine, AI, and the future of personalized health care. *Clinical and Translational Science*, 14(1), 86–93. https://doi.org/10.1111/cts.12884

Kayaalp, M. (2018). *Patient privacy in the era of big data. Balkan Medical Journal*. https://doi.org/10.4274/balkanmedj.2017.0966

Khan, B., Fatima, H., Qureshi, A., Kumar, S., Hanan, A., Hussain, J., & Abdullah, S. (2023). Drawbacks of artificial intelligence and their potential solutions in the healthcare sector. *Biomedical Materials and Devices*, 1(2), 1. https://doi.org/10.1007/S44174-023-00063-2

Lanotte, F., O'Brien, M. K., & Jayaraman, A. (2023). AI in rehabilitation medicine: Opportunities and challenges. *Annals of Rehabilitation Medicine*, 47(6), 444–458. https://doi.org/10.5535/arm.23131

Leoste, J., Strömberg-Järvis, K., Robal, T., Marmor, K., Kangur, K., & Rebane, A. M. (2024). Testing scenarios for using telepresence robots in healthcare settings. *Computational and Structural Biotechnology Journal*, 24, 105–114. https://doi.org/10.1016/j.csbj.2024.01.004

Li, J. (2023). Security implications of AI chatbots in health care. *Journal of Medical Internet Research*, 25, e47551. https://doi.org/10.2196/47551

Li, L. (2022). Reskilling and upskilling the future-ready workforce for industry 4.0 and beyond. *Information Systems Frontiers: A Journal of Research and Innovation*, 1–16. https://doi.org/10.1007/s10796-022-10308-y

Liao, J., Li, X., Gan, Y., Han, S., Rong, P., Wang, W., Li, W., & Zhou, L. (2023). Artificial intelligence assists precision medicine in cancer treatment. *Frontiers in Oncology*, 12, 998222. https://doi.org/10.3389/fonc.2022.998222

Mehta, J. (2023). The role of artificial intelligence in personalized medicine. Abmatic AI [Blog post]. https://abmatic.ai/blog/role-of-artificial-intelligence-in-personalized-marketing

Menash, G. (2023). Artificial Intelligence and Ethics: A Comprehensive Review of Bias Mitigation, Transparency, and Accountability in AI Systems [Unpublished manuscript]. Retrieved from https://www.researchgate.net/publication/375744287_

Artificial_Intelligence_and_Ethics_A_Comprehensive_Review_of_Bias_
Mitigation_Transparency_and_Accountability_in_AI_Systems

Mennella, C., Maniscalco, U., De Pietro, G., & Esposito, M. (2024). Ethical and regulatory challenges of AI technologies in healthcare: A narrative review. *Heliyon*, *10*(4), e26297. https://doi.org/10.1016/j.heliyon.2024.e26297

Mitchell, C., & Ploem, C. (2018). Legal challenges for the implementation of advanced clinical digital decision support systems in Europe. *Journal of Clinical and Translational Research*, *3*(Suppl 3), 424–430.

Mithany, R. H., Aslam, S., Abdallah, S., Abdelmaseeh, M., Gerges, F., Mohamed, M. S., Manasseh, M., Wanees, A., Shahid, M. H., Khalil, M. S., & Daniel, N. (2023). Advancements and challenges in the application of artificial intelligence in surgical arena: A literature review. *Cureus*, *15*(10), e47924. https://doi.org/10.7759/cureus.47924

Murdoch, B. (2021). Privacy and artificial intelligence: Challenges for protecting health information in a new era. *BMC Medical Ethics*, *22*(1), 1–5. https://doi.org/10.1186/S12910-021-00687-3

Mustafa, Z., & Nsour, H. (2023). Using computer vision techniques to automatically detect abnormalities in chest X-rays. *Diagnostics (Basel, Switzerland)*, *13*(18), 2979. https://doi.org/10.3390/diagnostics13182979

Naik, N., Hameed, B. M. Z., Shetty, D. K., Swain, D., Shah, M., Paul, R., Aggarwal, K., Ibrahim, S., Patil, V., Smriti, K., Shetty, S., Rai, B. P., Chlosta, P., & Somani, B. K. (2022). Legal and ethical consideration in artificial intelligence in healthcare: Who takes responsibility? *Frontiers in Surgery*, *9*, 862322. https://doi.org/10.3389/fsurg.2022.862322

Niazi, S. K. (2023). The coming of age of AI/ML in drug discovery, development, clinical testing, and manufacturing: The FDA perspectives. *Drug Design, Development and Therapy*, *17*, 2691–2725. https://doi.org/10.2147/DDDT.S424991

O'Neill, C. (2017). Is AI a threat or benefit to health workers? *CMAJ: Canadian Medical Association Journal = journal de l'Association medicale canadienne*, *189*(20), E732. https://doi.org/10.1503/cmaj.1095428

Padhan, S., Mohapatra, A., Ramasamy, S. K., & Agrawal, S. (2023). Artificial intelligence (AI) and robotics in elderly healthcare: Enabling independence and quality of life. *Cureus*, *15*(8), e42905. https://doi.org/10.7759/cureus.42905

Palaniappan, K., Lin, E. Y. T., & Vogel, S. (2024). Global regulatory frameworks for the use of artificial intelligence (AI) in the healthcare services sector. *Healthcare (Basel, Switzerland)*, *12*(5), 562. https://doi.org/10.3390/healthcare12050562

Parag, N., Govender, R., & Ally, S. B. (2023). Promoting cultural inclusivity in healthcare artificial intelligence: A framework for ensuring diversity. *Health Management, Policy & Innovation*. https://hmpi.org

Paul, D., Sanap, G., Shenoy, S., Kalyane, D., Kalia, K., & Tekade, R. K. (2021). Artificial intelligence in drug discovery and development. *Drug Discovery Today*, *26*(1), 80–93. https://doi.org/10.1016/j.drudis.2020.10.010

Petersson, L., Larsson, I., Nygren, J. M., Nilsen, P., Neher, M., Reed, J. E., Tyskbo, D., & Svedberg, P. (2022). Challenges to implementing artificial intelligence in healthcare: A qualitative interview study with healthcare leaders in Sweden. *BMC Health Services Research*, *22*(1), 850. https://doi.org/10.1186/s12913-022-08215-8

Peyroteo, M., Ferreira, I. A., Elvas, L. B., Ferreira, J. C., & Lapão, L. V. (2021). Remote monitoring systems for patients with chronic diseases in primary health care: Systematic review. *JMIR mHealth and uHealth*, *9*(12), e28285. https://doi.org/10.2196/28285

Quach, S., Thaichon, P., Martin, K. D., Weaven, S., & Palmatier, R. W. (2022). Digital technologies: Tensions in privacy and data. *Journal of the Academy of Marketing Science*, *50*(6), 1299–1323. https://doi.org/10.1007/s11747-022-00845-y

Qureshi, R., Irfan, M., Gondal, T. M., Khan, S., Wu, J., Hadi, M. U., Heymach, J., Le, X., Yan, H., & Alam, T. (2023). AI in drug discovery and its clinical relevance. *Heliyon*, 9(7), e17575. https://doi.org/10.1016/j.heliyon.2023.e17575

Rajkomar, A., Hardt, M., Howell, M. D., Corrado, G., & Chin, M. H. (2018). Ensuring fairness in machine learning to advance health equity. *Annals of Internal Medicine*, 169(12), 866–872. https://doi.org/10.7326/M18-1990

Ranev, D., & Teixeira, J. (2020). History of computer-assisted surgery. *Surgical Clinics of North America*, 100(2), 209–218. https://doi.org/10.1016/j.suc.2019.11.001

Reilly, J. (2024, April 24). Cost of AI in 2024: Estimating Development & Deployment Expenses. Akkio. https://www.digitalfirstmagazine.com/2024-the-year-artificial-intelligence-truly-takes-form/

Rossi, A., & Lenzini, G. (2020). Transparency by design in data-informed research: A collection of information design patterns. *Computer Law & Security Review*, 37, 105402. https://doi.org/10.1016/J.CLSR.2020.105402

Sahu, M., Gupta, R., Ambasta, R. K., & Kumar, P. (2022). Artificial intelligence and machine learning in precision medicine: A paradigm shift in big data analysis. *Progress in Molecular Biology and Translational Science*, 190(1), 57–100. https://doi.org/10.1016/bs.pmbts.2022.03.002

Sarker, S., Jamal, L., Ahmed, S. F., & Irtisam, N. (2021). Robotics and artificial intelligence in healthcare during COVID-19 pandemic: A systematic review. *Robotics and Autonomous Systems*, 146, 103902. https://doi.org/10.1016/j.robot.2021.103902

Sawik, B., Tobis, S., Baum, E., Suwalska, A., Kropińska, S., Stachnik, K., Pérez-Bernabeu, E., Cildoz, M., Agustin, A., & Wieczorowska-Tobis, K. (2023). Robots for elderly care: Review, multi-criteria optimization model and qualitative case study. *Healthcare (Basel, Switzerland)*, 11(9), 1286. https://doi.org/10.3390/healthcare11091286

Schork, N. J. (2019). Artificial intelligence and personalized medicine. *Cancer Treatment and Research*, 178, 265–283. https://doi.org/10.1007/978-3-030-16391-4_11

Seh, A. H., Zarour, M., Alenezi, M., Sarkar, A. K., Agrawal, A., Kumar, R., & Khan, R. A. (2020). Healthcare data breaches: Insights and implications. *Healthcare (Basel, Switzerland)*, 8(2), 133. https://doi.org/10.3390/healthcare8020133

Sloane, E. B., & J. Silva, R. (2020). Artificial intelligence in medical devices and clinical decision support systems. *Clinical Engineering Handbook*, 556–568. https://doi.org/10.1016/B978-0-12-813467-2.00084-5

Takács, Á, Nagy, D., Rudas, I., & Haidegger, T. (2016). Origins of surgical robotics: from space to the operating room. *Acta Polytechnica Hungarica*, 13(1). https://doi.org/10.12700/aph.13.1.2016.1.3

Thwaites, C. L., Ngoc Dinh, M., Nygate, J., Hoang Minh Tu, V., Van Cuong, N., Anh, T. T., McBride, A., Huynh, T., Chau, N. H., Lâm, H. M., Giang, D. D. H., Lam, P. K., Trinh, D. H. K., Nhat, L. T. H., & Vuong, N. L., et al. (2020). New technologies to improve healthcare in low- and middle-income countries: Global Grand Challenges satellite event, Oxford University Clinical Research Unit. University of Sussex. https://hdl.handle.net/10779/uos.23491634.v1

Vidhya, K. S., Sultana, A., Naveen Kumar M., & Rangareddy, H. (2023). Artificial Intelligence's impact on drug discovery and development from bench to bedside. *Cureus*, 15(10), e47486. https://doi.org/10.7759/cureus.47486

Wang, C., Zhang, J., Lassi, N., & Zhang, X. (2022). Privacy protection in using artificial intelligence for healthcare: Chinese regulation in comparative perspective. *Healthcare (Basel, Switzerland)*, 10(10), 1878. https://doi.org/10.3390/healthcare10101878

Ethics and governance of artificial intelligence for health: WHO guidance. Geneva: World Health Organization; 2021. License: CC BY-NC-SA 3.0 IGO.

Wosik, J., Fudim, M., Cameron, B., Gellad, Z. F., Cho, A., Phinney, D., Curtis, S., Roman, M., Poon, E. G., Ferranti, J., Katz, J. N., & Tcheng, J. (2020). Telehealth transformation: COVID-19 and the rise of virtual care. *Journal of the American Medical Informatics Association: JAMIA*, 27(6), 957–962. https://doi.org/10.1093/jamia/ocaa067

Yadav, S., Singh, A., Singhal, R., & Yadav, J. P. (2024). Revolutionizing drug discovery: The impact of artificial intelligence on advancements in pharmacology and the pharmaceutical industry. *Intelligent Pharmacy*. https://doi.org/10.1016/J.IPHA.2024.02.009

Yan, R. (2024). The impact of artificial intelligence on the labor market. *International Journal of Global Economics and Management*, 2(1), 233–238. https://doi.org/10.62051/ijgem.v2n1.29

13

THE FUTURE OF AI IN HEALTHCARE

Opportunities and Challenges

Olapeju A. Sam-Oyerinde, Oluwaremilekun O. Idowu, and Oluwagbenga P. Idowu

13.1 Introduction

The global market for artificial intelligence (AI) in healthcare is on an exponential growth trajectory, projected to skyrocket to an astonishing $148.4 billion by 2029 [1]. This represents a substantial increase from its already significant standing at $20.9 billion in 2024 [2]. The surge in demand for AI technologies within the healthcare sector underscores the industry's recognition of AI's transformative potential. From enhancing diagnostic accuracy to streamlining administrative processes and revolutionizing patient care, AI offers a multitude of benefits that healthcare providers are eager to leverage [3]. This rapid market expansion reflects not only the growing investment in AI solutions but also the increasing adoption and integration of AI-driven technologies across various healthcare settings globally [4]. As AI continues to demonstrate its value in improving healthcare outcomes, its market growth is expected to remain robust, reshaping the future of healthcare delivery on a global scale. This exponential growth underscores the rapid adoption of AI technologies and its profound impact on transforming healthcare worldwide.

AI presents a unique opportunity for health policy experts, physicians, and healthcare institutions to base their decisions on data, thereby improving patient treatment, disease management, and overall healthcare outcomes [5]. Many experts have leveraged internet tools for AI services and related applications [6]. This is evident from the data presented in Figure 13.1(a), showcasing the Google Trends analysis for "AI in healthcare" from 2019 to 2024. Additionally, Figure 13.1(b) provides global market statistics forecasted until 2029, sourced from Google Trends and MarketsandMarkets, respectively. The Google Trends data illustrates the level of interest in "AI in healthcare"

DOI: 10.1201/9781003481959-13

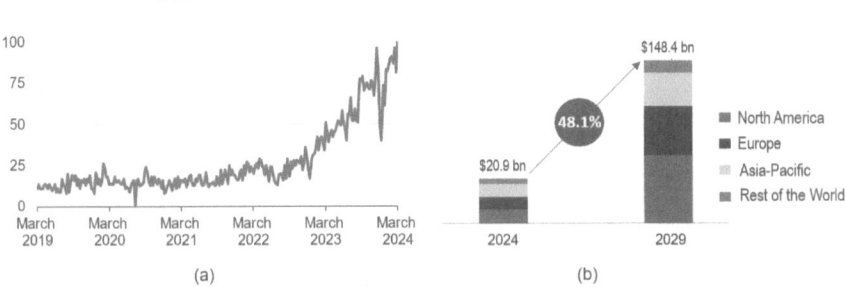

FIGURE 13.1   (a) Timeline showing occurrences of AI in healthcare from 2019 to 2024 based on Google Trends, and (b) projected market value of AI in healthcare, expected to reach USD 148.4 billion by 2029.

on a scale from 0 to 100, with 100 indicating the highest level of search and related activity for the topic. On the other hand, MarketsandMarkets predicts the market value to reach USD 148.4 billion by 2029. Google Trends is a free web service by Google Inc. that offers statistical insights into internet activities globally [7].

In recent years, there has been a rapid surge in advancements within AI, marking a significant potential for revolutionizing the healthcare sector [8]. This transformation has been primarily driven by the increasing availability and analysis of extensive datasets used for training AI systems. These AI applications have a profound impact on various aspects of healthcare [9], ranging from optimizing treatments to delivering personalized patient care, conducting diagnostics, monitoring health conditions, making prognostications, developing new drugs, and advancing medical research [10].

The field of AI in healthcare is multifaceted [11], with different technologies playing essential roles. As depicted in Figure 13.2, at the core of AI lies machine learning (ML), a fundamental aspect that utilizes data to create algorithms capable of determining variables, such as predicting disease onset [12]. Furthermore, deep learning (DL), an evolutionary subfield of ML, has gained prominence due to its utilization of neural networks with multiple layers, requiring substantial data inputs to achieve higher accuracy levels [13].

DL's progress has led to the discovery of correlations that were previously challenging to uncover using traditional ML approaches [14]. Another critical facet of AI is natural language processing (NLP) [15], which focuses on interpreting and translating human language into machine-readable information. In healthcare, NLP systems play a vital role in transcribing patient interactions, analyzing clinical notes, and generating comprehensive reports, including those related to radiological investigations [16].

Generative AI has further revolutionized healthcare by enhancing medical imaging, drug discovery, and personalized medicine. It improves image

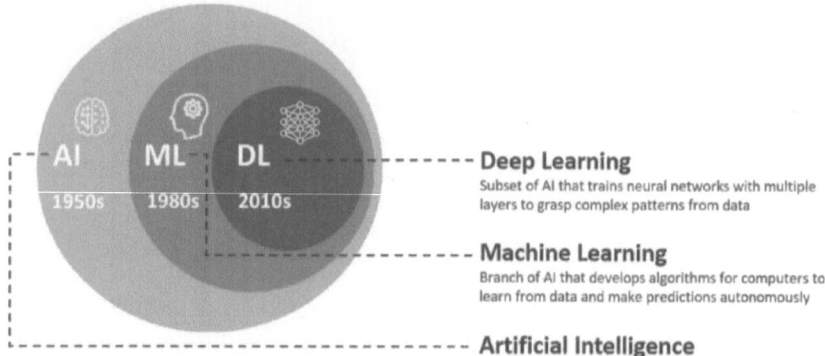

FIGURE 13.2   Three interconnecting layers illustrating the progression of AI, with ML and DL as subsets. The outermost layer represents AI from the 1950s, the middle layer represents ML as a branch of AI from the 1980s, and the innermost layer represents DL as a subset of ML from the 2010s.

quality for precise diagnoses and treatment planning [17], accelerates drug discovery by optimizing drug candidates [18], and analyzes vast patient datasets for personalized treatment strategies [19]. Generative AI's impact extends to medical training [20], healthcare analytics [21], virtual assistants [22], and genomic analysis [23], leading to more efficient healthcare delivery and better patient outcomes.

However, alongside these opportunities lie significant challenges that demand careful consideration and strategic mitigation. Data privacy and security concerns [24], biases in AI algorithms [25], lack of transparency in decision-making processes [26], regulatory ambiguities [27], and the need for better understanding among healthcare professionals and patients pose formidable hurdles in harnessing AI's full potential in healthcare [28].

This chapter delves into the future of AI in healthcare, exploring the myriad opportunities it presents and the challenges that must be overcome for its successful integration and utilization. By navigating through these opportunities and challenges, we aim to shed light on how AI can be leveraged ethically and effectively to shape a more efficient, patient-centric, and sustainable healthcare ecosystem.

13.2   Overview of AI in healthcare

The inception of AI traces back to 1950 when Alan Turing introduced the concept of using computers to mimic human intelligence and critical thinking abilities [29]. This groundbreaking idea paved the way for further exploration and development in the field. In 1956, John McCarthy provided a fundamental definition of AI as "the science and engineering of creating intelligent machines," encapsulating the essence of AI's purpose and functionality [30]. Originating as a basic set of rules, AI has advanced over many decades to encompass more sophisticated algorithms that mimic the functions of the human brain.

AI in healthcare involves the utilization of various technologies and algorithms to replicate human intelligence in machines [31]. These technologies enable computers and machines to perform tasks that typically necessitate human intelligence, such as analyzing medical data, making predictions, assisting in decision-making processes, and automating functions to enhance efficiency and accuracy.

Over the past few years, AI has seen extensive use in healthcare [32], spanning a multitude of domains such as medical imaging analysis, drug discovery, personalized medicine, predictive analytics, virtual health assistants, and healthcare management. These diverse applications aim to elevate patient care, refine medical decision-making processes, streamline healthcare operations, and foster innovation across the healthcare industry.

ML and AI are two of the most pervasive technologies globally. While they continually evolve and uncover novel applications, their presence in healthcare predates many other fields. Indeed, the debut of AI in healthcare dates back to the 1970s [33]. Since then, AI-powered applications have undergone significant advancement, reshaping the healthcare landscape by driving down costs, improving patient outcomes, and boosting overall productivity [34]. According to a survey conducted by AI in healthcare [35], more than 40% of industry experts already integrate AI and ML into their routine practices. The market for ML and AI in healthcare currently commands a value in the billions of dollars, with projections pointing toward remarkable growth in the coming years [36]. Healthcare professionals are increasingly relying on these technologies to sift through vast amounts of patient data, facilitating the development of more precise and personalized diagnoses and treatment strategies.

Figure 13.3 illustrates the evolution of AI in healthcare from 1950 to the present. The journey of AI in healthcare commenced in the 1950s with the introduction of ML and the coining of the term "Artificial Intelligence" in 1956 [37]. Recognition of AI's potential in healthcare followed, with milestones such as the development of the first chatbot, ELIZA, in 1964 [38]. ELIZA aimed to simulate human conversation and was a precursor to AI applications in healthcare. In 1972, MYCIN, an expert system for diagnosing patients based on symptoms and medical test results, demonstrated AI's capability in healthcare [39]. This was followed by the establishment of the SUMEX-AIM network in 1973 and the first AIM Workshop in 1975 [40], signaling a growing interest in AI applications for biomedical sciences. The introduction of clinical decision support systems like DXplain in 1986 further

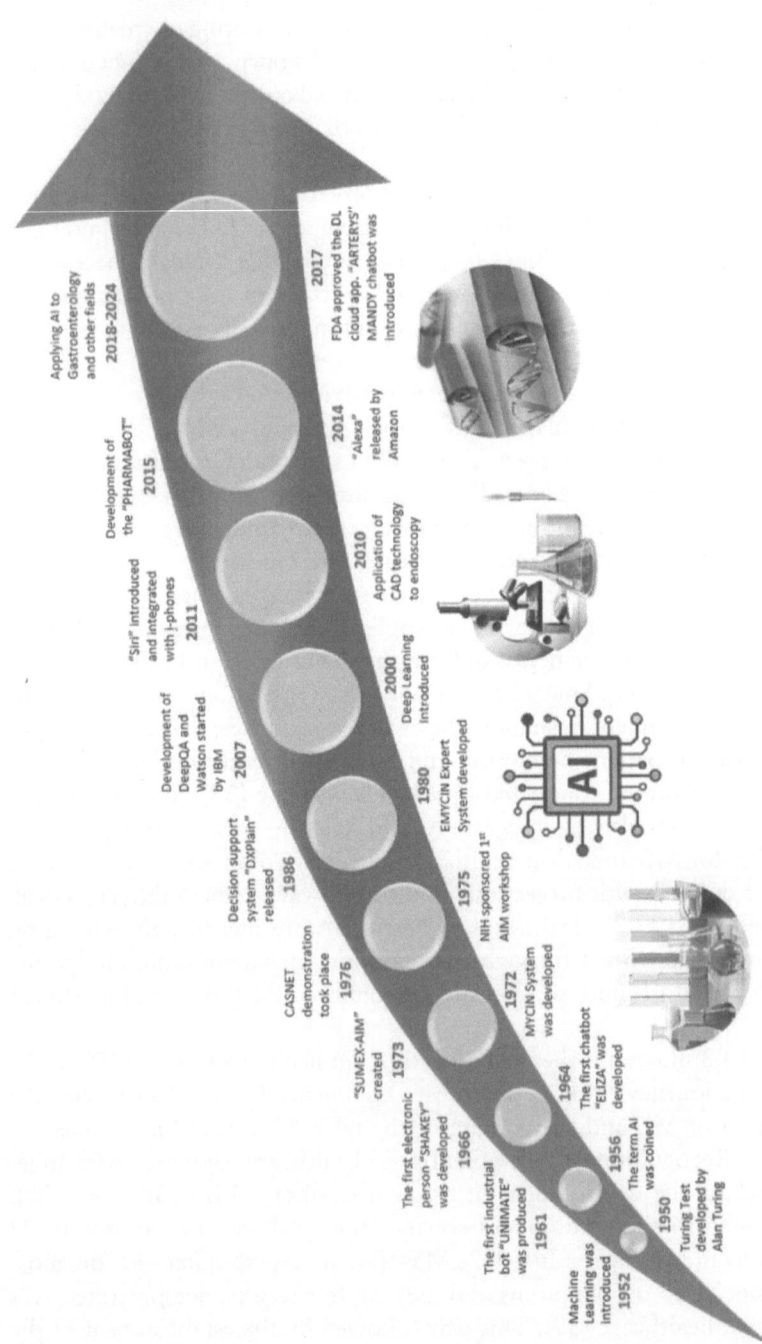

FIGURE 13.3 A chronological progression illustrating the evolution of AI in healthcare, highlighting key milestones and innovations from 1950 to 2024.

showcased AI's role in aiding clinicians with diagnostic processes and treatment decisions [41]. IBM's development of DeepQA and Watson systems in the 2000s marked a significant advancement in evidence-based reasoning and natural language interaction [42].

The subsequent decade witnessed a proliferation of AI-based assistants, such as Alexa and Siri, making AI technology more accessible to the public [43]. In healthcare, the introduction of PHARMABOT in 2015 and MANDY chatbot in 2017 exemplified AI's application in providing personalized medical recommendations and assistance [44]. Cloud technologies and DL have since been leveraged to expand AI's reach in various healthcare domains [45], with a focus on enhancing medical decision-making and patient care.

The ongoing efforts in applying AI to diverse healthcare fields underscore its potential to transform the delivery of healthcare services and improve patient outcomes. Between 2017 and the present, AI has significantly transformed healthcare, enhancing medical imaging, precision medicine, remote monitoring, telehealth, NLP, and drug discovery [46]. These advancements have improved diagnosis accuracy, personalized treatment, remote patient care, clinical decision-making, and drug development processes.

13.3 Introduction to the role and opportunities of AI in healthcare

AI is reshaping healthcare, offering groundbreaking solutions to persistent challenges and heralding a new era of medical advancement. As technology progresses, AI has emerged as a potent ally in the endeavor to enhance patient outcomes, refine clinical decision-making, and optimize healthcare delivery [47]. Spanning from enhancing diagnostic precision to revolutionizing patient care and simplifying administrative procedures, AI encompasses a wide array of applications poised to redefine the healthcare paradigm [48].

In this context, AI's role in healthcare is expansive and impactful. By leveraging sophisticated algorithms and data analysis techniques, AI empowers healthcare professionals to glean invaluable insights from extensive and intricate datasets [49]. This enables them to make more informed decisions and provide tailored care customized to the unique needs of each patient. Additionally, AI holds the promise of democratizing healthcare access by transcending geographical barriers and extending medical services to underserved communities [50].

As AI technologies evolve and mature, their influence on healthcare is set to intensify, fostering innovation, efficiency, and enhanced patient outcomes [51]. From early disease detection to precision medicine and patient engagement, AI presents a plethora of opportunities to revolutionize the healthcare landscape, paving the way for a future where healthcare is more accessible, efficient, and patient-centric than ever before [52].

13.3.1 Role of AI in healthcare

Figure 13.4 highlights the pivotal roles AI plays within the healthcare industry, including early detection of ailments, assistance in treatment, enhancement of decision-making processes, expansion of access to medical services, provision of superior patient experiences, facilitation of associated care, monitoring health through wearables, and support in end-of-life care [53].

13.3.1.1 Early detection of ailments

AI facilitates the early detection of diseases and medical conditions through advanced data analysis techniques applied to medical imaging, laboratory tests, and patient health records [54]. By identifying subtle signs of disease progression or abnormalities that may go unnoticed by human observers, AI algorithms enable healthcare providers to intervene at an earlier stage when treatment is most effective [55]. For example, AI-driven screening tools can analyze mammograms or MRI scans to detect early signs of breast cancer, allowing for prompt referral to oncologists for further evaluation and treatment.

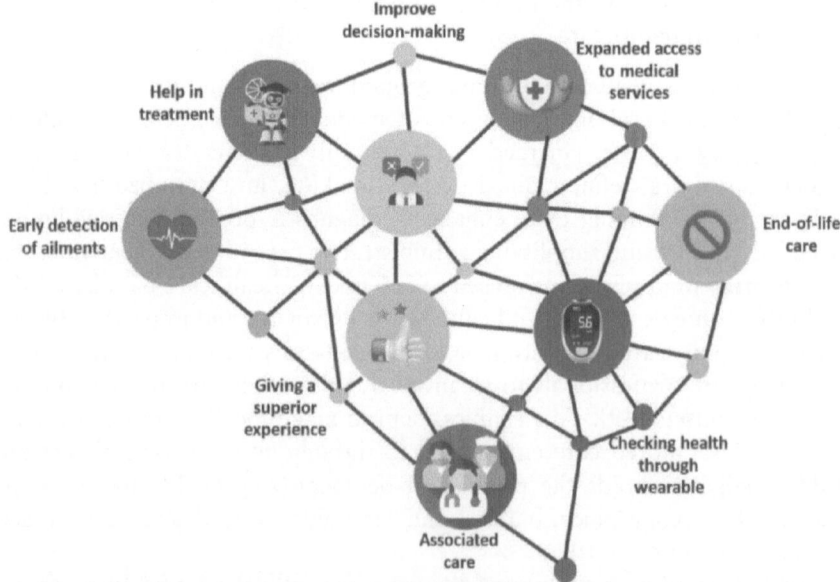

FIGURE 13.4 Graphical illustration of the roles of AI in modern healthcare, depicting interconnected aspects such as improving decision-making, expanding access to medical services, aiding in treatment, early detection of ailments, enhancing patient experience, associated care, monitoring health through wearables, and end-of-life care.

13.3.1.2   Help in treatment

AI aids healthcare providers in treatment planning and execution by analyzing vast amounts of patient data, including medical records, genetic information, and treatment outcomes [56]. By employing ML algorithms, AI can identify patterns and correlations within these datasets, enabling physicians to develop personalized treatment plans tailored to each patient's unique characteristics and needs [57]. For example, AI can analyze genetic markers to predict a patient's response to specific medications, allowing clinicians to prescribe the most effective and least harmful treatment regimen.

13.3.1.3   Improve decision-making

AI enhances clinical decision-making by providing healthcare professionals with actionable insights derived from data analysis [58]. By processing large datasets and identifying relevant patterns, AI algorithms can assist clinicians in diagnosing diseases, predicting patient outcomes, and selecting optimal treatment strategies [59]. For instance, AI-powered decision support systems can analyze electronic health records (EHRs) to alert physicians to potential drug interactions, adverse events, or deviations from clinical guidelines, enabling timely interventions and improved patient safety.

13.3.1.4   Expanding access to medical services

AI-powered telemedicine platforms and remote monitoring technologies improve access to healthcare services for individuals living in underserved or remote areas by enabling virtual consultations, remote monitoring, and telehealth interventions [60]. By leveraging AI algorithms to triage patients, analyze symptoms, and provide diagnostic recommendations, telemedicine platforms empower healthcare providers to deliver high-quality care remotely, reducing the need for in-person visits and minimizing barriers to access [61]. Additionally, AI-driven decision support systems can assist primary care providers and community health workers in diagnosing and managing common medical conditions, enhancing healthcare delivery in resource-constrained settings, and improving health outcomes for vulnerable populations [62].

13.3.1.5   Giving a superior experience

AI-powered virtual assistants and chatbots enhance the patient's experience by providing personalized, responsive, and convenient interactions [63]. These AI-driven interfaces can assist patients with scheduling appointments, accessing healthcare information, and answering medical questions in real-time. By automating routine administrative tasks and streamlining communication between patients and providers, AI improves patient satisfaction, reduces wait times, and enhances overall access to healthcare services [64].

13.3.1.6 Associated care

AI facilitates comprehensive and coordinated care for patients with chronic conditions or complex medical needs by integrating data from multiple sources and enabling seamless communication between healthcare providers [65]. AI-driven care coordination platforms can aggregate patient data from EHRs, wearables, and remote monitoring devices, enabling care teams to develop individualized care plans and monitor patients' progress in real-time [66]. By promoting collaboration and information sharing among providers, AI enhances care coordination, reduces medical errors, and improves patient outcomes.

13.3.1.7 Checking health through wearables

AI-enabled wearable devices continuously monitor patients' physiological parameters, such as heart rate, blood pressure, and activity levels, to detect early signs of health issues and provide personalized feedback and recommendations [67]. By analyzing data collected from wearables, AI algorithms can identify trends, patterns, and anomalies indicative of changes in health status, enabling timely interventions and proactive management of chronic conditions [68]. For example, AI-powered wearable devices can detect irregular heart rhythms suggestive of atrial fibrillation and alert users to seek medical attention, potentially preventing serious cardiac events.

13.3.1.8 End-of-life care

AI supports compassionate and personalized end-of-life care by assisting healthcare providers in addressing patients' physical, emotional, and spiritual needs during the final stages of life [69]. AI-driven decision support tools can help clinicians assess patients' symptoms, pain levels, and treatment preferences, allowing for tailored palliative care plans that prioritize comfort and dignity. Additionally, AI-powered communication platforms can facilitate sensitive discussions about end-of-life care goals and support patients and their families in making informed decisions about treatment options, advance directives, and hospice services [70].

13.3.2 Opportunities of AI in healthcare

Figure 13.5 showcases various significant opportunities presented by AI in the healthcare industry. These encompass early disease detection, diagnostic

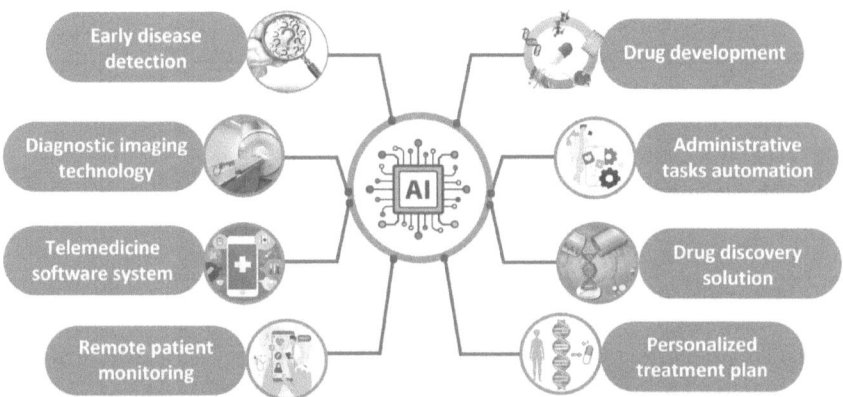

FIGURE 13.5 Diagram illustrating the opportunities of AI in modern healthcare, including early disease detection, diagnostic imaging technology, telemedicine software systems, remote patient monitoring, drug development, administrative tasks automation, drug discovery solutions, and personalized treatment plans.

imaging technology, telemedicine software systems, remote patient monitoring, drug development, automation of administrative tasks, drug discovery solutions, and personalized treatment plans [71].

13.3.2.1 Early disease detection

An ML model, trained on extensive mammogram data, can detect subtle patterns linked to breast cancer, prompting radiologists to conduct early evaluations for intervention [72]. For instance, AI algorithms analyze various data sources like EHRs, computed tomography (CT) scans, magnetic resonance imaging (MRI), ultrasound, mammography, X-ray radiography, and genetic information to identify early signs of conditions such as cancer, cardiovascular diseases, or neurological disorders.

This early detection significantly enhances patient outcomes by enabling timely treatment. By analyzing diverse datasets, including medical images, genetic information, and patient records, AI algorithms pinpoint subtle patterns or biomarkers indicating disease onset or progression. By facilitating early diagnosis, AI-driven detection systems can decrease healthcare costs, mitigate treatment complications, and save lives through timely intervention and preventive measures [73].

13.3.2.2 Diagnostic imaging technology

AI-enhanced imaging systems, such as those utilized in radiology or pathology, excel at highlighting abnormalities or areas of interest within medical images, thereby enhancing diagnostic accuracy and efficiency [74]. DL algorithms, for example, scrutinize MRI scans of the brain to identify indicators of Alzheimer's disease [75], such as alterations in brain structure or the presence of abnormal protein deposits. This aids in early diagnosis and intervention, crucial for effective management.

Diagnostic imaging assumes a pivotal role in diagnosing and managing diverse medical conditions. AI-enhanced imaging technologies are designed to refine diagnostic accuracy, minimize interpretation errors, and streamline workflow efficiency for radiologists and clinicians [76]. These algorithms meticulously analyze medical images, identifying abnormalities, classifying lesions, segmenting organs, and contributing to image reconstruction and enhancement. By learning from annotated image datasets, these algorithms become adept at recognizing patterns associated with specific diseases or conditions.

AI-powered diagnostic imaging systems expedite diagnosis, streamline treatment planning, and enhance patient outcomes by furnishing more precise and timely interpretations of medical images. Consequently, they reduce the need for unnecessary procedures and optimize resource allocation.

13.3.2.3 Telemedicine software systems

Telemedicine platforms, equipped with AI-powered chatbots or virtual assistants, streamline initial symptom assessments, offer medical advice, and triage patients based on their condition's severity [77]. For instance, a patient experiencing flu-like symptoms can utilize a telemedicine app to converse with a virtual assistant driven by NLP algorithms. The assistant can inquire about symptoms and medical history, provide self-care guidance, and advise whether further medical attention is necessary.

Telemedicine revolutionizes healthcare delivery by enabling remote access to services, enhancing patient convenience, and mitigating healthcare disparities, especially in underserved or rural regions [78]. AI-driven telemedicine platforms utilize technologies like video conferencing, chatbots, and remote monitoring devices to facilitate virtual consultations, symptom assessment, triage, and follow-up care. Through NLP algorithms, chatbots engage with patients, collect medical history, and dispense basic medical advice. By harnessing AI, telemedicine platforms bolster patient engagement, improve healthcare accessibility, optimize care delivery, and cut healthcare costs by minimizing unnecessary hospital visits and streamlining care coordination [79].

13.3.2.4 Remote patient monitoring

Wearable devices, including smartwatches or biosensors, outfitted with AI algorithms, provide continuous monitoring of physiological parameters such as heart rate, blood pressure, and glucose levels in individuals with chronic conditions [80]. For instance, a diabetes patient utilizes a continuous glucose monitoring (CGM) device to track real-time blood sugar levels. AI algorithms analyze the data, identifying trends, patterns, and deviations from target ranges, thereby alerting both the patient and their healthcare provider to potential issues or the necessity for medication adjustments.

Remote patient monitoring enables healthcare providers to monitor patients' health status and vital signs beyond traditional clinical settings, facilitating proactive management of chronic conditions, early detection of health deterioration, and timely intervention [81]. Wearable devices, equipped with sensors and AI algorithms, continually gather and analyze physiological data, including heart rate, blood pressure, glucose levels, and activity patterns. ML models process this information to detect deviations from baseline values, recognize trends, and issue alerts for healthcare providers [82].

AI-enabled remote patient monitoring systems empower patients to actively participate in managing their health, enhance adherence to treatment plans, diminish hospital readmissions, and improve patient-provider communication, ultimately leading to superior health outcomes and quality of life.

13.3.2.5 Drug development initiatives

AI-driven drug discovery platforms employ ML models to screen extensive databases of chemical compounds, forecast their biological activity, and pinpoint potential drug candidates with therapeutic promise [83]. For instance, a pharmaceutical firm utilizes AI algorithms to scrutinize genomic data from cancer patients, identifying specific genetic mutations fueling tumor growth. Guided by this analysis, the company formulates targeted therapies that selectively inhibit the activity of mutated proteins, resulting in more personalized and effective cancer treatments.

AI-powered drug discovery expedites the identification and development of novel therapeutics by harnessing computational methods to analyze biological data, predict drug-target interactions, and refine drug candidates [84]. AI algorithms analyze vast biological datasets encompassing genomic, proteomic, and chemical information to elucidate disease mechanisms, forecast drug efficacy and safety profiles, and craft molecules with desired pharmacological properties. Techniques like virtual screening, molecular docking, and quantitative structure-activity relationship (QSAR) modeling accelerate the drug discovery process [85].

AI-enabled drug discovery harbors the potential to truncate drug development timelines, slash costs, bolster the success rate of clinical trials, and uncover new treatments for challenging diseases, ultimately enhancing patient care and public health.

13.3.2.6 Automation of administrative tasks

AI-powered chatbots or virtual assistants streamline routine administrative tasks such as appointment scheduling, prescription refills, and insurance verification, enhancing operational efficiency and cutting administrative overhead [86]. When a patient contacts a healthcare provider's office to book an appointment, they no longer need to wait on hold to speak with a receptionist. Instead, they engage with an AI-powered chatbot equipped with natural language understanding (NLU), which swiftly schedules the appointment, verifies insurance coverage, and dispatches a confirmation email with appointment details.

Tasks like appointment scheduling, billing, and documentation can be both time-consuming and resource-intensive for healthcare providers. AI-powered automation systems aim to simplify administrative processes, boost efficiency, and elevate the overall patient experience [87]. These systems automate repetitive tasks by processing natural language inputs, extracting pertinent information from unstructured data, and executing decision-making tasks based on predefined rules or ML models. Virtual assistants, chatbots, and robotic process automation (RPA) platforms are widely utilized for administrative automation in healthcare settings [88].

By alleviating administrative burdens on healthcare staff, AI-driven automation systems liberate time for clinicians to dedicate to patient care. They enhance workflow efficiency, reduce errors, and elevate patient satisfaction, ultimately leading to a more streamlined and cost-effective healthcare delivery [89].

13.3.2.7 Innovative drug discovery solutions

AI algorithms analyze intricate biological data, encompassing protein structures, biochemical pathways, and gene expression profiles, to pinpoint novel drug targets and craft molecules with desired pharmacological attributes [90]. For instance, a biotech startup harnesses AI-powered drug discovery platforms to identify small molecules that bind to a specific protein implicated in Alzheimer's disease. Through computational screening of millions of chemical compounds and prediction of their binding affinity and selectivity, the startup identifies lead compounds for subsequent optimization and preclinical testing.

Conventional drug discovery methods are frequently time-consuming, costly, and plagued by high failure rates. AI-powered drug discovery offers a data-driven and hypothesis-free approach to uncover promising drug candidates, repurpose existing drugs, and refine therapeutic interventions [91]. AI algorithms scrutinize diverse biological data sources, including genomic, transcriptomic, and proteomic data, to unveil disease mechanisms, pinpoint druggable targets, and tailor molecules with desired pharmacological properties. DL models, generative adversarial networks (GANs), and reinforcement learning algorithms facilitate virtual screening, de novo molecule generation, and optimization of lead compounds [92].

AI-driven drug discovery holds the potential to transform the pharmaceutical industry by expediting the discovery of novel therapeutics, curbing development costs, and addressing unmet medical needs. By leveraging AI, researchers can explore broader chemical spaces, prioritize promising drug candidates, and efficiently introduce innovative treatments to the market.

13.3.2.8   Tailored personalized treatment plans

AI-driven predictive analytics models scrutinize patient data, spanning demographics, medical history, and genetic profiles, to forecast individual treatment responses and outcomes, informing personalized treatment decisions [93]. For instance, a hypertensive patient receives tailored treatment recommendations grounded in their genetic predisposition, lifestyle factors, and responses to previous medications. Through analysis of the patient's data, AI algorithms predict their risk of cardiovascular events and suggest specific medications, lifestyle adjustments, and monitoring protocols tailored to their unique needs and preferences.

Personalized medicine aims to individualize healthcare interventions based on patient characteristics, preferences, and genetic makeup, thereby maximizing treatment efficacy while minimizing adverse effects [94]. AI-driven predictive analytics models analyze a breadth of patient data, encompassing clinical variables, genomic profiles, imaging studies, and EHRs, to anticipate disease risk, treatment responses, and patient outcomes. ML algorithms harmonize and interpret multidimensional data to craft personalized treatment recommendations and refine therapeutic strategies.

By customizing treatment plans to individual patient profiles, AI-enabled personalized medicine approaches can bolster treatment outcomes, diminish adverse drug reactions, foster patient adherence, and optimize resource allocation in healthcare delivery [95]. Precision medicine holds the potential to revolutionize healthcare from a reactive to a proactive and preventive model, ultimately enhancing patient outcomes and population health.

13.4   Challenges of AI in healthcare

The integration of AI into healthcare presents multifarious challenges that demand meticulous resolution to fully realize its potential while simultaneously upholding patient safety, privacy, and ethical standards [96].

As AI permeates various facets of healthcare delivery, it encounters a spectrum of intricate challenges across technical, ethical, regulatory, and practical domains. These challenges, as depicted in Figure 13.6, include

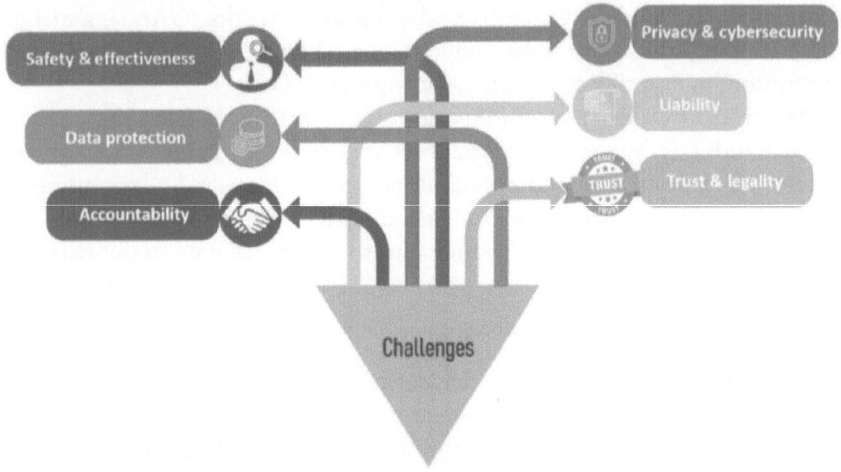

FIGURE 13.6 Diagram illustrating the challenges of AI in modern healthcare, including safety and effectiveness, data protection, accountability, privacy and cybersecurity, liability, and trust and legality.

ensuring the reliability and efficacy of AI algorithms, safeguarding patient confidentiality, addressing issues pertinent to accountability and trust, and navigating the intricate legal landscape. Addressing the multifaceted challenges inherent in integrating AI into healthcare demands a comprehensive approach that encompasses technical, ethical, regulatory, and practical considerations [97].

By prioritizing reliability, transparency, accountability, and legal compliance in AI-driven healthcare initiatives, stakeholders can effectively leverage the transformative potential of AI while concurrently preserving ethical standards and safeguarding patient safety and privacy. These challenges encompass safety and effectiveness, data protection, accountability, privacy and cybersecurity, liability, as well as trust and legality.

13.4.1 Safety and effectiveness

It is imperative to guarantee the safety and efficacy of AI algorithms in healthcare settings to avoid patient harm or adverse outcomes. Challenges encompass tackling algorithmic biases, reducing errors in clinical decision-making, and validating the accuracy of AI predictions [98]. For instance, if an AI algorithm employed for skin cancer diagnosis demonstrates bias toward specific skin types, it may lead to misdiagnoses and treatment delays for affected patients. Similarly, if an AI-powered decision support system suggests an inaccurate medication dosage, it could lead to adverse drug reactions or ineffective treatment.

13.4.2 Data protection

Safeguarding patient data and ensuring adherence to data protection regulations are pivotal challenges in AI-enabled healthcare environments. Issues such as data breaches, unauthorized access, and data misuse pose substantial risks to patient confidentiality and trust [99]. For instance, in the event of a data breach, wherein a healthcare organization's AI-powered EHR system is compromised, patient records may be exposed to unauthorized access. This could result in severe consequences for the organization, including financial penalties, reputational damage, and loss of patient trust.

13.4.3 Accountability

Establishing transparent lines of accountability for errors or adverse events in AI-based healthcare applications is essential to address legal, ethical, and regulatory concerns. Challenges include attributing responsibility and liability when errors occur and ensuring transparency in decision-making processes [100]. For instance, in the case of a life-threatening condition being missed by an AI-powered medical device due to a software glitch, determining whether the responsibility lies with the device manufacturer, healthcare provider, or regulatory agency can be intricate and contentious.

13.4.4 Privacy and cybersecurity

Protecting patient privacy and fortifying healthcare systems against cyber threats are pivotal challenges in AI-driven healthcare. Threats such as data breaches, ransomware attacks, and insider threats pose significant risks to patient data security and confidentiality [101]. For example, in a scenario where a cybercriminal gains unauthorized access to a hospital's AI-powered diagnostic imaging system and encrypts patient data, demanding a ransom for its release, patient care is disrupted, and sensitive medical information is exposed to unauthorized parties, leading to potential harm and breaches of confidentiality.

13.4.5 Liability

Assigning liability for errors or adverse outcomes arising from AI-based healthcare applications is a complex challenge that implicates multiple stakeholders. Challenges encompass uncertainties regarding liability frameworks, legal precedents, and insurance coverage for AI-related incidents [102]. For example, in the event of a malfunctioning AI-powered surgical robot causing patient injury during a procedure, determining the responsible party—whether it be the surgeon, hospital, robot manufacturer, or software developer—demands a meticulous examination of contractual agreements, regulatory standards, and industry norms.

13.4.6 Trust and legality

Cultivating trust and ensuring legal compliance in AI-driven healthcare solutions necessitates transparent communication, ethical conduct, and adherence to legal and regulatory mandates. Challenges encompass apprehensions regarding the reliability, fairness, and legality of AI algorithms, particularly in sensitive healthcare domains. For example, patients may harbor reservations about placing trust in AI-driven diagnostic tools if they perceive the algorithms as opaque or biased [103]. Moreover, healthcare providers may encounter legal and regulatory hurdles if AI applications fail to conform to privacy laws or medical regulations, potentially undermining patient confidence and compromising care quality.

13.5 AI in healthcare: Current trends and future outlook

AI is revolutionizing the healthcare industry by enhancing diagnostic accuracy, personalizing treatment plans, and improving patient outcomes. This section explores the current trends in AI healthcare adoption, showcasing how AI technologies are being integrated into medical practices today. Additionally, it delves into the future outlook for AI in healthcare, providing insights into the potential advancements and innovations that could further transform the field.

13.5.1 Current trends in AI healthcare adoption

The adoption of various AI techniques is progressively permeating diverse domains within healthcare applications. This proliferation is rooted in the commendable accomplishments observed in previously deployed applications. Figure 13.7 delineates the trajectories of utilization patterns for various AI methodologies over a 23-year period, from 2000 to the present year, ending in July 2024. The primary aim of constructing this trend analysis is to discern the evolving deployment patterns of AI techniques over time, focusing exclusively on publications employing methodologies within the healthcare application domain. These statistical insights are derived from a specialized repository, namely, the PubMed database [104], ensuring the reliability and relevance of the data. The observable pattern in Figure 13.7 reveals a consistent upward trend in AI adoption within the healthcare sector over the years, culminating in the present day.

The PubMed database alone records over 4000 publications in 2023 related to AI within the healthcare industry, underscoring the growing interest and significance of AI applications in healthcare research and practice.

Furthermore, Figure 13.8 depicts the trends in the utilization of AI, DL, and ML methodologies over the past seven years, from 2017 to the present year, ending in July 2024. The aim of constructing this trend analysis is to discern the deployment patterns of AI, DL, and ML techniques through

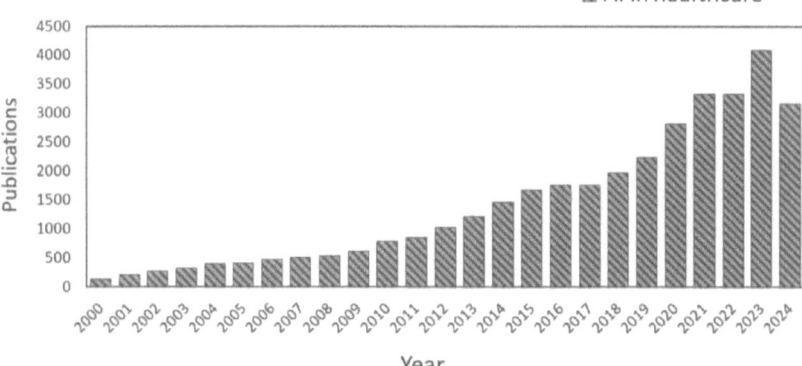

FIGURE 13.7 Statistical analysis of research publications on AI applications in healthcare, sourced from the PubMed database, based on title searches including "AI in Healthcare." The graph displays the number of research publications from 2000 to mid-2024.

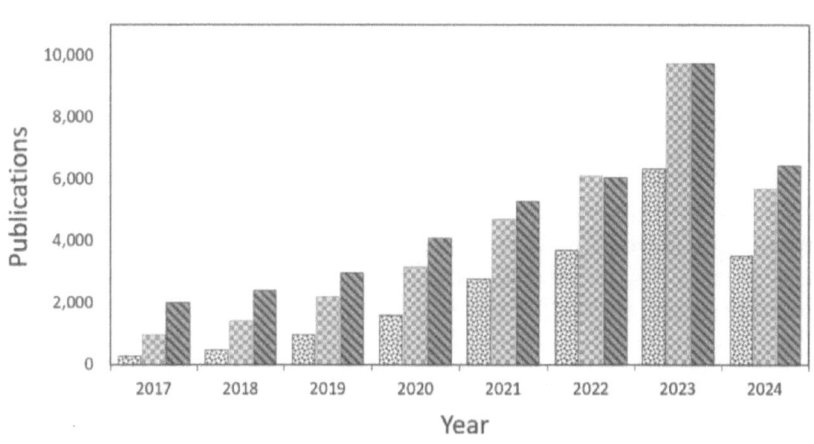

FIGURE 13.8 Comparison of research publications on the use of DL, ML, and AI in healthcare, spanning from 2017 to July 2024. The data, sourced from PubMed and IEEE databases, was compiled through title searches for "AI in Healthcare," "DL in Healthcare," and "ML in Healthcare."

comparative analysis over time, with the selection of publications based solely on the utilization of these three methodologies within the healthcare application domain. These statistical insights are derived from two distinct repositories, namely, the PubMed database and the Institute of Electrical and Electronics Engineers (IEEE) archive.

The observable pattern in Figure 13.8 indicates a clear upward trend in the adoption of DL, ML, and AI within the healthcare sector, suggesting a growing reliance on these technologies to address various healthcare challenges. The substantial increase in the number of publications related to DL, ML, and AI in healthcare reflects a heightened interest and investment in leveraging these technologies to enhance patient care, streamline processes, and advance medical research.

Specifically, the remarkable surge in publications for DL, ML, and AI in 2023 underscores the rapid pace at which these technologies are being embraced and integrated into healthcare systems. With over 9000 publications focusing on AI alone, alongside significant numbers for DL and ML, it is evident that researchers and practitioners are actively exploring the potential applications and benefits of these advanced technologies in healthcare settings.

This report, sourced from PubMed and IEEE, serves as a testament to the substantial interest and activity surrounding DL, ML, and AI research within the healthcare domain. It highlights the ongoing efforts to harness the capabilities of these technologies to revolutionize healthcare delivery, improve patient outcomes, and drive innovation in medical practice.

13.5.2 The future outlook for AI in healthcare

The current advancements in AI are poised to unlock a multitude of new research avenues and enhance existing applications, particularly in healthcare and its applications. These advancements pave the way for transformative changes in healthcare delivery, clinical decision-making, and patient outcomes [105]. The future outlook for AI in healthcare is exceptionally promising, with numerous predictions and projections indicating how AI will continue to revolutionize the industry. These trends are expected to accelerate in the coming years, reshaping healthcare delivery and driving innovation in patient care.

13.5.2.1 Application of generative AI in healthcare

Generative AI models, which aid in generating text and images, are viewed as a promising asset within the healthcare realm. This technology has the potential to revolutionize healthcare by enhancing diagnostic capabilities, cutting down on the time and expenses associated with healthcare delivery, and ultimately enhancing patient outcomes [106].

13.5.2.1.1 Synthetic data generation and data augmentation

Leveraged by generative AI models like GANs, synthetic data generation and augmentation offers a promising solution for harmonizing the accessibility of valuable data with the imperative of safeguarding patient privacy [107]. These advanced models facilitate the creation of realistic and anonymized patient data, specifically tailored for research and training endeavors, thereby unlocking a wide spectrum of versatile applications. GANs demonstrate exceptional proficiency in synthesizing EHR data by acquiring a deep understanding of the underlying data distributions. This not only ensures outstanding performance but also addresses concerns regarding data privacy. Such an approach holds significant value, especially in scenarios where access to genuine patient data is constrained or restricted due to privacy considerations. Additionally, leveraging synthetic data contributes significantly to bolstering the accuracy and resilience of ML models, as it introduces a more varied and representative dataset during the training phase [108]. Furthermore, the capability to generate synthetic data encompassing diverse characteristics and parameters empowers researchers and clinicians to delve into and validate a myriad of hypotheses, thereby fostering new insights and discoveries.

13.5.2.1.2 Drug discovery

Generative AI models are instrumental in drug discovery as they generate novel small molecules, nucleic acid sequences, and proteins with precise structures or functions, thus advancing drug discovery [109]. These models analyze the chemical structures of successful drugs and simulate variations, facilitating the swift creation of potential drug candidates compared to conventional methods. This expedited process not only conserves time and resources but also unveils potential drugs that may have been overlooked using traditional approaches. Moreover, generative AI assists in forecasting the efficacy and safety of new drugs, a pivotal aspect of drug development. Through extensive dataset analysis, generative AI identifies potential issues that could emerge during clinical trials, resulting in reduced time and costs in drug development [110].

Furthermore, generative AI plays a role in identifying specific biological processes pertinent to diseases, aiding in the discovery of new drug targets. This can ultimately lead to the formulation of more efficacious treatments, fostering advancements in healthcare.

13.5.2.1.3 Medical diagnosis

Generative models trained on extensive medical datasets, including MRI and CT scan imagery, excel in identifying disease-related patterns. For example, GANs are adept at tasks like image reconstruction, synthesis, segmentation, registration, and classification. They can also generate synthetic medical images to train ML models for image-based diagnosis or enhance medical datasets [111]. Likewise, large language models (LLMs) contribute to enhancing the output of various computer-aided diagnosis (CAD) networks, such as those for diagnosis, lesion segmentation, and report generation, by converting and organizing information into natural language text [112]. This transformation makes the system more user-friendly and accessible for patients compared to traditional CAD systems.

EHRs and patient records offer rich data sources, and LLMs analyze them with sophistication. They can process and understand medical terminologies, extract complex medical data, and derive meaning from incomplete information. LLMs integrate data from multiple EHR sources, such as lab results, physician's notes, and medical imaging reports, to provide a holistic view of a patient's health. This is especially useful in complex cases with multiple conditions or related symptoms.

Despite lacking formal medical training, LLMs such as GPT-4 exhibit significant medical knowledge and perform well in decision-making tasks. They can propose potential diagnoses, recommend tests, and suggest treatment plans based on patient symptoms. Some studies indicate that these models achieve performance levels comparable to those of medical students on medical exams. However, it is important to acknowledge their limitations: while they support decision-making, they cannot fully replace the clinical judgment of outpatient physicians.

13.5.2.1.4 Large language models in healthcare administration and documentation

LLMs such as OpenAI's GPT-4 and Google's PALM-2 are transforming clinical documentation and healthcare administration by producing concise summaries of patient data, which are essential for quick and accurate interpretation. Integrated within EHR systems, these models efficiently handle extensive patient information, including medical history, medications, allergies, and lab results. They highlight critical details such as diagnoses, prescribed treatments, and health trends, thereby enhancing communication between healthcare providers and patients [113].

Integrating LLMs into documentation processes alleviates physicians' workloads in managing EHRs and helps mitigate burnout. These models automate routine tasks and generate draft documents for clinician review, thereby improving efficiency and time management. Furthermore, their incorporation into EHR systems enhances patient safety by reducing medical errors. LLMs offer decision support by identifying discrepancies, care gaps, potential adverse interactions, and contraindications, thereby ensuring more accurate and reliable patient care.

Furthermore, generative AI extends its capabilities to automate other healthcare tasks such as appointment scheduling, claims processing, and patient record management. AI-driven scheduling systems optimize appointment schedules based on doctor availability, patient preferences, and urgency, while automated insurance claims processing minimizes errors and enhances the patient experience with faster services. This comprehensive integration of generative AI streamlines healthcare operations, improves accuracy, and ultimately leads to better patient care outcomes [114].

13.5.2.1.5 Personalized medicine

Generative AI revolutionizes personalized medicine by analyzing genetic profiles, lifestyle data, and medical histories to predict treatment responses. Through extensive data training, AI identifies complex patterns and correlations, such as heightened medication responsiveness linked to specific genetic markers. This knowledge informs tailored treatment plans, optimizing efficacy by accounting for individual factors [115]. In mental health, Generative AI aids in creating interactive tools for cognitive behavioral therapy (CBT). CBT focuses on modifying maladaptive thought patterns and behaviors. AI generates personalized scenarios to provoke and guide patient responses, allowing for controlled practice of coping strategies and potentially improving mental health outcomes.

13.5.2.1.6 Medical education and training

Generative AI enhances medical education by creating diverse virtual patient cases, spanning various medical conditions and demographics. This technology fosters a safe learning environment where students can interact, diagnose, and propose treatments without risks to real patients. It offers opportunities to practice rare or complex cases, preparing students for unexpected clinical scenarios and improving problem-solving skills [116]. Moreover, AI tailors learning experiences to individual students' needs, adapting pace and content accordingly.

Furthermore, generative AI simulates conversations between healthcare professionals and patients, aiding in communication skill development and delivering difficult news sensitively. It also provides valuable data for educators by tracking student performance, identifying areas for improvement, and offering feedback to refine teaching strategies and curricula.

13.5.2.1.7 Patient education

Generative AI significantly enhances patient education by crafting personalized materials tailored to individual conditions, symptoms, and inquiries [117]. For example, in diabetes management, it generates content on blood sugar regulation, diet, exercise, and medication adherence, improving patient understanding and engagement. Furthermore, Generative AI fosters interactive learning by allowing patients to ask questions and receive informative responses, deepening their comprehension of medical conditions. This feature is especially helpful for patients uncomfortable discussing certain topics with healthcare providers. Moreover, Generative AI creates visual aids like diagrams or infographics to explain complex medical concepts, aiding patient comprehension. It also adjusts content to different reading levels, promoting health literacy among patients. Additionally, Generative AI supports ongoing education through follow-up content and reminders, emphasizing medication adherence and overall health maintenance [118]. Furthermore, it addresses mental health concerns by providing responses to patients' anxieties, fostering support throughout their healthcare journey. Lastly, Generative AI's multilingual capabilities ensure accessibility for non-English speakers, promoting inclusivity in healthcare education.

13.6 Conclusion

AI is profoundly transforming healthcare by enhancing diagnostics, treatment precision, and patient monitoring. Generative AI, in particular, promises to revolutionize the field through its ability to create personalized treatment plans and improve patient outcomes. Other AI subfields such as ML and DL are also making substantial contributions, offering advanced data analysis, predictive modeling, NLP, and robotic automation. DL, with its capability to handle vast datasets, has surpassed traditional ML and feature engineering methods in tackling complex data challenges.

The integration of AI in healthcare requires a careful balance between innovation and responsibility. Addressing key challenges including safety, data protection, accountability, privacy, cybersecurity, and legal issues is essential. This report has examined AI's impact on various aspects of healthcare, including disease detection, diagnostic imaging, telemedicine, remote monitoring, drug development, and administrative automation. Data from PubMed and IEEE shows a significant increase in AI adoption, highlighting its growing role in addressing healthcare challenges.

Looking forward, AI's future in healthcare is promising, especially with generative models that can personalize treatment and enhance outcomes. Continued research and collaboration are crucial for optimizing AI's potential while ensuring ethical and effective applications.

References

1 MarketsandMarkets. Global AI Healthcare Market Size Estimated to Reach $148.4 Billion by 2029. GlobeNewswire, 20 Mar. 2024, https://www.globenewswire.com/en/news-release/2024/03/20/2849384/0/en/Global-A-I-Healthcare-Market-Size-Estimated-To-Reach-148-4-Billion-By-2029.html.

2 MarketsandMarkets. Artificial Intelligence in Healthcare Market. Marketsand-Markets, Dec. 2024. https://www.marketsandmarkets.com/Market-Reports/artificial-intelligence-healthcare-market-54679303.html.

3 Alowais SA, Alghamdi SS, Alsuhebany N. et al. Revolutionizing Healthcare: The Role of Artificial Intelligence in Clinical Practice. *BMC Med Educ.* 2023; 23:689. Doi: 10.1186/s12909-023-04698-z.

4 Bohr A., Memarzadeh K. The Rise of Artificial Intelligence in Healthcare Applications. In: Bohr A. & Memarzadeh K. (eds.), *Artificial Intelligence in Healthcare*, 2020; 25–60. Doi: 10.1016/B978-0-12-818438-7.00002-2.

5 Davenport T, Kalakota R. The Potential for Artificial Intelligence in Healthcare. *Future Healthc J.* 2019 Jun; 6(2):94–98. Doi: 10.7861/futurehosp.6-2-94.

6 Miller DD, Brown EW. Artificial Intelligence in Medical Practice: The Question to the Answer? *Am J Med.* 2018; 131(2):129–133.

7 Springer S, Strzelecki A, Zieger M. Maximum Generable Interest: A Universal Standard for Google Trends Search Queries. *Healthc Anal (N Y).* 2023 Nov; 3:100158. Doi: 10.1016/j.health.2023.100158.

8 Combi C, Pozzani G, Pozzi G. Telemedicine for Developing Countries. *Appl Clin Inform.* 2016; 07(04):1025–1050.

9 Singhal S, and Carlton S. The Era of Exponential Improvement in Healthcare? McKinsey & Company Review. 2019. https://www.mckinsey.com/industries/healthcare/our-insights/the-era-of-exponential-improvement-in-healthcare

10 Monica M Bertagnolli, Advancing Health Through Artificial Intelligence/Machine Learning: The Critical Importance of Multidisciplinary Collaboration. *PNAS Nexus.* 2023; 2(12):pgad356. Doi: 10.1093/pnasnexus/pgad356.

11 Zhang L, Tan J, Han D, Zhu H. From Machine Learning to Deep Learning: Progress in Machine Intelligence for Rational Drug Discovery. *Drug Discov Today.* 2017; 22(11):1680–1685.

12 Paul D, Sanap G, Shenoy S, Kalyane D, Kalia K, Tekade RK. Artificial Intelligence in Drug Discovery and Development. *Drug Discov Today.* 2021 Jan; 26(1):80–93. Doi: 10.1016/j.drudis.2020.10.010.

13 Taye MM. Understanding of Machine Learning with Deep Learning: Architectures, Workflow, Applications and Future Directions. *Computers.* 2023; 12(5):91.

14 Ahmed SF, Alam MSB, Hassan M. et al. Deep Learning Modelling Techniques: Current Progress, Applications, Advantages, and Challenges. *Artif Intell Rev.* 2023; 56:13521–13617.

15 Khurana D, Koli A, Khatter K. et al. Natural Language Processing: State of the Art, Current Trends and Challenges. *Multimed Tools Appl.* 2023; 82:3713–3744.

16 Aramaki E, Wakamiya S, Yada S, Nakamura Y. Natural Language Processing: From Bedside to Everywhere. *Yearb Med Inform.* 2022 Aug; 31(1):243–253. Doi: 10.1055/s-0042-1742510.

17 Pinto-Coelho L. How Artificial Intelligence Is Shaping Medical Imaging Technology: A Survey of Innovations and Applications. *Bioengineering (Basel).* 2023 Dec 18; 10(12):1435. Doi: 10.3390/bioengineering10121435.

18 Gangwal A, Lavecchia A. Unleashing the Power Of Generative AI in Drug Discovery. *Drug Discov Today.* 2024; 29(6):103992. Doi: 10.1016/j.drudis. 2024.103992.

19 Wallace MP, Moodie EEM. Personalizing Medicine: A Review of Adaptive Treatment Strategies. *Pharmacoepidemiol Drug Saf.* 2014; 23(6):580–585. Doi: 10.1002/pds.3606.

20 Moritz S, Romeike B, Stosch C, Tolks D. Generative AI (gAI) in Medical Education: Chat-GPT and Co. *GMS J Med Educ.* 2023; 40(4):Doc54. Doi: 10.3205/zma001636.

21 Reddy S. Generative AI in Healthcare: An Implementation Science Informed Translational Path on Application, Integration and Governance. *Implement Sci.* 2024 Mar 15; 19(1):27. Doi: 10.1186/s13012-024-01357-9.

22 Samala AD, Rawas S. Generative AI as Virtual Healthcare Assistant for Enhancing Patient Care Quality. *Int J Online Biomed Eng.* 2024; 20(05):174–187. Doi: 10.3991/ijoe.v20i05.45937.

23 Quazi S. Artificial Intelligence and Machine Learning in Precision and Genomic Medicine. *Med Oncol.* 2022 Jun 15; 39(8):120. Doi: 10.1007/s12032-022-01711-1.

24 National Research Council (US) Committee on Maintaining Privacy and Security in Health Care Applications of the National Information Infrastructure. *For the Record Protecting Electronic Health Information*, National Academies Press (US), 1997.

25 Ferrara E. Fairness and Bias in Artificial Intelligence: A Brief Survey of Sources, Impacts, and Mitigation Strategies. *Sci.* 2024; 6(1):3. Doi: 10.3390/sci6010003.

26 Felzmann H, Fosch-Villaronga E, Lutz C et al. Towards Transparency by Design for Artificial Intelligence. *Sci Eng Ethics.* 2020; 26:3333–3361. Doi: 10.1007/s11948-020-00276-4.

27 Zaidan E, Ibrahim IA. AI Governance in a Complex and Rapidly Changing Regulatory Landscape: A Global Perspective. *Humanit Soc Sci Commun.* 2024; 11:1121. Doi: 10.1057/s41599-024-03560-x.

28 Jeyaraman M, Balaji S, Jeyaraman N, Yadav S. Unraveling the Ethical Enigma: Artificial Intelligence in Healthcare. *Cureus.* 2023 Aug 10; 15(8):e43262. Doi: 10.7759/cureus.43262.

29 Turing AM. Computing Machinery and Intelligence. *Mind.* 1950; *LIX*:433–460.

30 Lifschitz V ed., *Artificial Intelligence and Mathematical Theory of Computation, Papers in Honor of John McCarthy*, Academic Press, San Diego, 1991.

31 Zhang Z. Predictive analytics in the era of big data: opportunities and challenges. *Ann Transl Med.* 2020; 8(4):68. Doi: 10.21037/atm.2019.10.97.

32 Hirani R, Noruzi K, Khuram H, Hussaini AS, Aifuwa EI, Ely KE, Lewis JM, Gabr AE, Smiley A, Tiwari RK, et al. Artificial Intelligence and Healthcare: A Journey through History, Present Innovations, and Future Possibilities. *Life.* 2024; 14(5):557. Doi: 10.3390/life14050557.

33 Kaul V, Enslin S, Gross SA. History of Artificial Intelligence in Medicine. *Gastrointest Endosc.* 2020 Oct; 92(4):807–812. Doi: 10.1016/j.gie.2020.06.040.

34 Wang F, Casalino LP, Khullar D. Deep Learning in Medicine—Promise, Progress, and Challenges. *JAMA Intern Med.* 2019; 179:293–294.

35 Pedro AR, Dias MB, Laranjo L, Cunha AS, Cordeiro JV. Artificial Intelligence in Medicine: A Comprehensive Survey of Medical doctor's Perspectives in Portugal. *PLoS One.* 2023 Sep 7; 18(9):e0290613. Doi: 10.1371/journal.pone.0290613.

36 Blease C, Kaptchuk TJ, Bernstein MH, Mandl KD, Halamka JD, DesRoches CM. Artificial Intelligence and the Future of Primary Care: Exploratory Qualitative Study of UK General Practitioners' Views. *J Med Internet Res.* 2019; 21(3):e12802. Doi: 10.2196/12802.

37 Amisha, Malik P, Pathania M, Rathaur VK. Overview of Artificial Intelligence in Medicine. *J Family Med Prim Care.* 2019; 8(7):2328–2331. Doi:10.4103/jfmpc.jfmpc_440_19.

38 Bekbolatova M, Mayer J, Ong CW, Toma M. Transformative Potential of AI in Healthcare: Definitions, Applications, and Navigating the Ethical Landscape and Public Perspectives. *Healthcare (Basel).* 2024; 12(2):125. Doi:10.3390/healthcare12020125.

39 Henning PA, Henning J, Glück K. Artificial Intelligence: Its Future in the Health Sector and Its Role for Medical Education. *J Eur CME*. 2021;10(1):2014099. Doi:10.1080/21614083.2021.2014099.

40 Kulikowski CA. An Opening Chapter of the First Generation of Artificial Intelligence in Medicine: The First Rutgers AIM Workshop, June 1975. *Yearb Med Inform*. 2015; 10(1):227–233. Doi:10.15265/IY-2015-016.

41 Gomez-Cabello CA, Borna S, Pressman S, Haider SA, Haider CR, Forte AJ. Artificial-Intelligence-Based Clinical Decision Support Systems in Primary Care: A Scoping Review of Current Clinical Implementations. *Eur J Investig Health Psychol Educ*. 2024; 14(3):685–698. Doi:10.3390/ejihpe14030045.

42 Ferrucci DA, Brown EW, Chu-Carroll J, Fan J, Gondek D, Kalyanpur A, Lally A, Murdock JW, Nyberg E, Prager JM, Schlaefer N, Welty C. Building Watson: An Overview of the DeepQA Project. AI Mag. 2010; 31:59–79.

43 Brill TM, Munoz L, Miller RJ. Siri, Alexa, and other digital assistants: a study of customer satisfaction with artificial intelligence applications. *J Mark Manag*. 2019; 35(15–16):1401–1436. Doi: 10.1080/0267257X.2019.1687571.

44 Abd-Alrazaq A, Safi Z, Alajlani M, Warren J, Househ M, Denecke K. Technical Metrics Used to Evaluate Health Care Chatbots: Scoping Review. *J Med Internet Res*. 2020 Jun 5; 22(6):e18301. Doi: 10.2196/18301.

45 Bajwa J, Munir U, Nori A, Williams B. Artificial Intelligence in Healthcare: Transforming the Practice of Medicine. *Future Healthc J*. 2021 Jul; 8(2):e188–e194. Doi: 10.7861/fhj.2021-0095.

46 Alowais SA, Alghamdi SS, Alsuhebany N et al. Revolutionizing Healthcare: The Role of Artificial Intelligence in Clinical Practice. *BMC Med Educ*. 2023; 23:689. Doi: 10.1186/s12909-023-04698-z.

47 Gala D, Behl H, Shah M, Makaryus AN. The Role of Artificial Intelligence in Improving Patient Outcomes and Future of Healthcare Delivery in Cardiology: A Narrative Review of the Literature. *Healthcare (Basel)*. 2024; 12(4):481. Doi:10.3390/healthcare12040481.

48 Alhur A. Redefining Healthcare with Artificial Intelligence (AI): The Contributions of ChatGPT, Gemini, and Co-pilot. *Cureus*. 2024; 16(4):e57795. Doi:10.7759/cureus.57795.

49 Bhagat SV, Kanyal D. Navigating the Future: The Transformative Impact of Artificial Intelligence on Hospital Management – A Comprehensive Review. *Cureus*. 2024 Feb 20; 16(2):e54518. Doi: 10.7759/cureus.54518.

50 Sun G, Zhou YH. AI in Healthcare: Navigating Opportunities and Challenges in Digital Communication. *Front Digit Health*. 2023 Dec 19; 5:1291132. Doi: 10.3389/fdgth.2023.1291132.

51 Ritoré Á, Jiménez CM, González JL, Rejón-Parrilla JC, Hervás P, et al. The Role of Open Access Data in Democratizing Healthcare AI: A Pathway to Research Enhancement, Patient Well-Being and Treatment Equity in Andalusia, Spain. *PLOS Digital Health*. 2024; 3(9):e0000599. Doi: 10.1371/journal.pdig.0000599.

52 Polevikov S. Advancing AI in Healthcare: A Comprehensive Review of Best Practices. *Clin Chim Acta*. 2023; 548:117519.

53 Al Kuwaiti A, Nazer K, Al-Reedy A, Al-Shehri S, Al-Muhanna A, Subbarayalu AV, Al Muhanna D, Al-Muhanna FA. A Review of the Role of Artificial Intelligence in Healthcare. *J Pers Med*. 2023 Jun 5; 13(6):951. Doi: 10.3390/jpm13060951.

54 Kumar Y, Koul A, Singla R, Ijaz MF. Artificial Intelligence in Disease Diagnosis: A Systematic Literature Review, Synthesizing Framework and Future Research Agenda. *J Ambient Intell Humaniz Comput*. 2023; 14(7):8459–8486. Doi: 10.1007/s12652-021-03612-z.

55 Stafie CS, Sufaru IG, Ghiciuc CM, Stafie II, Sufaru EC, Solomon SM, Hancianu M. Exploring the Intersection of Artificial Intelligence and Clinical Healthcare: A Multidisciplinary Review. *Diagnostics (Basel)*. 2023 Jun 7; 13(12):1995. Doi: 10.3390/diagnostics13121995.

56 Krishnan G, Singh S, Pathania M, Gosavi S, Abhishek S, Parchani A, Dhar M. Artificial Intelligence in Clinical Medicine: Catalyzing a Sustainable Global Healthcare Paradigm. *Front Artif Intell*. 2023 Aug 29; 6:1227091. Doi: 10.3389/frai.2023.1227091.

57 Taib BG, Karwath A, Wensley K, Minku L, Gkoutos GV, Moiemen N. Artificial Intelligence in the Management and Treatment of Burns: A Systematic Review and Meta-Analyses. *J Plast Reconstr Aesthet Surg*. 2023; 77:133–161. Doi:10.1016/j.bjps.2022.11.049.

58 Khosravi M, Zare Z, Mojtabaeian SM, Izadi R. Artificial Intelligence and Decision-Making in Healthcare: A Thematic Analysis of a Systematic Review of Reviews. *Health Serv Res Manag Epidemiol*. 2024 Mar 5; 11:23333928241234863. Doi: 10.1177/23333928241234863.

59 Rao A et al. "Evaluating GPT as an Adjunct for Radiologic Decision Making: GPT-4 Versus GPT-3.5 in a Breast Imaging Pilot." *Journal of the American College of Radiology: JACR*. 2023; 20(10):990–997. Doi:10.1016/j.jacr.2023.05.003.

60 Bekbolatova M, Mayer J, Ong CW, Toma M. Transformative Potential of AI in Healthcare: Definitions, Applications, and Navigating the Ethical Landscape and Public Perspectives. *Healthcare*. 2024; 12(2):125. Doi: 10.3390/healthcare12020125.

61 Rahman MM et al. The Evolving Roles and Impacts of 5G Enabled Technologies in Healthcare: The World Epidemic COVID-19 Issues. *Array (New York, N.Y.)*. 2022; 14:100178. doi:10.1016/j.array.2022.100178.

62 Baron R, Haick H. Mobile Diagnostic Clinics. *ACS Sensors*. 2024; 9(6):2777–2792. Doi: 10.1021/acssensors.4c00636.

63 Jadczyk T, Wojakowski W, Tendera M, Henry TD, Egnaczyk G, Shreenivas S. Artificial Intelligence Can Improve Patient Management at the Time of a Pandemic: The Role of Voice Technology. *J Med Internet Res*. 2021 May 25; 23(5):e22959. Doi: 10.2196/22959.

64 Harada Y, Shimizu T. Impact of a Commercial Artificial Intelligence-Driven Patient Self-Assessment Solution on Waiting Times at General Internal Medicine Outpatient Departments: Retrospective Study. *JMIR Medical Informatics*. 2020; 8(8):e21056. Doi: 10.2196/21056.

65 Karalis VD. The Integration of Artificial Intelligence into Clinical Practice. *Appl. Biosci*. 2024; 3(1):14–44. Doi: 10.3390/applbiosci3010002.

66 Rony MKK, Parvin MR, Ferdousi S. Advancing Nursing Practice with Artificial Intelligence: Enhancing Preparedness for the Future. *Nurs Open*. 2024 Jan; 11(1):10.1002/nop2.2070. Doi: 10.1002/nop2.2070.

67 Shajari S, Kuruvinashetti K, Komeili A, Sundararaj U. The Emergence of AI-Based Wearable Sensors for Digital Health Technology: A Review. *Sensors (Basel)*. 2023 Nov 29; 23(23):9498. Doi: 10.3390/s23239498.

68 Manickam P et al. "Artificial Intelligence (AI) and Internet of Medical Things (IoMT) Assisted Biomedical Systems for Intelligent Healthcare." *Biosensors*. 2022 Jul 25; 12(8):562. Doi: 10.3390/bios12080562.

69 Ng JY, Cramer H, Lee MS, Moher D. Traditional, Complementary, and Integrative Medicine and Artificial Intelligence: Novel Opportunities in Healthcare. *Integr Med Res*. 2024 Mar; 13(1):101024. Doi: 10.1016/j.imr.2024.101024.

70 Srivastava R, Srivastava S. Can Artificial Intelligence Aid Communication? Considering the Possibilities of GPT-3 in Palliative Care. *Indian J Palliat Care*. 2023 Oct–Dec; 29(4):418–425. Doi: 10.25259/IJPC_155_2023.

71 Maleki Varnosfaderani S, Forouzanfar M. The Role of AI in Hospitals and Clinics: Transforming Healthcare in the 21st Century. *Bioengineering (Basel)*. 2024 Mar 29; 11(4):337. Doi: 10.3390/bioengineering11040337.

72 Carriero A, Groenhoff L, Vologina E, Basile P, Albera M. Deep Learning in Breast Cancer Imaging: State of the Art and Recent Advancements in Early 2024. *Diagnostics (Basel)*. 2024 Apr 19; 14(8):848. Doi: 10.3390/diagnostics14080848.

73 Ul Rehman S et al. AI-Based Tool for Early Detection of Alzheimer's Disease. *Heliyon*. 2024 Apr 9; 10(8):e29375. Doi:10.1016/j.heliyon.2024.e29375.

74 Hosny A, Parmar C, Quackenbush J, Schwartz LH, Aerts HJWL. Artificial Intelligence in Radiology. *Nat Rev Cancer*. 2018 Aug; 18(8):500–510. Doi: 10.1038/s41568-018-0016-5.

75 Pruthviraja D, Nagaraju SC, Mudligiriyappa N, Raisinghani MS, Khan SB, Alkhaldi NA, Malibari AA. Detection of Alzheimer's Disease Based on Cloud-Based Deep Learning Paradigm. *Diagnostics (Basel)*. 2023 Aug 15; 13(16):2687. Doi: 10.3390/diagnostics13162687.

76 Najjar R. Redefining Radiology: A Review of Artificial Intelligence Integration in Medical Imaging. *Diagnostics (Basel)*. 2023 Aug 25; 13(17):2760. Doi: 10.3390/diagnostics13172760.

77 Villafuerte N, Manzano S, Ayala P, García MV. Artificial Intelligence in Virtual Telemedicine Triage: A Respiratory Infection Diagnosis Tool with Electronic Measuring Device. *Future Internet*. 2023; 15(7):227. Doi: 10.3390/fi15070227.

78 Haleem A, Javaid M, Singh RP, Suman R. Telemedicine for Healthcare: Capabilities, Features, Barriers, and Applications. *Sens Int*. 2021; 2:100117. Doi: 10.1016/j.sintl.2021.100117.

79 Kiburg KV. et al. Telemedicine and Delivery of Ophthalmic Care in Rural and Remote Communities: Drawing from Australian Experience. *Clin Exp Ophthalmol*. 2022; 50(7):793–800. Doi: 10.1111/ceo.14147.

80 Zahedani AD, McLaughlin T, Veluvali A et al. Digital Health Application Integrating Wearable Data and Behavioral Patterns Improves Metabolic Health. *npj Digit*. 2023; 6:216. Doi: 10.1038/s41746-023-00956-y.

81 Peyroteo M, Ferreira IA, Elvas LB, Ferreira JC, Lapão LV. Remote Monitoring Systems for Patients with Chronic Diseases in Primary Health Care: Systematic Review. *JMIR Mhealth Uhealth*. 2021 Dec 21; 9(12):e28285. Doi: 10.2196/28285.

82 Christopoulou SC. Machine Learning Models and Technologies for Evidence-Based Telehealth and Smart Care: A Review. *Biomed Informatics*. 2024; 4(1):754–779.

83 Visan AI, Negut I Integrating Artificial Intelligence for Drug Discovery in the Context of Revolutionizing Drug Delivery. *Life*. 2024; 14(2):233. https://doi.org/10.3390/life14020233

84 Han R, Yoon H, Kim G, Lee H, Lee Y. Revolutionizing Medicinal Chemistry: The Application of Artificial Intelligence (AI) in Early Drug Discovery. *Pharmaceuticals (Basel)*. 2023 Sep 6; 16(9):1259. Doi: 10.3390/ph16091259.

85 Lin X, Li X, Lin X. A Review on Applications of Computational Methods in Drug Screening and Design. *Molecules*. 2020 Mar 18; 25(6):1375. Doi: 10.3390/molecules25061375.

86 Zhou G, Rusnac DV, Park H et al. An Artificial Intelligence Accelerated Virtual Screening Platform for Drug Discovery. *Nat Commun*. 2024; 15:7761. Doi: 10.1038/s41467-024-52061-7.

87 Davenport TH, Hongsermeier TM, McCord KA. Using AI to Improve Electronic Health Records. Harvard Business Review. December 13, 2018. Available at: https://hbr.org/2018/12/using-ai-to-improve-electronic-health-records.

88 Langer C. Decision-Making Power and Responsibility in an Automated Administration. *Discov Artif Intell*. 2024; 4:59. Doi: 10.1007/s44163-024-00152-1.

89 Vilaza GN, McCashin D. Is the Automation of Digital Mental Health Ethical? Applying an Ethical Framework to Chatbots for Cognitive Behaviour Therapy. *Front Digital Health*. 2021 Aug 6; 3:689736. Doi: 10.3389/fdgth.2021.689736.

90 Vora LK, Gholap AD, Jetha K, Thakur RRS, Solanki HK, Chavda VP. Artificial Intelligence in Pharmaceutical Technology and Drug Delivery Design. *Pharmaceutics*. 2023 Jul 10; 15(7):1916. Doi: 10.3390/pharmaceutics15071916.

91 Qureshi R, Irfan M, Gondal TM, Khan S, Wu J, Hadi MU, Heymach J, Le X, Yan H, Alam T. AI in Drug Discovery and Its Clinical Relevance. *Heliyon*. 2023 Jul; 9(7):e17575. Doi: 10.1016/j.heliyon.2023.e17575.

92 Chen Y, Wang Z, Wang L et al. Deep Generative Model for Drug Design from Protein Target Sequence. *J Cheminform*. 2023; 15(38). Doi: 10.1186/s13321-023-00702-2.

93 Yelne S, Chaudhary M, Dod K, Sayyad A, Sharma R. Harnessing the Power of AI: A Comprehensive Review of Its Impact and Challenges in Nursing Science and Healthcare. *Cureus*. 2023 Nov 22; 15(11):e49252. Doi: 10.7759/cureus.49252.

94 Mathur S, Sutton J. Personalized Medicine Could Transform Healthcare. *Biomed Rep*. 2017 Jul; 7(1):3–5. Doi: 10.3892/br.2017.922.

95 Bhargava K. Chinni, Cedric Manlhiot. Emerging Analytical Approaches for Personalized Medicine Using Machine Learning in Pediatric and Congenital Heart Disease, *Can J Cardiol*. 2024; 40(10):1880–1896. ISSN 0828-282X. Doi: 10.1016/j.cjca.2024.07.026.

96 Mennella C, Maniscalco U, De Pietro G, Esposito M. Ethical and Regulatory Challenges of AI Technologies in Healthcare: A Narrative Review. *Heliyon*. 2024 Feb 15; 10(4):e26297. Doi: 10.1016/j.heliyon.2024.e26297.

97 Gerke S, Minssen T, Cohen G. Ethical and Legal Challenges of Artificial Intelligence-Driven Healthcare. *Artif Intell Healthc*. 2020; 295–336. Doi: 10.1016/B978-0-12-818438-7.00012-5.

98 Norori N, Hu Q, Aellen FM, Faraci FD, Tzovara A. Addressing Bias in Big Data and AI for Health Care: A Call for Open Science. *Patterns (N Y)*. 2021 Oct 8; 2(10):100347. Doi: 10.1016/j.patter.2021.100347.

99 Seh AH, Zarour M, Alenezi M, Sarkar AK, Agrawal A, Kumar R, Khan RA. Healthcare Data Breaches: Insights and Implications. *Healthcare (Basel)*. 2020 May 13; 8(2):133. Doi: 10.3390/healthcare8020133.

100 Tahri Sqalli M, Aslonov B, Gafurov M, Nurmatov S. Humanizing AI in Medical Training: Ethical Framework for Responsible Design. *Front Artif Intell*. 2023 May 16; 6:1189914. Doi: 10.3389/frai.2023.1189914.

101 Yeo LH, Banfield J Human Factors in Electronic Health Records Cybersecurity Breach: An Exploratory Analysis. *Perspect Health Inf Manag*. 2022 Mar 15; 19(spring).

102 Bottomley D, Thaldar D. Liability for Harm Caused by AI in Healthcare: An Overview of the core Legal Concepts. *Front Pharmacol*. 2023 Dec 14; 14:1297353. Doi: 10.3389/fphar.2023.1297353.

103 Asan O, Bayrak AE, Choudhury A. Artificial Intelligence and Human Trust in Healthcare: Focus on Clinicians. *J Med Internet Res*. 2020 Jun 19; 22(6):e15154. Doi: 10.2196/15154.

104 Ossom Williamson P, Minter CIJ. Exploring PubMed as a Reliable Resource for Scholarly Communications Services. *J Med Libr Assoc*. 2019 Jan; 107(1):16–29. Doi: 10.5195/jmla.2019.433.

105 Iyortsuun NK, Kim SH, Jhon M, Yang HJ, Pant S. A Review of Machine Learning and Deep Learning Approaches on Mental Health Diagnosis. *Healthcare (Basel)*. 2023 Jan 17; 11(3):285. Doi: 10.3390/healthcare11030285.

106 Noorbakhsh-Sabet N et al. Artificial Intelligence Transforms the Future of Health Care. *Am J Med.* 2019; 132(7):795–801. Doi: 10.1016/j.amjmed.2019.01.017.

107 Cacciamani GE et al. "Generative Artificial Intelligence in Health Care." *J Urol.* 2023; 210(5):723–725. Doi:10.1097/JU.0000000000003703.

108 Giuffrè M, Shung DL. Harnessing the Power of Synthetic Data in Healthcare: Innovation, Application, and Privacy. *NPJ Digit Med.* 2023 Oct 9; 6(1):186. Doi: 10.1038/s41746-023-00927-3.

109 Arvanitis TN et al. A Method for Machine Learning Generation of Realistic Synthetic Datasets for Validating Healthcare Applications. *Health Inform J.* 2022; 28(2):14604582221077000. Doi: 10.1177/14604582221077000.

110 Jiménez-Luna J et al. Artificial Intelligence in Drug Discovery: Recent Advances and Future Perspectives. *Expert Opinion on Drug Discovery.* 2021; 16(9):949–959.

111 Skandarani Y, Jodoin P-M, Lalande A. GANs for Medical Image Synthesis: An Empirical Study. *J Imaging.* 2023; 9(3):69. Doi: 10.3390/jimaging9030069.

112 Ullah E, Parwani A, Baig MM et al. Challenges and Barriers of Using Large Language Models (LLM) Such as ChatGPT for Diagnostic Medicine With a Focus on Digital Pathology – A Recent Scoping Review. *Diagn Pathol.* 2024; 19(43). Doi: 10.1186/s13000-024-01464-7.

113 Pawelek J, Baca-Motes K, Pandit JA, Berk BB, Ramos E. The Power of Patient Engagement with Electronic Health Records as Research Participants. *JMIR Med Inform.* 2022 Jul 8; 10(7):e39145. Doi: 10.2196/39145.

114 Decker H et al. "Large Language Model-Based Chatbot vs Surgeon-Generated Informed Consent Documentation for Common Procedures." *JAMA Network Open.* 2023 Oct 2; 6(10):e2336997. Doi: 10.1001/jamanetworkopen.2023.36997.

115 Giannakopoulos K, Kavadella A, Aaqel Salim A, Stamatopoulos V, Kaklamanos EG. Evaluation of the Performance of Generative AI Large Language Models ChatGPT, Google Bard, and Microsoft Bing Chat in Supporting Evidence-Based Dentistry: Comparative Mixed Methods Study. *J Med Internet Res.* 2023; 25:e51580. Doi: 10.2196/51580.

116 Johnson KB, Wei WQ, Weeraratne D, Frisse ME, Misulis K, Rhee K, Zhao J, Snowdon JL. Precision Medicine, AI, and the Future of Personalized Health Care. *Clin Transl Sci.* 2021; 14(1):86–93. Doi: 10.1111/cts.12884.

117 Karabacak M, Ozkara BB, Margetis K, Wintermark M, Bisdas S. The Advent of Generative Language Models in Medical Education. *JMIR Med Educ.* 2023; 9:e48163. Doi: 10.2196/48163.

118 Campbell DJ, Estephan LE, Sina EM, et al. Evaluating ChatGPT Responses on Thyroid Nodules for Patient Education. *Thyroid.* 2024; 34(3):371–377.

INDEX

Note: Page references in *italics* denote figures and in **bold** tables.